FOURTH EDITION

Qualitative Research in Nursing

Advancing the Humanistic Imperative

Helen J. Streubert Speziale, EdD, RN
Special Assistant to the President
for Sponsored Research and
National Programs

Dona Rinaldi Carpenter, EdD, RN
Professor
Department of Nursing
University of Scranton
Scranton, Pennsylvania

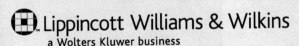
. Lippincott Williams & Wilkins
a Wolters Kluwer business
Philadelphia · Baltimore · New York · London
Buenos Aires · Hong Kong · Sydney · Tokyo

Acquisitions Editor: Margaret Zuccarini
Managing Editor: Michelle Clarke
Production Editor: Audrey Lickwar
Director of Nursing Production: Helen Ewan
Senior Managing Editor / Production: Erika Kors
Creative Director: Doug Smock
Senior Manufacturing Manager: William Alberti
Indexer: Nancy Newman
Compositor: TechBooks
Printer: RR Donnelley—Crawfordsville

4th Edition

9 8 7 6

Library of Congress Cataloging-in-Publication Data

Speziale, Helen Streubert.
  Qualitative research in nursing : advancing the humanistic imperative /
Helen J. Streubert Speziale, Dona R. Carpenter. – 4th ed.
    p. ; cm.
  Includes bibliographical references and index.
  ISBN 0-7817-6313-4 (alk. paper)
    1. Nursing–Research–Methodology.   2. Sociology–Research–Methodology.
  I. Carpenter, Dona Rinaldi.   II. Title.
  [DNLM: 1. Nursing Research–methods.   2. Qualitative Research.
3. Quality Assurance, Health Care.   4. Research Design.   WY 20.5
S915q 2007]
RT81.5.S78 2007
610.73072–dc22

                                            2005031053

LWW.com

This book is dedicated first and foremost to my wonderful husband, Michael, a man who loves me tirelessly and knows when to make me move beyond "my work" to enjoy life more fully. To my wonderful sons, Michael and Matthew, who are a constant source of pride and wonderment. Finally, to my four dear friends, Fran, Mary Ellen, Michael, and Paul, who have supported me in my darkest hours...reminding me always that life is to be savored.
HJS

This 4th edition is dedicated to my family, whose love and support give me strength and courage. To my parents, Elaine and Vito Rinaldi, for a lifetime of love and strength. To my children, Emily Joy and Brian Wells Jr., for your unconditional love and the tremendous happiness you bring to your mother's life. And last but not least, to my husband, Brian, for making my world safe, for always being there for me, and for making me laugh, even in the face of disaster. I love you all.
DRC

About the Authors

*H*elen J. Streubert Speziale, EdD, RN, is Special Assistant to the President for Sponsored Research and National Programs. In this role, she supports faculty in development of sponsored research projects. She has authored and co-authored articles and book chapters on qualitative research and nursing education. In addition, she has presented her work nationally and internationally.

Dona Rinaldi Carpenter, EdD, RN, is Professor of Nursing at the University of Scranton, Scranton, Pennsylvania, where she teaches medical-surgical nursing and nursing research to undergraduate and graduate students. Her research interests focus on nursing education and professional commitment. She has authored and co-authored several articles and book chapters and has presented her work at national and international meetings.

Contributor

Sandra Beth Lewenson, EdD, RN, FAAN, is Associate Dean of Academic Affairs at the Lienhard School of Nursing at Pace University, Pleasantville, New York. She teaches in both the undergraduate and graduate programs. Her areas of expertise include community health and the history of nursing. Her research focus is nursing's historical relationship with the women's suffrage movement at the beginning of the 20th century. She has published several books and articles on the topic

Reviewers

Annie M. Carson
Professor
Cambrian College of Applied Arts and
   Technology
Sudbury, Ontario, Canada

Sarah C. Fogel, PhD, RN
Assistant Professor in Nursing
Vanderbilt University
Nashville, Tennessee

**Lucille C. Gambardella, PhD, RN, CS,
APN-BC**
Chair/Professor, Department of Nursing
Wesley College
Dover, Delaware

Janet T. Ihlenfeld, PhD, RN, BSN, MS
Professor, Department of Nursing
D'Youville College
Buffalo, New York

Françoise Pradel, PhD
Assistant Professor
University of Maryland School of Pharmacy
Baltimore, Maryland

Deanna L. Reising, PhD, APRN, BC
Assistant Professor
Indiana University School of Nursing
Bloomington, Indiana

Judith A. Strasser, DNSc, RN
Professor
Wesley College
Dover, Delaware

Sheila Cox Sullivan, PhD, RN
Associate Professor and Associate Dean
College of Nursing
Harding University
Searcy, Arkansas

Dr. Joan Tilghman
Division of Nursing
Howard University
Washington, DC

Diane M. Tomasic, EdD, RN
Professor of Nursing
West Liberty State College
West Liberty, West Virginia

Robin K. Tomin, MSN, RN
Associate Professor of Nursing
Malone College, School of Nursing
Canton, Ohio

Preface

*T*he fourth edition of *Qualitative Research in Nursing: Advancing the Humanistic Imperative* presents major revisions and updated material essential to qualitative research methods and publications. The organization of the text has been modified to address ethical issues earlier in the text, as they have applicability to all methodologies presented. This edition also includes a complete and expansive look at the actual process of conducting a qualitative research study, writing a qualitative research proposal, and clinical application of qualitative methods. Each companion chapter has been completely revised and includes a new research article applicable to the method addressed with accompanying critiques. Further, a new peer reviewed research proposal and critique follows Chapter 16. These are included as examples for readers preparing qualitative grant proposals. We continue to work diligently to bring to the reader the latest in qualitative thinking by nurses and those who have supported nurses' work. Therefore, major revisions and updates have been included, as they were available during the preparation of this fourth edition. Finally, this edition continues to include the same strong philosophical and methodological principles that have been important to our readers over the years.

The purpose of this book has, from it's inception, been to assist those new to qualitative inquiry to discover the fundamental characteristics of a set of methods that have been critical to the advancement of nursing's scientific body of knowledge. The text provides a strong and organized reference for understanding qualitative methodology. We continue to believe strongly, however, that it is only through engagement in the methods that those new to qualitative inquiry will begin to appreciate the value of the methods (approaches) for studying the human condition as it is revealed in nursing practice.

Clearly qualitative research methods have been recognized and valued as legitimate methods of scientific inquiry. This is a major change since the first writing of this text. There is still work to be done, however. Although qualitative research methods have come into their own, with significant numbers of journal pages dedicated to the publication of qualitative work and journals solely dedicated to qualitative research, we continue to be heartened by the fact that more qualitative researchers are able to become panel members of grant review teams and are now securing more research dollars for this exciting and enlightening research paradigm.

Those of you familiar with our text know that our original work arose from our own experiences with trying to develop a qualitative research agenda based on reading the works of, and studying with, those outside of the nursing discipline. This text continues to build on our experiences and shares with the reader the expansion of our own thinking over the years, but also the works of those who have been significant in opening our collective vision in the field of qualitative study.

Our personal lives as nurses, nurse educators, and nurse researchers are built on the common understanding that individuals are integrated wholes who share in common experiences with other individuals. It is for this reason that qualitative inquiry supports our commitment to understanding the human condition. We fully believe that we live lives that recognize the interconnectedness of our humanness and we strive to assist others to join in the mutual understanding that we derive from being part of the human experience. The skills for understanding the human experience are found in the pages of this text. We believe that the understanding that is gleaned from participating in qualitative inquiry gives each nurse researcher the opportunity to see his or her practice through a unique lens. To fully realize the skills of a qualitative researcher, we believe that fundamental understanding of the history, elements, context, and outcomes of each approach presented in the text is essential. Further, those who find qualitative inquiry supportive of their personal research philosophy are encouraged to use the primary references documented in the text to explore more deeply the basic ideologies that were responsible for the development of the qualitative research paradigm.

As in our previous editions, the text introduces the historical background of each approach, shares the fundamental elements, how one decides whether to use a particular approach, and the expected outcomes. Knowing these parts will help the reader begin to integrate and synthesize the research paradigm that we have found so successful in bringing about an understanding of a whole and authentic human experience.

Organization

This text is organized to facilitate the reader's comprehension of each approach and to provide examples of how the approaches have been used in nursing practice, education, and administration.

In Chapter 1, Philosophy and Theory: Foundations of Qualitative Research, the reader is introduced to the traditions of science, the interpretations of what constitutes science, perceptions of reality, and the influences of critical and feminist theory on the discipline of qualitative research.

In Chapter 2, the Conduct of Qualitative Research: Common Essential Elements, the development of a qualitative study is examined. The characteristics common to all qualitative studies are offered, including selection of the method, understanding the philosophic underpinnings of the approach selected, and use of a literature review, explicating the researcher's beliefs, choosing a setting, selecting the informant, and achieving saturation.

Chapter 3, Designing Data Generation and Management Strategies, offers the reader ideas about how to select and use specific data collection strategies, including interviews, focus groups, narratives, chat rooms, participant observation, and field notes. In addition, an explanation is provided for managing data including the common elements of data analysis, demonstrating trustworthiness, and presentation of the findings.

Chapter 4, Ethical Consideration in Qualitative Research, represents an expanded revision to the information presented in the last edition. A significant amount of literature has been published with regard to ethical issues in qualitative research. This information is offered to assist the reader in fully understanding the unique and sensitive relationship that occurs in the process of a qualitative study and suggests ways to maximize protection of human subjects while engaged in the relationship.

Chapter 5, Phenomenology as Method offers an in-depth description of philosophy and methodological conceptualizations of this approach to qualitative inquiry. An overview of the phenomenological perspective, with descriptive and interpretive views of the process, is offered. The reader is given an exceptional guide to the process of phenomenological inquiry, including an expansion of previously presented hermeneutics. Table 5-1 lists the procedural step for implementing a phenomenological study from the perspective of six phenomenologists. It is an exceptional reference for the would-be phenomenological researcher.

Chapter 6, Phenomenology in Practice, Education, and Administration, as in previous editions, offers the reader the opportunity to understand the presentation of the method offered in Chapter 5 by giving examples of published phenomenological research from practice, education, and administration. Critique guidelines and formal critique by the chapter author also are provided to assist in understanding the application and quality of the work that is published. To facilitate the integration of the information presented, a reprint of one of the critiqued studies is included. Finally, a table of recently published phenomenological research gives the reader a ready reference of work using this specific approach.

Chapter 7, Grounded Theory as Method; Chapter 9, Ethnography as Method; Chapter 11, Historical Research Method; and Chapter 13, Action

Research Method follow the format found in Chapter 5. This includes in-depth discussion of the philosophic and methodological issues specific to the approach. Data generation and treatment as well as ethical issues specific to the particular approach are discussed in detail.

Chapters 8, 10, 12, and 14 repeat the format found in Chapter 6, incorporating a detailed examination of published studies that illustrate a particular approach followed by guidelines for critiquing the approach used. These chapters include tables that offer a substantial resource list of recent studies completed in the areas of education, administration, and practice. Finally, each of these chapters includes a reprinting of a selected study that illustrates the qualitative method discussed in that particular chapter.

Chapter 15, Triangulation as a Qualitative Research Strategy, expands on information related to data, investigator, theory, and methodological triangulation. It is intended to enhance the reader's understanding of the difference ways triangulation can be used in a qualitative research study.

Chapter 16, Writing a Qualitative Research Proposal, introduces the reader to the concept of developing a qualitative research agenda, as well as the elements of developing a qualitative research proposal. An example of a peer reviewed funded grant and critique is included in the chapter.

Chapter 17, A Practical Guide for Sharing Qualitative Research Results, provides a full description of issues related to developing qualitative research projects and dissemination of qualitative research findings. It details for the reader the potential triumphs and the pitfalls in moving qualitative research into a public forum.

Key Features and Benefits

The following features are included in the philosophical and methodological framework.

- Description of the philosophical underpinnings of each approach. This description provides more than the "how" of the approach; it presents the underlying assumptions of the approaches.

- Detailed description of the procedural steps used in each of the approaches. This offers the reader the opportunity to learn step by step how the approach is implemented.

- Completely revised tables profiling studies conducted using each of the approaches. These tables offer the reader an excellent resource for further exploring the existing body of knowledge specific to the approach being discussed.

- In-depth discussion of published research studies that have used the approaches under discussion. This examination shares with the reader not only what has been published but also the strengths and weaknesses of the studies reviewed.

- Specific critiquing guidelines available in all companion chapters for each of the approaches. These guidelines help the reader understand the specific question that should be asked of research studies that have used or will be using the approach.

- Inclusion of completely revised companion chapters. Comparison chapters describing application of each of the approaches included in the text provide strong evidence of the impact these qualitative research methods are having on the discipline of nursing and the potential benefits they will continue to have. These chapters all provide neophyte qualitative researchers with clear descriptions of what is accepted from the researchers who will evaluate their work.

- Inclusion of a sample of a funded qualitative research grant, including the critique offered by the grant review panel.

- Chapters on ethical consideration in qualitative research and triangulation.

- Table highlighting the methods described as they have been used to study nursing practice issues.

We hope that his book will continue to serve as both a starting point for the new researcher and a reference for more experienced nurses. It is expected that each approach detailed will offer the reader a sound understanding of qualitative research methods. Finally, we are grateful for the support of our readership over the years, and hope that the fourth edition of this textbook exceeds your expectations.

Helen J. Streubert Speziale
Dona Rinaldi Carpenter

Acknowledgments

*T*he fourth edition of this textbook has been an important undertaking, with major changes since we first began writing about qualitative research methods. As always our life experiences with friends and colleagues who have supported and valued our work continue to influence our writing. We wish to acknowledge all those people who continue to shape our thinking and our way of being in the world...our friends, our families, our teachers, our students, and our colleagues.

Specifically, we wish to acknowledge those who have been most closely involved in the production of the fourth edition of this text, Margaret Zuccarini, Michelle Clarke, and Audrey Lickwar, and the research assistance of Lori A. Paolowsky and Melissa A. Kalinowski, University of Scranton nursing students.

Contents

Chapter 8

Grounded Theory in Practice, Education, and Administration   153
Dona Rinaldi Carpenter

Chapter 9

Ethnography as Method   195
Helen J. Streubert Speziale

Chapter 10

Ethnography in Practice, Education, and Administration   227
Helen J. Streubert Speziale

Chapter *11*

Historical Research Method 251
Sandra B. Lewenson

Chapter *12*

Historical Research in Practice, Education, and Administration 273
Sandra B. Lewenson

Chapter *13*

Action Research Method 327
Helen J. Streubert Speziale

Chapter *14*

Action Research in Practice, Education, and Administration 349
Helen J. Streubert Speziale

Chapter *15*

Triangulation as a Qualitative Research Strategy 379
Dona Rinaldi Carpenter

Chapter *16*

Writing a Qualitative Research Proposal 393
Dona Rinaldi Carpenter

Chapter
17

A Practical Guide for Sharing Qualitative Research Results   441
Helen J. Streubert Speziale

1

Philosophy and Theory: Foundations of Qualitative Research

When the first edition of this textbook was published in 1995, the world of qualitative research in nursing looked very different than it does today. At that time, there were few qualitative studies being published, few qualitative papers being given, and few nurses who called themselves qualitative researchers. Most of the qualitative researchers of that time were trained by sociologists, psychologists, and anthropologists who taught nurses how to use their methods and procedures to generate nursing knowledge. Since that time, qualitative nurse researcher pioneers have adapted what they learned and have helped to create a new generation of researchers. As a result of this early work, nursing knowledge can now be derived from the qualitative paradigm. Journals and conferences are now much richer because of the work of those early scholars in bringing to the mainstream a philosophy of science that demonstrates an investment in understanding the humanistic imperative. In the introductory remarks for the third edition, I addressed the fact that there have been debates about the rigor, value, and utility of qualitative research. There are now, as then, continued debates about the qualifications necessary to conduct qualitative research, how it is funded, and its place in advancing nursing science. What is even more striking today are the questions about whether the path we are on is the right one. "Increases in number of journal articles, proliferation of journals or conferences focused on qualitative research, and the number of doctorally prepared qualitative researchers we now have are only an advance if qualitative research, and not other external drivers, remains the focus" (Cheek, 2002, p. 1135).

Cheek (2002) states "more articles and more students 'doing' qualitative research does not necessarily mean that qualitative research is advancing, neither does it ensure the advancement of scholarship in qualitative research" (p. 1137). She further suggests, we need to ask questions about what is being promoted in terms of the preparation and advancement of the next generation of qualitative researchers, who will assume the teaching responsibilities of further generations, examination and credentialing of qualitative researchers, and editorship of journals. (p. 1137)

The presence of the debate about the future development of qualitative research and preparation of qualitative researchers is a strong indicator of the value placed on the paradigm. The deliberations are important and useful and demonstrate the critical assessment that surrounds the field. The goal of this text is to offer nurse researchers an introduction to the philosophies, approaches, strategies, and outcomes that are categorized as qualitative research. This introduction to qualitative research should stimulate its readers to want to learn more about the specific approaches included in the text and facilitate the use of them to discover new nursing knowledge.

The tradition of science is uniquely quantitative. The quantitative approach to research has been justified by its success in measuring, analyzing, replicating, and applying knowledge gained from this paradigm. The inability to quantitatively measure some phenomena and the dissatisfaction with the results of measurement of other phenomena have led to an intense interest in using other approaches to study particularly human phenomena. This interest has led to an acceptance of qualitative research approaches as another way to discover knowledge.

The tradition of using qualitative methods to study human phenomena is grounded in the social sciences. The tradition arose because aspects of human values, culture, and relationships were unable to be described fully using quantitative research methods. Krasner (2000) states that the early philosophers "argued that human phenomena could not and should not be reduced to mathematical formulas" (p. 70). The practice of qualitative research has expanded to clinical settings because "empirical approaches have proven to be of limited service in answering some of the challenging and pressing clinical questions, especially where human subjectivity and interpretation are involved" (Thorne, 1997, p. 288). The appeal for nurses is that qualitative research methods attempt to describe and interpret perplexing human phenomena: phenomena that are not easily quantifiable (Krasner, 2000, p. 70). Nurses and other health care professionals clearly want to grasp the lived experience of their clients, to enter into the world their clients inhabit, and to understand the basic social processes that illuminate human health and illness events (Thorne, 1997).

This chapter shares with the reader the foundations of qualitative research. Its purpose is to present qualitative knowledge structure and generate excitement for the qualitative research approach as an alternative to quantitative inquiry.

PHILOSOPHIC UNDERPINNINGS OF QUALITATIVE RESEARCH

*F*rom a philosophic viewpoint, the study of humans is deeply rooted in descriptive modes of science. Human scientists have been concerned with describing the fundamental patterns of human thought and behavior since early times. Descartes' view of science was long held as the only approach to new knowledge. His ideas were grounded in an objective reality, a position that supported the idea that cause and effect could explain all things. Kant is attributed with questioning the fundamental nature of reality as seen through a Cartesian lens. He opened discussion about human rationality. Kant proposed that perception was more than the act of observation. For him, all reality was not explainable by cause and effect. He raised issues supporting the notion that nature was not independent of thought or reason (Hamilton, 1994). What was observed, therefore, was not the only reality.

The concept of scientific versus practical reason was born of Kant's ideas about nature, specifically as the concept relates to perception (Ermath, 1978; Hamilton, 1994). Later existentialists advanced Kant's ideas to explore reality as it is perceived rather than as an observed phenomenon only. Kant's ideas about freedom and practical reasoning emancipated science. Scientists questioned whether empiricism was the only way to gain knowledge. Later philosophers such as Husserl furthered Kant's propositions, and, eventually, the German school of philosophy developed and expanded the ideas about self, self-consciousness, reality, and freedom.

The early debates about science and reality established the foundations of the qualitative paradigm that many social scientists use today. Qualitative research offers the opportunity to focus on finding answers to questions centered on social experience, how it is created, and how it gives meaning to human life (Denzin & Lincoln, 1994). Knowing how social experiences construct an individual's reality is an important criterion for developing science. Based on this idea, an exploration of ways of knowing is appropriate.

If one takes the ontologic position that reality is apprehensible, then the positivist or empiricist framework becomes one's reference point. However, it seems inconceivable that individuals can believe they are able to fully apprehend reality. According to Denzin and Lincoln (1994), post-positivists believe there is a reality to be known but have conceded that this reality only will be "imperfectly or probabilistically apprehendable [sic]" (p. 109). Critical theorists and constructivists see reality from a dynamic standpoint. The critical theorist perspective is that reality is "shaped by social, political, cultural, economic, ethnic, and gender values" (Denzin & Lincoln, 1994, p. 109). Further, feminist critical theorists believe that knowledge is co-created by researcher and those researched. The constructivist, however, sees reality as "relativism—local and specific" (Denzin & Lincoln, 1994, p. 109). Therefore, "reality is actually realities" (Lincoln, 1992, p. 379). Clearly, it is a post-positivist viewpoint that supports the notion of a dynamic reality.

In a human enterprise such as nursing, it is imperative that nurses accept the utility of a research tradition that provides for the most meaningful way to describe and understand human experiences. Recognizing that reality is dynamic is the first step in establishing a truly humanistic perspective of research.

WAYS OF KNOWING

" *T*he term *knowing* refers to ways of perceiving and understanding the self and the world. Knowing is an ontologic, dynamic changing process" (Chinn & Kramer, 2004, p. 2). There are many ways that we come to know information. One way is through experts—someone we view as an authority tells us what to know. As children, this is usually our parent(s). As we grow up, the experts in our lives may be teachers, extended family, employers, or formal authority figures such as law enforcement officials. This has been called the *received view*.

Trial and error is another way that individuals learn about the world. Through trying out new ideas or actions and determining the value of the response or outcome, we learn what is *correct*. There are other ways that individuals come to know what it is they value. Although it is important to know how it is we come to know, it is equally important to know how what we come to value is created or validated.

For many years, women in particular were told what to know. This limited debate and dialogue about information. Much of what was known and valued was professed by empirical scientists who supported a Cartesian framework that espoused a belief that if objective measurement could not be assigned to a phenomenon, the importance and thus the existence of the phenomenon was in question. Many contemporary scientists and philosophers question the value of this system, particularly in situations that include humans and their interactions with other humans. There is much debate about the relative value of information that is derived from a purely objective standpoint when it comes to human phenomena within a social context. The concepts of objectivity, reduction, and manipulation, which are fundamental to empirical science, defy the authentic fiber of humans and their social interactions. Too many intervening or confounding variables can influence the findings of empirical science when the focus is human social context or interaction.

With the belief that science should inform the lives of people who interact and function in society, researchers need to examine all parts of reality—subjective reality as well as its objective counterpart. Researchers should acknowledge knowing in the subjective sense and value it equally so that scientific knowledge will represent the views of people who experience life. The early phenomenologists believed that the only reality was the one that is perceived. Thus, the measurement of perception challenges the empirical scientist. Perception is not objective; rather, perception is a way of observing and processing those things that are present to the self within the context of one's lived experience. For example, two individuals may observe the same lecture and leave the classroom with different interpretations of what the lecturer said. Each individual's interpretation is based on what that person perceived to be reality—a reality that is developed and constructed over a lifetime of receiving, processing, and interpreting information, as well as engaging in human interaction. The internalization of what becomes known as belief systems comes from perception and construction of what is real for the individual.

WAYS OF KNOWING IN NURSING

*I*n her seminal work on ways of knowing in nursing, Carper (1978) identified four fundamental patterns that emerge as the way nurses come to know: empirical knowing, aesthetic knowing, personal knowing, and moral knowing. *Empirical knowing* represents the traditional, objective, logical, and positivist tradition of science. Empirical knowing and thus empirical science is committed to providing explanations for phenomena and then controlling them. An example of empirical knowing is the knowledge derived from the biologic sciences that describes and explains human function. Biologic scientists have been able to predict and control certain aspects of human structure and function. Treatment of diabetes mellitus is an example of empirical research being applied in the health care field. From their empirical studies, biologic scientists know that providing insulin to individuals with diabetes mellitus controls the symptoms created by the nonfunctioning pancreas. The nursing profession's alignment with empirical knowing and its subsequent pursuit of this mode of inquiry follows the positivist paradigm, which believes that objective data, measurement, and generalizability are essential to the generation and dissemination of knowledge. This type of nursing knowledge is critical in situations in which control and generalizability are important. More recently, Chinn and Kramer (2004) have expanded on the traditional meaning of empirics to include theory development and the use of research methods that are not based strictly on hypothesis testing, such as phenomenology and ethnography.

Aesthetic knowing is the art of nursing. The understanding and interpretation of subjective experience and the creative development of nursing care are based on an appreciation of subjective expression. Aesthetic knowing is abstract and defies a formal description and measurement. According to Carper (1978),

> The aesthetic pattern of knowing in nursing involves the perception of abstract particulars as distinguished from the recognition of abstracted universals. It is the knowing of the unique particular rather than an exemplary class. (p. 16)

Aesthetic knowing in nursing provides the framework for the exploration of qualitative research methodologies. Qualitative research calls for recognition of patterns in phenomena rather than the explication of facts that will be controllable and generalizable. An example of aesthetic knowing is the way a nurse would provide care differently for two elderly women who are preparing for cataract surgery, based on the nurse's knowledge of each woman's particular life patterns.

Wainwright (2000) states, "a nursing aesthetic can provide us with an essential set of tools to help answer the question of what amounts to good nursing. It may also provide us with additional insights into the nature of nursing ethics" (p. 755). "Nursing knowledge as defined in nursing theories and when lived by nurses creates the art of nursing" (Mitchell, 2001, p. 207).

Personal knowing requires that the individual—in this case, the nurse—know the self. The degree to which an individual knows oneself is determined by his or her abilities to self-actualize. Movement toward knowledge of the self and self-actualization requires comfort with ambiguity and a commitment to patience in understanding. Personal knowing is a commitment to authentication of relationships and a *presencing* with others, that is, the enlightenment and sensitization people bring to genuine human interactions. Personal knowing deals with the fundamental *existentialism* of humans, that is, the capacity for change and the value placed on becoming.

Personal knowing also supports the qualitative research paradigm. In the conduct of qualitative inquiry, researchers are obligated by the philosophic underpinnings of the methodologies they use to accept the self as part of the research enterprise and to approach research participants in a genuine and authentic manner. An awareness of one's beliefs and understandings is essential to fully discover the phenomena studied in a qualitative research inquiry. Furthermore, qualitative researchers believe there is always subjectivity in their pursuit of the truth. The very nature of human interactions is based on subjective knowledge. In the most objective research endeavor, subjective realities will affect what is studied. "Scientific research, as a human endeavor to advance knowledge, is influenced by the sociocultural and historical context in which it takes place and is considered neither value free, objective, nor neutral" (Henderson, 1995, p. 59).

Moral knowing reflects our ethical obligations in a situation or our ideas about what should be done in a given situation. Through the moral way of knowing, individuals come to a realization of what is right and just. As with personal knowing and aesthetic knowing, moral knowing is another abstract dimension of how it is that individuals come to know a situation. Moral knowing is based on traditional principles and codes of ethics or conduct. This type of knowing becomes most important when humans face situations in which decisions of right and wrong are blurred by differences in values or beliefs. Moral knowing requires an openness to differences in philosophic positions. Ethics and logic are required to examine the intricacies of human situations that do not fit standard formulas for conduct.

Munhall (2001) states, "all of the foregoing patterns are rich and essential sources of nursing knowledge that can be studied from various perspectives of science" (p. 41). The importance of sharing these ways of knowing is to offer the reader a context in which to judge the appropriateness of nursing knowledge and the way that nurses develop that knowledge. It is only through examinations of current belief structures that people are able to achieve their own standards of what will be best in a given situation. Moreover, when we select our research methods, we should choose them based on the questions we are asking (Burnard & Hannigan, 2000) within the context of what is known and what we believe.

May (1994) and Sandelowski (1994) expanded on the idea of knowing as it relates to nursing knowledge. May (1994) used the term *abstract knowing* to describe the analytic experience of knowing:

> The rigorous implementation and explication of method alone never explains the process of abstract knowing, regardless of which paradigm the scientist espouses and which method is chosen. Method does not produce insight or understanding or the creative leap that the agile mind makes in the struggle to comprehend observation and to link them together. Regardless of the paradigmatic perspective held by the scientist, the process of knowing itself cannot be observed and measured directly, but only by its product. (p. 13)

May (1994) further suggested that knowledge is "shaped *but not completely defined* by the process through which it is created" (p. 14). Based on her ideas about knowing, she gave credibility to what she called "magic," which is similar to the intuitive connections discussed in Benner's (1984) work on expert clinical judgment. Based on her conversations with and observations of qualitative researchers, May determined that, at a certain point, pattern recognition creates the insight into the phenomenon under study. She believes that the ability to see knowledge is a result of intellectual rigor and readiness (magic). Her ideas support the concept of intuition or, as she labeled it, "abstract knowing" in nursing research.

Sandelowski (1994) took a position on knowing similar to the aesthetic knowing described by Carper (1978): We must accept the art as well as the science of research. Sandelowski believed that the two are not mutually exclusive.

> What differentiates the arts from the sciences is not the search for truth per se, but rather the kinds of truths that are sought. Science typically is concerned with propositional truths, or truth about something. Art is concerned with universal truths, with being true to: even with being more true to life than life itself. (Hospers, as cited in Sandelowski, 1994, p. 52)

Both May (1994) and Sandelowski (1994) provide us with an expansion of the original positions on knowing offered by Carper (1978). These authors provide a validation for knowing other than in the empirical sense. Most important, they offer nurse researchers a way to discover knowledge that complements the positivist paradigm and gives voice to other ways of knowing. In the case of qualitative research and nursing practice, it is only through examination of the prevailing ideologies that nurses will be able to decide which ideology most reflects their personal patterns of discovery and creation of meaning.

MEANING OF SCIENCE

Science is defined in a number of ways. According to Siepmann (1999), "science is the field of study which attempts to describe and understand the nature of the universe in whole or part." Aristotle described three types of science: (1) acquisition of knowledge as a path to truth for its own sake; (2) practical science, aimed at action based on truth; and (3) productive science, that which is aimed at making according to true principles (Guiliano, 2003, p. 45). Guba (1990), in sharing a view of empirical science, articulated the meaning of science as it is practiced within the premise of value-neutral, logical, empirical methods that promise "the growth of rational control over ourselves and our worlds" (p. 317). Parse (2001) offers the term *sciencing* to describe "coming to know and understand the meaning of a phenomena [sic] of concern to a discipline" (p. 1). Each of these definitions or descriptions gives a different lens through which to view truth.

Much of what individuals know about science in the nursing profession is based on the empirical view of science, which places significant value on rationality, objectivity, prediction, and control. The question arises: Is this view of science consistent with the phenomena of interest to nurses? The empirical view of science permeates many aspects of human activity. In adopting this view, one adopts a value system. Many empiricists believe that if a phenomenon is not observable, then it is not real. If a particular phenomenon does not conform to reality as it is currently known, empiricists could judge it to be irrational and therefore unimportant. If a phenomenon is studied without controls protecting the objectivity of the study, then it is said to lack rigor or to be "soft" science and therefore results in unusable data. If the findings from an inquiry do not lead to generalization that contributes to prediction and control of the phenomena under study, some empiricists would argue that it is not "good" science.

For many years, an empiricist view of science has permeated society and has structured what is valued. Feminist scholars have suggested that the scientific paradigm that focuses on prediction and control has gained wide acceptance because of its roots in a male paradigm. Historically, women have played only a small role in the creation of knowledge. Therefore, male scientists who valued prediction and control over description and understanding have largely created the definitions and values of science. According to Anderson (2004),

> Various practitioners of feminist epistemology and philosophy of science argue that dominant knowledge practices disadvantage women by (1) excluding them from inquiry, (2) denying them epistemic authority, (3) denigrating their "feminine" cognitive styles and modes of knowledge, (4) producing theories of women that represent them as inferior, deviant, or significant only in the ways they serve male interests, (5) producing theories of social phenomena that render women's activities and interests, or gendered power relations, invisible, and (6) producing knowledge (science and technology) that is not useful for people in subordinate positions, or that reinforces gender and other social hierarchies.

An empirical, objective, rational science has significant value when the phenomenon of interest is other than human behavior. However, the goals of this type of science—prediction and control—are less valuable when the subject of the inquiry is unable to be made objective.

As a result of the limitations that come from a positivist view of science, philosophers and social scientists have offered an alternative path to discovery that places value on the study of human experiences. In this model, researchers acknowledge and value subjectivity as part of any scientific inquiry. Human values contribute to scientific knowledge; therefore, neutrality is impossible. Prediction is thought to be limiting and capable of creating a false sense of reality. In a human science framework, the best scientists can hope for in creating new knowledge is to provide understanding and interpretation of phenomena within context. Human science and the methods of inquiry that accompany it offer an opportunity to study and create meaning that enriches and informs human life.

Burnard and Hannigan (2000) state that regardless of the paradigm, "research is nearly always a searching for patterns, similarities and differences" (p. 5).

Induction Versus Deduction

Knowledge is generated from either an inductive or deductive posture. *Inductive reasoning* is a process that starts with the details of the experience and moves to a more general picture of the phenomenon of interest (Liehr & Smith, 2002, p. 110). For example, a nurse interested in studying the experiences of women in labor would interview women who have undergone labor to discover their experiences of it. Within context, the nurse could make statements about the labor experience that might be applicable to understanding the labor experience for women not in the study. Hence, qualitative research methods are inductive.

Deductive reasoning moves from general to specific. A researcher interested in conducting research within a deductive framework would develop a hypothesis about a phenomenon and then would seek to prove it. For example, a nurse wanting to know about the labor experience might hypothesize that women in labor experience more pain when they do not use visualization techniques during transition. The researcher's responsibility in such a study would be to identify a pain measure and then collect data on women in the transition phase of labor to determine whether they experience more or less pain based on the use of visualization techniques. Within a deductive framework, the researcher can use the study findings to predict and ultimately attempt to control the pain experience of laboring women. Deductive reasoning is the framework for quantitative research studies.

Both frameworks are important in the development of knowledge. Based on the question being asked, the researcher will select either an inductive or deductive stance.

RELATIONSHIP OF THEORY TO RESEARCH

*I*n addition to understanding the framework from which the researcher enters the research enterprise, it is important to be aware of the relationship of theory to research—specifically, qualitative research. The issue of theory and qualitative research comes up regularly in the literature. The difficulty for the neophyte qualitative researcher is determining what is meant when the statement is made that qualitative research is atheoretical when, on further reading, the researcher discovers debates in the literature that speak to all knowledge being theoretically based. The best way to begin to understand the debate is to understand the language. What exactly is theory? According to Chinn and Kramer (2004), a theory is "a creative and rigorous structuring of ideas that projects a tentative, purposeful, and systematic view of phenomena" (p. 91). The purpose of research is to explain, predict, or control outcomes. In the qualitative research paradigm, the focus is on understanding. Consequently, many qualitative researchers espouse the importance of maintaining an atheoretical stance to their research. The question to be raised is this: Is there a debate, or is there reason to believe that the debate arises from differences in interpretation?

Thomas (2002) offers that the definitional boundaries of the term *theory* have been expanded to the point that any *reasoned* discussion is labeled theory (p. 420). Some would argue that the debate is better described as a conflict of definitions or interpretations. Fawcett (2000) defined *philosophy* as "a statement encompassing ontological claims about the phenomena of central interest to a discipline, epistemic claims about how those phenomena come to be known, and ethical claims about what the members of a discipline value" (p. 6). Fawcett's definition supports philosophy as a higher level of abstraction than theory. Fawcett further shares that the purpose of a philosophy is "to inform the members of disciplines and the general public about the beliefs and values of a particular discipline" (p. 6). One of the ways to manage the interpretive debate is to adopt Fawcett's hierarchical structure regarding philosophy and theory.

Often, to further illustrate the point, qualitative researchers subscribe to a particular school of thought regarding their research based on the specific philosophical position they believe most closely aligns with their personal understanding. For instance, in phenomenology there are two sets of ideas about approaching understanding phenomena: descriptive and hermeneutic. Both of these traditions arise out of a rich history of inquiry into understanding the human phenomena by different phenomenologists. The purpose of subscribing to one school or the other is not to explain, predict, or control particular phenomena but rather to understand the phenomena using a particular set of guiding principles. The purpose of these principles is to structure the design of the inquiry, not to prove that they are right or wrong.

Chinn and Kramer's (2004) definition of theory is not useful in qualitative research if it is viewed as the "creative and rigorous structuring of ideas that projects a tentative, purposeful, and systematic view of phenomena" (p. 91). Not everything studied by qualitative researchers can be viewed in this systematized way. However, the information discovered as part of a qualitative inquiry may lead to the development of yet unknown theories. Not all qualitative research studies lead to theory development, but certainly specific approaches used in qualitative research can lead to theory development. Grounded theory is an example of such an approach (see

Chapter 7). In grounded theory, the researcher's goal is to develop theory to describe a particular social process.

As an example of how a study may lead to theory development, Keating-Lefler and Wilson (2004) used grounded theory methodology to develop a substantive theory of becoming a mother for the first time while being single, unpartnered, and Medicaid eligible. This example clearly demonstrates the potential use of qualitative research for theory development.

The point of offering the debate about theory to the reader is to place the role of theory development within the context of qualitative research and to help the nurse new to qualitative research begin to understand what on the surface appears to be a contradiction. It is generally accepted that qualitative research findings have the potential to create theory. In the instance of grounded theory, the method is dedicated to the discovery of theory.

With regard to theoretical points of view attributed to specific methods, the reader needs to understand that the term *theory* is used by a variety of authors in many different ways. The term *theory* requires the same degree of scrutiny that many other frequently used and misused terms require. In addition, full disclosure by those using the term is needed so that those interested in understanding the debate have the information required to approach it logically.

Objective Versus Subjective Data Within a Nursing Context

Empirical scientists believe that the study of any phenomena must be devoid of subjectivity (Namenwirth, 1986). Furthermore, they have contended that objectivity is essential in guiding the way to truth. The problem with this position is that no human activity can be performed without subjectivity. Researchers, as well as those being studied, think and act based on their subjective interpretations of the world. It is important in quantitative research to make the study as objective as possible. However, it is critical to understand that no research activity is ever totally without its subjective components.

Based on his reading and interpretation of Hanson (1958), Phillips (1987) suggested that objectivity is impossible: "The theory, hypothesis, framework, or background knowledge held by an investigator can strongly influence what he sees" (p. 9). Kerlinger (1979) also proposed that "the procedures of science are objective and not the scientists. Scientists, like all men and women, are opinionated, dogmatic, and ideological" (p. 264). Therefore, the idea of objectivity loses its meaning. On some level, all research endeavors have the subjective influence of the scientist. Procedural objectivity is the goal; however, even it is biased because the scientist will interpret the findings. Even if the findings of a study are statistical (thought to be an objective measure), the scientist interprets the statistical data through a lens of opinions and biases about what the numbers say (MacKenzie, 1981; Taylor, 1985).

Humanistic scientists value the subjective component of the quest for knowledge. They embrace the idea of subjectivity, recognizing that humans are incapable of total objectivity because they have been situated in a reality constructed by subjective experiences. Meaning, and therefore the search for the truth, is possible only through social observation and interaction. The degree to which the scientist is part of the development of scientific knowledge is debated even by the humanistic scientists. Post-empiricists accept the subjective nature of inquiry but still support rigor and objective study through method. The objectivity post-empiricists speak of is one of context. For example, post-empiricist scientists would acknowledge their subjective realities and then, always being aware of them, seek to keep them apart from data collection but to include them in the analysis and the final report.

Constructivist humanistic scientists believe that "knowledge is the result of a dialogical process between the self-understanding person and that which is encountered—whether a text, a work of art, or the meaningful expression of another person" (Smith, 1990, p. 177). Clearly, subjectivity is acknowledged, but the degree to which it is embraced is based on philosophic beliefs.

Humanistic scientists see objectivity in its empirical definition to be impossible. The degree to which a researcher can be objective, and therefore unbiased, is determined by the philosophic tradition to which the human scientist ascribes. That subjectivity which is included in the discussion of human science conveys an understanding that participation in the world prohibits humans from ever being fully objective.

Nurse researchers engaged in qualitative research recognize the subjective reality inherent in the research process and embrace it. They are bound by method to acknowledge their subjectivity and to place it in a context that permits full examination of the effect of subjectivity on the research endeavor and description of the phenomenon under study.

GROUNDING RESEARCH IN THE REALITIES OF NURSING

*N*urse scientists have the responsibility of developing new knowledge. Fawcett (1999) offers that nursing needs three types of research: basic, applied, and clinical. The question that needs answering will drive the research type and paradigm selected. If a nurse scientist is interested in discovering the most effective way to suction a tracheostomy tube, then a quantitative approach will be the appropriate way to study the problem. But, if the nurse scientist is interested in discovering what the experience of suctioning is for people who are suctioned, qualitative research methods are more appropriate. What the nurse scientist must do is clearly define the problem and then identify whether it requires an inductive or deductive approach. Only the researcher can determine what the explicit question is and how best to answer it. As Lincoln (1992) pointed out, the area of health research is open to inquiry, and the qualitative model is a superior choice over conventional methods.

Emancipation

In recent years, much has been written about "emancipatory research" (Henderson, 1995). Two predominant paradigms permeate what is published: critical theory and feminist theory. *Critical theory*, as described by Habermas (1971), is a way to develop knowledge that is free, undistorted, and unconstrained. According to Habermas, the predominant paradigm in science was not reflective of people's reality. He found that empiricism created cognitive dissonance. The goal of critical theory is to "unfreeze lawlike structures and to encourage self reflections for those whom the laws are about" (Wilson-Thomas, 1995, p. 573). "Critical [theorists] . . . sought to expose oppressive relationships among groups and to enlighten those who are oppressed" (Bent, 1993, p. 296).

Similarly, *feminist theory* takes the idea of emancipation further and speaks specifically to women's lives. Feminist theorists value women and women's experiences (Hall & Stevens, 1991). Feminist scholars believe that the traditional laws of science limit and preclude the discovery of what is uniquely feminist. Seibold (2000) identifies feminist research as being focused first and foremost on women's experiences. Feminist researchers attempt to see the world from the view of the women studied and to be critical in examination of the issues and active in improving the condition of those studied.

In both paradigms, the predominant themes are liberating the study participants and making their voices heard. Sigsworth (1995) identified seven fundamental conditions that are necessary for feminist research that, when editorialized, are appropriate for critical theorist ideas about research as well. These conditions are as follows: (1) the research should be focused on the experiences of the population studied, their perceptions, and their truths; (2) "artificial dichotomies and sharp boundaries are suspect in research involving human beings" (Sigsworth, 1995, p. 897); (3) history and concurrent events are always considered when planning, conducting, analyzing, and interpreting findings; (4) the questions asked are as important as the answers discovered; (5) research should not be hierarchical; (6) researchers' assumptions, biases, and presuppositions are part of the research enterprise; and (7) researchers and research participants are partners whose discoveries lead to understanding.

According to Hall and Stevens (1991), qualitative methods are more in line with the feminist perspective, as well as with critical theorist ideas. The tenets offered earlier are primary in conducting a study regardless of the methodology used. However, by their stated purposes, the methods of qualitative research are far more accommodating to the ideas supported by critical and feminist theorists. Researchers who wish their work to be emancipating and liberating should consider the methods of qualitative research described in this text.

SUMMARY

*I*n this chapter, the fundamentals of qualitative research as a specific research paradigm have been described. Every attempt has been made to offer to the reader varied ideas on each of the topics covered. An explanation of science, philosophy, and theory grounds some of the more rigorously debated ideas in qualitative research. Understanding how individuals acquire knowledge and use their experience to develop their approaches to inquiry helps the reader to value differing research paradigms. Equally important is an understanding that no single paradigm will answer all the questions important to nursing. It is only through use of both qualitative and quantitative research methods that we will come to a better understanding of human beings and their health. The information presented in this chapter also included the relationship of historical, practical, and theoretical ideas about qualitative research. It is hoped that these ideas have piqued the reader's interest and will lead to exploration of the specifics of qualitative research as they are developed in this text.

References

Anderson, E. (2004). Feminist epistemology and philosophy of science. In E. N. Zalta (Ed.), *The Stanford Encyclopedia of Philosophy* (Summer 2004 Edition). Retrieved August 10, 2005, from http://plato.stanford.edu/archives/sum2004/entries/feminism-epistemology/

Benner, P. (1984). *From novice to expert.* Menlo Park, CA: Addison-Wesley.

Bent, K. N. (1993). Perspectives on critical and feminist theory in developing nursing praxis. *Journal of Professional Nursing, 9*(5), 296-303.

Burnard, P., & Hannigan, B. (2000). Qualitative and quantitative approaches in mental health nursing: Moving the debate forward. *Journal of Psychiatric and Mental Health Nursing, 7*, 1-6.

Carper, B. (1978). Fundamental patterns of knowing in nursing. *Advances in Nursing Science, 1*(1), 13-23.

Cheek, J. (2002). Advancing what? Qualitative research, scholarship, and the research imperative. *Qualitative Health Research, 12*(8), 1130-1140.

Chinn, P. L., & Kramer, M. K. (2004). *Integrated knowledge development in nursing* (6th ed.). St. Louis: Mosby.

Denzin, N. K., & Lincoln, Y. S. (Eds.). (1994). *Handbook of qualitative research.* Thousand Oaks, CA: Sage.

Ermath, M. (1978). *Wilhelm Dilthey: The critique of historical reason.* Chicago: University of Chicago Press.

Fawcett, J. (1999). The state of nursing science: Hallmarks of the 20th and 21st centuries. *Nursing Science Quarterly, 12*(4), 311-318.

Fawcett, J. (2000). Analysis and evaluation of contemporary nursing knowledge: Nursing theories and models. Philadelphia: F.A. Davis.

Guba, E. G. (1990). *The paradigm dialogue.* Newbury Park, CA: Sage.

Guiliano, K. K. (2003). Expanding the use of empiricism in nursing: Can we bridge the gap between knowledge and clinical practice? *Nursing Philosophy, 4*, 44-52.

Habermas, J. (1971). *Knowledge and human interests* (J. J. Strapiro, trans.). Boston: Beacon Press.

Hall, J. M., & Stevens, P. E. (1991). Rigour in feminist research. *Advances in Nursing Science, 22*(3), 16-29.

Hamilton, D. (1994). Traditions, preferences, and postures in applied qualitative research. In N. K. Denzin & Y. S. Lincoln (Eds.), *Handbook of qualitative research* (pp. 60-69). Thousand Oaks, CA: Sage.

Hanson, N. R. (1958). *Patterns of discovery.* Cambridge: Cambridge University Press.

Henderson, D. J. (1995). Consciousness raising in participatory research: Method and methodology for emancipatory inquiry. *Advances in Nursing Science, 17*(3), 58-69.

Keating-Lefler, R., & Wilson, M. E. (2004). The experience of becoming a mother for single, unpartnered, Medicaid-eligible, first-time mothers. *Journal of Nursing Scholarship, 36*(1), 23-29.

Kerlinger, F. N. (1979). *Behavioral research: A conceptual approach.* New York: Holt, Rinehart & Winston.

Krasner, D. L. (2000). Qualitative research: A different paradigm—part 1. *Journal of Wound, Ostomy and Continence Nursing, 28*, 70-72.

Liehr, P., & Smith, M. J. (2002). Theoretical frameworks. In G. LoBiondo-Wood & J. Haber (Eds.), *Nursing research: Methods, critical appraisal, and utilization* (5th ed., pp. 107-120). St. Louis: Mosby.

Lincoln, Y. S. (1992). Sympathetic connections between qualitative methods and health research. *Qualitative Health Research, 2*(4), 375-391.

MacKenzie, D. (1981). *Statistics in Great Britain: 1885-1930.* Edinburgh, UK: Edinburgh University Press.

May, K. A. (1994). Abstract knowing: The case for magic in method. In J. Morse (Ed.), *Critical issues in qualitative research methods* (pp. 10-21). Thousand Oaks, CA: Sage.

Mitchell, G. J. (2001). Prescription, freedom, and participation: Drilling down into theory-based nursing practice. *Nursing Science Quarterly, 14*(3), 205-210.

Munhall, P. L. (2001). Epistemology in nursing. In P. L. Munhall (Ed.), *Nursing research: A qualitative perspective* (pp. 37-64). Boston: Jones and Bartlett.

Namenwirth, M. (1986). Science seen through a feminist prism. In R. Bleier (Ed.), *Feminist approaches to science* (pp. 18-41). New York: Pergamon Press.

Parse, R. R. (2001). *Qualitative inquiry: The path of sciencing*. Boston: Jones and Bartlett.

Phillips, D. C. (1987). *Philosophy, science, and social inquiry*. New York: Pergamon Press.

Sandelowski, M. (1994). The proof is in the pottery: Toward a poetic for qualitative inquiry. In J. Morse (Ed.), *Critical issues in qualitative research methods* (pp. 44-62). Thousand Oaks, CA: Sage.

Seibold, C. (2000). Qualitative research from a feminist perspective in the postmodern era: Methodological, ethical and reflexive concerns. *Nursing Inquiry, 7*(3), 147-155.

Siepmann, J. P. (1999). What is science? *Journal of Theoretics, 1-3*. Retrieved August 5, 2004, from http://www.journaloftheoretics.com/Editorials/Vol-1/e1-3.htm

Sigsworth, J. (1995). Feminist research: Its relevance to nursing. *Journal of Advanced Nursing, 22*, 896-899.

Smith, J. K. (1990). Alternative research paradigms and the problem of criteria. In E. G. Guba (Ed.), *The paradigm dialogue* (pp. 167-187). Newbury Park, CA: Sage.

Taylor, C. (1985). *Human agency and language*. Cambridge, UK: Cambridge University Press.

Thomas, G. (2002). Theory's spell-on qualitative inquiry and educational research. *British Educational Research Journal, 28*(3), 419-434.

Thorne, S. (1997). Phenomenological positivism and other problematic trends in health science research. *Qualitative Health Research, 7*(2), 287-293.

Wainwright, P. (2000). Towards an aesthetics of nursing. *Journal of Advanced Nursing, 32*(3), 750-756.

Wilson-Thomas, L. (1995). Applying critical social theory in nursing education to bridge the gap between theory, research and practice. *Journal of Advanced Nursing, 21*, 568-575.

CHAPTER 2

The Conduct of Qualitative Research: Common Essential Elements

*A*s the emphasis in the clinical arena has moved toward evidenced-based practice, it has become increasingly important to examine how and why nurses make the decisions that they do with regard to their research. To fully comprehend the importance of this examination, the following question is offered: Are research foci selected to address research dissertation advisors' agendas, class objectives, employers' agendas, funding agency priorities, or promotion and tenure criteria, or to meet the needs of the patients nurses serve? This question is not meant to suggest that conducting research for "practical" reasons is not legitimate. It is also not meant to suggest that the findings will ultimately not serve patients. However, it remains primary that nurses focus on development of nursing knowledge. And because the time and energy required to conduct research are significant, it should be work that nurse researchers are deeply invested in.

One of the differences in nursing research presently that may have not been as true in the past is that nurse researchers spend more time developing their research questions and clarifying what it is they are planning to study. It becomes increasingly more important that research studies be based on sound rationale and a clear understanding of the research question. Denzin (2000) suggests that in addition to carefully developing the research question, researchers must also examine the political nature of their work. All research represents a political enterprise that carries significant implications. The more nurses understand the motivating factors involved in their work, the more explicit they can be about its benefits.

Once the research question is clearly articulated and the researcher has an understanding of the problem and what impact the research activity will have on those studied, the discipline, and those to whom the results may be meaningful, the researcher will need to decide which research paradigm will most appropriately answer the question. This chapter offers the reasons for choosing a qualitative approach to inquiry, describes the common elements of the qualitative research process, and shares with the reader very practical information regarding how to enter the field. Based on this overview of the important aspects of qualitative research, readers will be able to assess whether qualitative inquiry offers an opportunity to explore the questions that arise from their practice.

Undoubtedly, to fully engage in one of the methods discussed in this book, the reader will need a solid understanding of the method and its assumptions. In addition, it is essential to engage a research mentor (Morse, 1997). As Morse has offered, one cannot learn to drive a car by reading the manual; hence, the researcher should not assume that one could conduct a qualitative study by reading this or any other qualitative research text. A mentor will make "shifting gears" a more effective process.

INITIATING THE STUDY: CHOOSING A QUALITATIVE APPROACH

Exploring the Common Characteristics of Qualitative Research

In the conduct of research, certain attributes are common to the discovery process. This is true of both qualitative and quantitative designs. This section explores those common characteristics of qualitative research. Table 2.1 offers a comparison of qualitative and quantitative methods.

Table 2.1 • Comparison of Quantitative and Qualitative Research Methods	
Quantitative	*Qualitative*
Objective	Subjectivity valued
One reality	Multiple realities
Reduction, control, prediction	Discovery, description, understanding
Measurable	Interpretative
Mechanistic	Organismic
Parts equal the whole	Whole is greater than the parts
Report statistical analyses	Report rich narrative
Researcher separate	Researcher part of research process
Subjects	Participants
Context free	Context dependent

Qualitative researchers emphasize six significant characteristics in their research: (1) a belief in multiple realities; (2) a commitment to identifying an approach to understanding that supports the phenomenon studied; (3) a commitment to the participant's viewpoint; (4) the conduct of inquiry in a way that limits disruption of the natural context of the phenomena of interest; (5) acknowledged participation of the researcher in the research process; and (6) the reporting of the data in a literary style rich with participant commentaries.

The idea that multiple realities exist and create meaning for the individuals studied is a fundamental belief of qualitative researchers. "Qualitative researchers direct their attention to human realities rather than to the concrete realities of objects" (Boyd, 2001, p. 76). Instead of searching for one reality—one truth—researchers committed to qualitative research believe that individuals actively participate in social actions, and through these interactions that occur based on previous experiences, individuals come to know and understand phenomena in different ways. Because people do understand and live experiences differently, qualitative researchers do not subscribe to one truth but, rather, to many truths. Qualitative researchers believe that there are always multiple realities (perspectives) to consider when trying to fully understand a situation (Boyd, 2001).

Qualitative researchers are committed to discovery through the use of multiple ways of understanding. These researchers address questions about particular phenomena by finding an appropriate method or approach to answer the research question. The discovery leads the choice of method rather than the method leading the discovery. In some cases, more than one qualitative approach or more than one data collection strategy may be necessary to fully understand a phenomenon. For example, in her work on end-of-life decisions by hemodialysis patients, Calvin (2004) used interviews, transcripts, and field notes to determine how dialysis patients made end-of-life decisions. The interviews provided the researcher with individual perceptions of the decision-making process. The transcripts and field notes offered additional data to further the understanding of how individuals on dialysis make decisions about end-of-life treatments. In this instance and in other qualitative research studies, researchers are committed to *discovery.* The discovery process in qualitative research provides the opportunity for variation in the use of data collection strategies. Method and data collection strategies may change as needed, rather than being prescribed before the inquiry begins. As Maggs-Rapport (2000) suggests, "there are benefits to be derived from an approach which combines . . . methods and methodologies, provided that methodological rigor is applied without compromising the underlying value of any one methodology" (p. 224). This process differs from the way traditional or positivist science is developed.

Commitment to participants' viewpoints is another characteristic of qualitative research. Use of unstructured interview, observation, and artifacts grounds researchers in the real life of study participants. Researchers are co-participants in discovery and understanding of the realities of the phenomena studied. Qualitative researchers will conduct extensive interviews and observations, searching documents and artifacts of importance to fully understand the context of what is researched. The purpose of the extensive investigation is to provide a view of reality that is important to the study participants, rather than to the researchers. For example, in a grounded theory study focused on becoming a mother, Keating-Lefler and Wilson (2004) offered only one introductory question to study participants to engage them in describing what it is like to become a first-time mother given the special circumstances of being single, unpartnered, and Medicaid eligible. Instead of using an instrument to examine the women's perceptions, which would include pre-established ideas about what the women's experiences were, Keating-Lefler and Wilson used the following: "Please tell me what the experience of becoming a mother has been like for you and how it has affected your life?" This open-ended prompt allowed the participants to share *their* experiences, in *their own* words, rather than being forced into pre-established lines of thinking developed by researchers.

Another characteristic of qualitative research is conduct of the inquiry in a way that does not disturb the natural context of the phenomena studied. Researchers are obligated to conduct a study in a manner that least disturbs the natural setting. Using ethnographic research to illustrate this characteristic, the ethnographer would study a particular culture with as little intrusion as possible. Living among study participants is one way to minimize the intrusion and maintain the natural context of the setting. It is unrealistic to believe that the introduction of an unknown individual will not change the nature of the relationships and activities observed; however, the researcher's prolonged presence should minimize the effect of the intrusion.

All research affects the study participants in some way. The addition of any new person or experience changes the way people think or act. The important factor in qualitative research that makes the difference is the serious attention to discovering the *emic view,* that is, the insider's perspective. What is it like for the participant? Qualitative researchers explore the insider's view with utmost respect for the individual's perspective and his or her space. As stated earlier, prolonged engagement by the researcher has the effect of reducing overt changes in behavior of those studied. Therefore, a nurse interested in conducting a qualitative study must provide adequate time for building a trusting relationship and eliminating the distractions created by introducing someone new in the setting.

Researcher as instrument is another characteristic of qualitative research. The use of the researcher as instrument requires an acceptance that the researcher is part of the study. Because the researcher is the observer, interviewer, or the interpreter of various aspects of the inquiry, objectivity serves no purpose. Qualitative investigators accept that all research is conducted with a subjective bias. They further believe that researcher participation in the inquiry has the potential to add to the richness of data collection and analysis. Objectivity is a principle in quantitative research that documents the rigor of the science. In qualitative research, rigor is most often determined by the study participants and consumers of the study. From the participants' points of view: Do they recognize what the researcher has reported to be their culture or experience? From the consumer's perspective: Does the researcher stay true to the participants' expressions of their experience? Is enough evidence provided so that the consumer can assess this? The acknowledgment of the subjective nature of qualitative research and the understanding that researchers affect what is studied are fundamental to the conduct of qualitative inquiry.

Regardless of the approach, qualitative researchers will report the study findings in a rich literary style. Participants' experiences are the findings of qualitative research. Therefore, it is essential these experiences be reported from the perspective of the people who have lived them. Inclusion of quotations, commentaries, and narratives adds to the richness of the report and to the understanding of the experience and context in which they occur. Table 2.1 describes the contrasts between quantitative and qualitative research.

These six characteristics guide qualitative researchers on a journey of exploration and discovery. Doing qualitative research is similar to reading a good novel. When conducted in the spirit of the philosophy that supports it, qualitative research is rich and rewarding, leaving researchers and consumers with a desire to understand more about the phenomena of interest.

Selecting the Method Based on Phenomenon of Interest

Agreement with the basic tenets of qualitative research is the first step in deciding whether to initiate a qualitative research study. Once researchers understand that these essential elements will guide all that they do, they can begin to explore various qualitative methods. It is important to note that all qualitative approaches "share a similar goal in that they seek to arrive at an understanding of a particular phenomenon from the perspective of those experiencing the phenomenon" (Woodgate, 2000, p. 194). What the researcher will need to determine is which approach will answer the research question. The choice of method depends on the question being asked.

Because each method is explained in depth in the following chapters, the examples that follow serve only as an introduction to method selection based on the phenomena of interest. While reading the examples, keep in mind that the qualitative nurse researcher is more concerned with values, beliefs, and meaning attached to health and illness than to aggregates of conditions (Hayes, 2001).

For example, while working in a nursing home, a nurse might observe individuals who seem to be very happy in their setting while others are not. The nurse is interested in discovering what the experience of living in the nursing home is for those who seem to be well adjusted. In this case, the nurse would use phenomenology to learn more about the experience of living in a nursing home from those who seem to enjoy being there. The purpose of phenomenology is to explore the lived experience of individuals. Phenomenology provides researchers with the framework for discovering what it is like to live an experience.

If the nurse researcher is interested in the nursing home as an institution that cares for the elderly in a particular community, as well as its political antecedents, a historical inquiry is the research approach of choice. For a historical study, review of institutional documents such as meeting minutes, policy manuals in addition to community meeting minutes, personal documents, diaries, research papers and proceedings, newspaper articles, commentaries, narratives, and personal interviews will provide the necessary information to chronicle the contribution the institution has made in the care of elderly.

Another question that might be important to answer is the following: What is it like to make the decision to become a nursing home resident? Based on the preceding comments, phenomenology may be the method of choice; however, assume that it is not the experience of being a resident that is of interest to the researcher but, rather, the process that the individual goes through to arrive at the decision that the nursing home is the right place to be. In this case, the research method selected would be grounded theory. The researcher is more interested in understanding the process of choosing to leave one's home and enter a nursing home rather than the actual experience of being a nursing home resident. The purpose is what determines the method. More specifically, the grounded theory researcher interested in the process of choosing to leave one's residence to be cared for in a nursing home is committed to developing a theory—understanding the process that an individual goes through to arrive at that decision.

In a related situation, a nurse might be interested in studying the culture of family support groups for those with loved ones in a nursing home. The nurse researcher would want to observe and collect information about group members, their activities, values, meaningful artifacts, and life ways, as well as participate in group sessions. In doing so, a full understanding of the culture of the support group studied would become evident. In this case, ethnography would be the method of choice.

If a nurse researcher is interested in social change as it relates to nursing home residents and their ability to participate in the setting, an action research study might be the appropriate choice. By working with residents to study those who have been active in maintaining an independent environment, the researcher and residents have the potential to learn from the experiences of those residents who have been most involved, to learn how they maintain their independence, and to help to co-create structures to ensure full participation for those living in the facility. If the researcher is committed to a collaborative research approach that facilitates participation and action, then action research is an appropriate choice. When researchers choose action research, they serve two masters: theory and practice (Jenks, 1995).

This limited description demonstrates that there are a number of research methods to address specific practice questions. Researchers need to clearly identify the focus of the inquiry and then choose the method that will most effectively answer the question.

Understanding the Philosophic Position

After researchers have identified the research question and have made explicit the approach to studying the question, a thorough understanding of the philosophic assumptions that are the foundation of the method is essential. Too frequently, novice qualitative researchers develop and implement research studies without having a solid understanding of the philosophic underpinnings of the chosen method. This lack of understanding has the potential of leading to sloppy science, resulting in misunderstood findings. For instance, phenomenology is an approach that can be used to study lived experience. Based on the philosophic position supported by the researcher, different interpretations might occur. To further illustrate this point, phenomenologists who support Edmund Husserl—a prominent leader of the phenomenological movement—and his followers believe that the purpose of phenomenology is to provide pure understanding. Supporters of the philosophic positions of Martin Heidegger and his colleagues believe that phenomenology is interpretive. Neither group is incorrect; rather, each approaches the study of lived experience with different sets of goals and expectations.

The comments offered here should help the reader develop an appreciation for the importance of understanding the method chosen and its philosophic underpinnings. Making explicit the school of thought that guides an inquiry will help researchers to conduct a credible study and help those people who use the findings apply the results within the appropriate context.

Using the Literature Review

In the development of a quantitative research study, an interested researcher would begin with an extensive literature search on the topic of interest. This review documents the necessity for the study and provides a discussion of the area of interest and related topics. It helps the researcher determine whether the planned study has been conducted, and if so, whether significant results were discovered. Furthermore, it helps the researcher refine the research question, select a theoretical framework, and build a case for why the topic of interest should be studied and how the researcher will approach the topic.

Qualitative researchers do not generally begin with an *extensive* literature review. Some qualitative researchers would suggest that no literature review should be conducted before the inquiry begins. Others accept that a cursory review of the literature may help focus the study or provide an orienting framework (Creswell, 2003, p. 30). The reason for not conducting the literature review initially is to reduce the likelihood that the investigator will develop suppositions or biases about the topic under consideration. Further, by not developing preconceived ideas about the topic, it is assumed that the researcher will be protected from leading the participants during the interviewing process in the direction of the researcher's beliefs. For instance, if a researcher is interested in developing a theory about the process a client goes through in accepting the necessity of an amputation, a review of the literature before the study might lead to the development of preconceived notions about amputees. The researcher may not have held these beliefs before the review, but, following it, now has information that could affect how he or she collects and analyzes data. Creswell states, "in a qualitative study, use the literature sparingly in the beginning of the plan in order to convey an inductive design, unless the qualitative strategy-type requires a substantial literature orientation at the outset" (p. 33).

It is, however, essential to conduct the literature review after analyzing the data. The purpose of reviewing the literature in a qualitative study is to place the findings of the study in the context of what is already known. Generally, qualitative researchers do not use the literature review to establish grounds for the study or to suggest a theoretical or conceptual framework. The purpose of the literature review in a qualitative study is to tell the reader how the findings fit into what is already known about the phenomena. It is not meant to confirm or argue existing findings.

Explicating the Researcher's Beliefs

Before starting a qualitative study, it is in the researcher's best interest to make clear his or her thoughts, ideas, suppositions, or presuppositions about the topic, as well as personal biases. The purpose of this activity is to bring to consciousness and reveal what is believed about a topic. By bringing to consciousness the researcher's beliefs, he or she is in a better position to approach the topic honestly and openly. Explication of personal beliefs makes the investigator more aware of the potential judgments that may occur during data collection and analysis based on the researcher's belief system rather than on the actual data collected from participants. One of the best ways to make one's beliefs known is to write them down. Writing out what one believes before actually conducting the study gives the author a frame of reference. Journaling during the time that one is engaged in the research also helps to keep an open mind and differentiate what the researcher's thoughts are versus the ideas, comments, and activities of the participants. As qualitative researchers conduct their studies, they can use their journal to "reality-test" what is being observed or heard against what they have written down (the researcher's ideas or presuppositions).

As an example, let's say that the topic of interest is quality of life for individuals diagnosed with multiple sclerosis (MS). The researcher has an interest in the topic based on a long history of working with individuals with end-stage disease. Based on the researcher's experience, his or her perception is that people with MS live sad, limited existences. If researchers do not explicate these perceptions, they may lead informants to describe their experiences in the direction of the researchers' own beliefs about what is real or important. This can occur as a result of the questions asked. In asking questions, the researcher might try to validate his or her ideas about MS without really discovering the meaning of MS for those who live with it. Remember, the way the questions are worded can affect the outcome of the interview and sometimes impose answers on respondents (McDougall, 2000). The act of expressing one's ideas should help remind the researcher to listen and see what is real for the informants rather than what is real for the researcher. Schutz (1970) recommended that researchers follow this process of describing personal beliefs about their assumptions to help them refrain from making judgments about phenomena based on personal experiences.

Once the researcher has explicated his or her thoughts, feelings, and perceptions about phenomena, it is recommended that the researcher bracket those thoughts, feelings, and perceptions. *Bracketing* is the cognitive process of putting aside one's own beliefs, not making judgments about what one has observed or heard, and remaining open to data as they are revealed. Specifically, in descriptive phenomenology, this activity is carried out before the beginning of the study and is repeated throughout data collection and analysis. In ethnographic work, keeping a diary of personal thoughts and feelings is an excellent way to make clear the researcher's ideas. Once revealed, the researcher can set them aside. *Setting them aside* means to be constantly aware of what the researcher believes and trying to keep it separate from what is being shared by the informant. By conducting this self-disclosure, researchers are more likely to be able to keep their eyes open and to remain cognizant of when data collection and analysis reflect their own personal beliefs rather than informants' beliefs.

Ahern (1999) states that the process of bracketing is iterative and part of a reflexive journey. She states that it is important to process your thoughts about the phenomenon of interest. As suggested earlier, writing down your thoughts is one of the best ways to be aware of what you believe. Once they have been written down, you should reflect on what you have written and try to understand why you have written what you have, what values are inherent in your statements, and how they affect the study. It is essential that the researcher be aware of the potential impact that imposing personal agendas can have on the process of data collection and analysis. Bracketing is essential if the researcher is to share the informants' views of the studied phenomena.

Choosing the Setting for Data Collection

The setting for qualitative research is the field. The *field* is the place where individuals of interest live—where they experience life. The inquiry will be conducted in the homes, neighborhoods, classrooms, or sites selected by the study participants. The reason for conducting data collection in the field is to maintain the natural settings where phenomena occur. For instance, if an investigator is interested in studying the culture of an intensive care unit (ICU), he or she will visit an ICU. If a researcher is interested in studying the clinical decision-making skills of nurses, he or she will go to nurses who use this process and ask them where they want to be interviewed or observed.

Being in the field requires reciprocity in decision making. The researcher is not in control of the study setting or those who inform the inquiry. Participants will decide what information they share with the researcher. For instance, if the researcher is interested in studying the experiences of people who have received a cancer diagnosis, he or she would need access to people who have had this life situation. The researcher may make the decision to enter the setting and may select appropriate individuals to interview. However, participants may not wish to share their thoughts or feelings in one sitting or at all. Visiting frequently and building a trusting relationship can help the participant feel more comfortable in sharing sensitive information and provide the element of control that may be very important to the participant. It is essential to remember that using qualitative research methods requires good interpersonal skills and a willingness to relinquish control. The mutual trust that develops based on the reciprocal nature of decision making will enhance the discovery process by allowing access to personal information and private spaces usually reserved for significant people in the lives of informants. The conduct of qualitative research with its requirement of close social interaction may create situations that can either limit or enhance access to information. The close social interaction also has the potential to create ethical dilemmas that need careful attention (see Chapter 4). Only by being aware of the distinctive nature of the interactions and being in the field will the researcher be truly aware of the strengths and potential weaknesses of this form of research.

Selecting Participants

Qualitative researchers generally do not label the individuals who inform their inquiries as *subjects*. The use of the terms *participants* or *informants* illustrates the status those studied play in the research process. "Individuals cooperating in the study play an active rather than a passive role and are therefore referred to as informants or study participants" (Polit, Beck, & Hungler, 2001, p. 31). The participants' active involvement in the inquiry helps those who are interested in their experiences or cultures to better understand their lives and social interactions.

Individuals are selected to participate in qualitative research based on their first-hand experience with a culture, social process, or phenomenon of interest. For instance, if a phenomenologist is interested in studying the culture of a woman who has anorexia, then the informants for the study must be those women who are anorexic. The participants are selected for the purpose of describing an experience in which they have participated. Unlike quantitative research, there is no need to randomly select individuals because manipulation, control, and generalization of findings are not the intent of the inquiry. The outcome of a qualitative study should be greater understanding of the phenomena (Krasner, 2001). Therefore, the researcher interested in women who are anorexic should interview as many anorexic women as possible to obtain a clear understanding of the culture. This type of sampling has been labeled *purposeful sampling* (Lincoln & Guba, 1995; Patton, 1990). It has also been called *purposive sampling* (Field & Morse, 1985). A similar type of sampling is *theoretical sampling* (Glaser & Strauss, 1967; Patton, 1980). Theoretical sampling, used primarily in grounded theory, is one particular type of purposeful sampling (Coyne, 1997). Theoretical sampling is a complex form of sampling based on concepts that have proven theoretical relevance to the evolving theory (Coyne, 1997; Strauss & Corbin, 1990). More specifically, Glaser (1978) states,

> Theoretical sampling is the process of data collection for generating
> theory whereby the analyst jointly collects, codes, and analyses his data
> and decides what data to collect next and where to find them in order
> to develop his theory as it emerges. (p. 36)

Theoretical sampling "is a valuable way of encouraging studies to develop and
build on theory at an early stage" (Thompson, 1999, p. 816).

What both purposeful and theoretical sampling represent is a commitment to observing and interviewing people who have had experience with
or are part of the culture or phenomenon of interest. The goal for researchers
is to develop a rich or dense description of the culture or phenomenon,
rather than using sampling techniques that support generalizability of the
findings. A particular purposeful sampling technique is *snowballing*.
Snowballing uses one informant to find another. This technique is especially
useful when those you wish to interview are difficult to locate. For example,
if you were interested in studying the experience of adoptive parents of
Romanian children who have chronic health problems, it would be difficult
to locate these parents in one place. However, if you know one set of parents
who are willing to refer you to another set of parents, you are able to use this
contact method to find other parents. Sixsmith, Boneham, and Goldring
(2003) offer that although this strategy may be very helpful, it also has the
drawback of potentially limiting those in your study who are from similar
backgrounds.

Cohen, Phillips, and Palos (2001) discuss the value of including cultural
minorities in qualitative research studies. They share that it is not only
valuable to include minorities but also mandated by the National Institutes of
Health. Therefore, when studying a particular culture or phenomenon, the
qualitative nurse researcher should be aware of the importance and overall
benefits of including minorities in the study when appropriate. Cohen and
colleagues discuss the potential skepticism that may be encountered when
nurses of different cultural backgrounds try to enlist members of other
cultures. They suggest that nurse researchers engage diverse populations by
using some of the following strategies: (1) seek endorsement and support
from community leaders; (2) commit to giving back something to the group
you wish to study; (3) develop an ongoing relationship of trust and respect;
(4) develop cultural competence and sensitivity; (5) become well acquainted
with the group before you approach them; (6) recognize the heterogeneous
nature of a group; and (7) use anthropologic strategies when conducting the
research (Cohen et al., 2001, p. 194).

Choosing the setting and participants appropriately will assist in
developing a successful research study. Knowing how to access the site,
knowing what to expect from those who are part of a particular group,
and knowing how to most effectively develop a trusting relationship with

those from whom you intend to learn will support achievement of the research goals.

Achieving Saturation

A feature that is closely related to the topic of sampling is saturation. *Saturation* refers to the repetition of discovered information and confirmation of previously collected data (Morse, 1994). This means that rather than sampling a specific number of individuals to gain significance based on statistical manipulation, the qualitative researcher is looking for repetition and confirmation of previously collected data. For example, Rew (2003) was interested in developing a theory to explain how homeless youth engage in self-care behaviors. Her sample included homeless youth living temporarily in an urban area. Rew stated that saturation was reached at the end of 12 interviews; three additional participants were recruited to verify the findings. At the end of 12 interviews, Rew was able to recognize the repetition in the data and determined that the addition of new informants confirmed her findings rather than added new information. The repetitive nature of data is the point at which the researcher determines that saturation has been achieved.

Morse (1989), however, warned that saturation may be a myth. She believes that if another group of individuals were observed or interviewed at another time, new data might be revealed. The best that a qualitative researcher can hope for in terms of saturation is to saturate the specific culture or phenomenon at a particular time.

SUMMARY

*I*n this chapter, an explanation of the commonalities of qualitative research have been offered to provide an informed framework for deciding whether qualitative research best suits you as the researcher and the research question you wish to pursue. Introduction to the process is offered to help the reader understand what the similarities and differences are between quantitative and qualitative research paradigms. The intent is to offer the reader an exposure to the processes and terms that are important to qualitative research approaches. It is essential that the reader understand and then embrace the similarities and differences in research paradigms before launching into implementation of a qualitative study. In the next chapter, a description of qualitative data generation and management will be provided to ground the reader in the language and processes of qualitative research. The intent is to offer the reader of this chapter and Chapter 3 a general understanding of qualitative research. In the chapters that follow, a more intensive description of specific approaches will be offered to more completely engage the reader in understanding many of the important qualitative research approaches.

References

Ahern, K. J. (1999). Ten tips for reflexive bracketing. *Qualitative Health Research,* *9*(3), 407–412.

Boyd, C. O. (2001). Philosophical foundations of qualitative research. In P. L. Munhall (Ed.), *Nursing research: A qualitative perspective* (pp. 65–89). Sudbury, MA: Jones and Bartlett.

Calvin, A. O. (2004). Haemodialysis patients and end-of-life decisions: A theory of personal preservation. *Journal of Advanced Nursing, 46*(5), 558–567.

Cohen, M. Z., Phillips, J. M., & Palos, G. (2001). Qualitative research with diverse populations. *Seminars in Oncology Nursing, 17*(3), 190–196.

Coyne, I. T. (1997). Sampling in qualitative research. Purposeful and theoretical sampling: Merging or clear boundaries? *Journal of Advanced Nursing, 26*, 623–630.

Creswell, J. W. (2003). *Research design: Qualitative, quantitative, and mixed methods approaches* (2nd ed.). Thousand Oaks, CA: Sage.

Denzin, N. K. (2000). Aesthetics and the practice of qualitative inquiry. *Qualitative Inquiry, 6*(2), 253–265.

Field, P. A., & Morse, J. M. (1985). *Nursing research: The application of qualitative approaches.* Rockville, MD: Aspen.

Glaser, B. G. (1978). *Theoretical sensitivity: Advances in the methodology of grounded theory.* Mill Valley, CA: Sociology Press.

Glaser, B. G., & Strauss, A. (1967). *The discovery of grounded theory.* Chicago: Aldine.

Hayes, P. (2001). Diversity in a global society. *Clinical Nursing Research, 10*(2), 99–101.

Jenks, J. M. (1995). New generation research approaches. In H. J. Streubert & D. R. Carpenter (Eds.), *Qualitative research in nursing* (pp. 242–268). Philadelphia: J. B. Lippincott.

Keating-Lefler, R., & Wilson, M. E. (2004). The experience of becoming a mother for single, unpartnered, Medicaid-eligible, first-time mothers. *Journal of Nursing Scholarship, 36*(1), 23–29.

Krasner, D. L. (2001). Qualitative research: A different paradigm—part 1. *Journal of Wound, Ostomy and Continence Nurses Society, 28*(2), 70–72.

Lincoln, Y. S., & Guba, E. G. (1985). *Naturalistic inquiry.* Beverly Hills, CA: Sage.

Maggs-Rapport, F. (2000). Combining methodological approaches in research: Ethnography and interpretive phenomenology. *Journal of Advanced Nursing, 31*(1), 219–225.

McDougall, P. (2000). In-depth interviewing: The key issues of reliability and validity. *Community Practitioner, 73*(8), 722–724.

Morse, J. M. (1989). Strategies for sampling. In J. M. Morse (Ed.), *Qualitative nursing research: A contemporary dialogue* (pp. 117–131). Rockville, MD: Aspen.

Morse, J. M. (1994). Designing funded qualitative research. In N. K. Denzin & Y. S. Lincoln (Eds.), *Handbook of qualitative research* (pp. 220–235). Thousand Oaks, CA: Sage.

Morse, J. M. (1997). Learning to drive from a manual? *Qualitative Health Research*, 7(2), 181-183.

Patton, M. Q. (1980). *Qualitative evaluation methods*. Beverly Hills, CA: Sage.

Patton, M. Q. (1990). *Qualitative evaluation and research methods*. Newbury Park, CA: Sage.

Polit, D. F., Beck, C. T., & Hungler, B. P. (2001). *Essentials of nursing research: Methods, appraisal, and utilization* (5th ed.). Philadelphia: Lippincott Williams & Wilkins.

Rew, L. (2003). A theory of taking care of oneself grounded in experiences of homeless youth. *Nursing Research*, 52(4), 234-241.

Schutz, A. (1970). *On phenomenology and social relations*. Chicago: University of Chicago Press.

Sixsmith, J., Boneham, M., & Goldring, J. E. (2003). Accessing the community: Gaining insider perspectives from the outside. *Qualitative Health Research*, 13(4), 578-589.

Strauss, A., & Corbin, J. (1990). *Basics of qualitative research: Grounded theory procedures and techniques*. Newbury Park, CA: Sage.

Thompson, C. (1999). Qualitative research into nurse decision making: Factors for consideration in theoretical sampling. *Qualitative Health Research*, 9(6), 815-828.

Woodgate, R. (2000). Part 1: An introduction to conducting qualitative research in children with cancer. *Journal of Pediatric Oncology Nursing*, 17(4), 192-206.

3

Designing Data Generation and Management Strategies

"*I*nquiry is . . . a dialogical process. It is a dialogue with the participants, the data [themselves], the events surrounding the research process, and the investigators as introspective individuals or as interacting team members (Hall, 2003, p. 494). Therefore, to implement a high-quality qualitative research study, a researcher must make sure that the research question is clear, that the method selected to answer the question is appropriate, and that the people and data sources needed are available. Once this has been achieved, the researcher then will begin collecting data. Once data are collected, they must be analyzed and synthesized; conclusions will need to be drawn and practice implications stated. This chapter explores the strategies for collecting and managing data. General concepts of qualitative research are offered. The specifics of data generation and management to be used for particular qualitative approaches are offered in the chapter that follows.

GENERATING DATA

A variety of strategies can be used to generate qualitative research data: interviews, observations, narrative, and focus groups. "The reconstruction of social phenomena can come in a number of forms: video, photography, film and text" (Maggs-Rapport, 2000, p. 221). The strategies offered in this chapter are not meant to be exhaustive but rather descriptive of the more common data collection techniques. Each researcher will need to determine, based on the question asked, the research approach selected, the sensitivity of the subject matter, and available resources, which methods of data generation are most appropriate. For example, if the researcher is interested in investigating the experiences of comfort for clients living in a nursing home, those who agree to be interviewed may be more willing to speak in a focus group than face-to-face. As the researcher, you will need to carefully assess the research goals and then match those with the best data collection strategy.

Conducting Interviews

"Before entering the field to conduct interviews, researchers have to be open to their influence on the inquiry. An important term to be aware of in discussion of the researcher's role in qualitative inquiry is *reflexivity*. According to Carolan (2003), "reflexivity is a term that is widely used, with a diverse range of connotations, and sometimes with virtually no meaning at all" (p. 8). For the purpose of this chapter, reflexivity is defined as the responsibility of researchers to examine their influence in all aspects of qualitative inquiry— self-reflection. Primeau (2003) states, "reflexivity enhances the quality of research through its ability to extend our understanding of how our positions and interests as researchers affect all stages of the research process" (p. 9). As researchers, it is our responsibility to reflect on our influence, critically analyze it, and use it to enhance our work, always being aware of the fact that no research is without its subjective aspects. Once researchers develop a mechanism to maintain a self-reflective stance, they are ready to enter the field and collect data.

One of the most frequently used data collection strategies is the open-ended interview. According to Robinson (2000), it is the mainstay of qualitative nursing research. Formally defined, "the formal qualitative interview is an unstructured conversation with a purpose that usually features audiotape and verbatim transcription of data, and use of an interview guide rather than a rigid schedule of questions" (p. 18). According to Bianco and Carr-Chellman (2002), "interviews range in type and length and are used for different purposes but are present in virtually all qualitative traditions" (p. 254). It is increasingly popular to conduct qualitative interviews through discussion boards or e-mail.

For interviews to be successful, they must be interdependent by nature. Accessing closely held information will only occur if there is mutual trust and respect between researcher and informant (Perry, Thurston, & Green, 2004). When preparing to enter into the interview, the researcher must be cognizant of the fact that the outcome of the interview is an understanding of the meaning of the experience for those who are part of it. Hence, "meaning is not 'just the facts' but rather the understandings one has that are specific to the individual (what was said) yet transcendent of the specific (what is the relationship between what was said, how it was said, what the listener was attempting to ask or hear, what the speaker was attempting to convey or say)" (Dilley, 2004, p. 128). Essential to comprehend is the complexity of the interview process and the importance of committing oneself to fully engaging in it. Interviews should not be conducted without adequate preparation and understanding of the process, its intent, and the desired outcome.

Before entering the field to conduct an interview, it is important for the researcher to consider the social and cultural context in which data will be collected (McDougall, 2000). Interviewers come with histories and cultural value systems; on many levels, the cultural and social expectations of both individuals—interviewer and interviewee—will affect what is said and what is heard. At the extreme, "differences in age, social class, race and ethnicity between the interviewer and interviewee may inhibit rapport" (p. 722). To facilitate dialogue during data collection, the researcher needs to be aware of cultural differences and work to reduce their impact as much as possible. One of the ways suggested earlier in this text is to use the researcher's journal as a place to chronicle feelings, attitudes, and values relative to the interview process and those who will be interviewed. Another suggestion is to take the time to build rapport with those from whom you will be soliciting information. In the process of building a relationship, the researcher can assure the informants that their confidentiality will be protected.

Open-ended interviews provide participants with the opportunity to fully describe their experience. Interviews generally are conducted face-to-face. To facilitate sharing by the research participants, it is a good practice to conduct the interview in a place and at a time that is most comfortable and convenient for the participants. The more comfortable each participant is, the more likely he or she will share important information.

The actual interviews can be brief with a specific objective, such as verifying previously reported information. Or interviewing can cover a longer period, either in one sitting or over a prolonged time. A life history is an example of data collection that may continue for a long time at each sitting and also over weeks, months, or even years.

The *structured interview* is one in which researchers use a set of preselected questions that they wish to have answered. Structured interviews are more likely to occur in quantitative rather than qualitative research studies. An *unstructured interview* provides the opportunity for greater latitude in the answers provided. In the unstructured interview, the researcher asks open-ended questions, such as "What is it like to care for an abusive client? Can you describe your experience for me?" In this example, there is no defined response. Using these questions, the respondent is able to move about freely in his or her description of caring for an abusive client. The unstructured interview is the preferred technique in a qualitative study.

When engaging in interviews, there are special population-specific concerns that you should be aware of. One in particular that has gained significant attention is age. Robinson (2000) and Docherty and Sandelowski (1999) have addressed interviewing the elderly and children. Robinson found in her work with institutionalized elderly that the interview had six distinct phases. These included (1) introducing; (2) personalizing; (3) reminiscing; (4) contextualizing; (5) closing; and (6) reciprocating. In describing these phases, Robinson clearly states the relevance and importance of allowing the aged individual to lead the conversation. Although interviews may take longer with the elderly, the time for sharing is well worth the richness of the data collected.

Docherty and Sandelowski (1999) offer advice on interviewing children based on an extensive review of the literature. Based on their review, researchers should be aware that "developmental age, the target event under investigation, interview structure, multiple interviewers, and research design" (p. 183) are all factors requiring the interviewer's attention. In addition, Docherty and Sandelowski raise the issue of attention span and recall, both of which may not be directly linked to developmental age.

Regardless of the data collection strategies used, researchers need to gain access to participants. Access is an extremely important consideration when designing data collection strategies. When interviewing is the major way the researcher will collect data, it is important to determine how he or she will achieve access. The way in which researchers present themselves to prospective study participants will affect the level and type of participation provided. Sixsmith, Boneham, and Goldring (2003) suggest specific strategies for large-scale studies that may assist with access. These include (1) stakeholder analysis; (2) identification of gatekeepers; (3) snowballing; (4) advertising; (5) dispersing questionnaires in public areas that can be used by the subjects to contact researchers for interviews; (6) street interviews; and (7) the ethnographic technique of "being there."

After the researcher gains access, it is important to establish rapport by conveying a sense of interest and concern for the research informant. The research participant must trust the researcher before he or she will feel comfortable revealing information.

Using Focus Groups

Using focus groups for data collection is another valuable strategy for qualitative researchers. A *focus group* is "a semi-structured group session, moderated by a group leader, held in an informal setting, with the purpose of collecting information on a designated topic" (Carey, 1994, p. 226). Although focus groups as a method of data collection did not arise from a qualitative tradition, they have been found to be most useful in a number of settings, but most importantly when dealing with sensitive topics. Focus groups are particularly suited to the collection of qualitative data because they have the advantages of being inexpensive, flexible, stimulating, cumulative, elaborative, assistive in information recall, and capable of producing rich data (Fontana & Frey, 1994; MacDougall & Baum, 1997). The major disadvantage of focus groups is *groupthink*, a process that occurs when stronger members of a group or segments of the group have major control or influence over the verbalizations of other group members (Carey & Smith, 1994). Generally, a good group leader can overcome the tendency of *groupthink* if he or she is attentive to its potential throughout data collection. The advantages of a focus group as a data collection strategy outweigh the disadvantages.

Focus groups have been used to collect information on a variety of topics. They are thought to be most useful when the topic of inquiry is considered sensitive. Although the use of focus groups for sensitive topic inquiry is well documented, its overall popularity as a qualitative research data collection strategy is increasing based on many of the advantages cited earlier. Moloney, Dietrich, Strickland, and Myerburg (2003) recommend virtual focus groups, which use computer-mediated communications such as e-mail. Moloney and colleagues differentiate virtual focus groups into two types: discussion boards and chat rooms. Discussion boards refer to "an ongoing site where participants are free to log on at any time, read others' postings, and post their own thoughts" (p. 275). Chat rooms refer to "a discussion site that functions in real time, where participants log on at a specific time and converse back and forth . . . instant messenger is a type of a chat room" (p. 275). Researchers should exercise caution, however, when using e-mail as an information exchange medium because anonymity can be compromised. (See Chapter 4 for an expanded discussion of the ethical issues relevant to data collected through the Internet).

It is important to point out that the focus group is not a data collection strategy that should be engaged in without serious attention to its elements. A good focus group session has the potential for learning about both the *focus* and the *group* (Kidd & Parshall, 2000). To do so, the group facilitator must have a solid understanding of group process (Joseph, Griffin, & Sullivan, 2000) and should collect data with at least one other researcher/facilitator (Kidd & Parshall, 2000). Hudson (2003) offers three distinct segments of focus groups: introducing the group, conducting the group, and closing the group. Those planning to use focus groups should be well versed in what each part requires.

In addition, when deciding who should attend a focus group, the researcher must be certain that the people invited to participate "have a shared trait or experience on which the discussion can build" (Lucasey, 2000). Group size should be between 6 and 10 members. Larger group size may preclude everyone from having a chance to speak. Smaller group size may make group members feel as though they cannot speak freely or have to speak when they have nothing to offer.

Recording of focus group data can be problematic and is another area that should be seriously considered before the decision is made to use this strategy for data collection. A number of authors address the complexity of transcribing recorded data when the data are being generated during a focus group. Location of the microphone, intonation, participants talking at the same time, and mechanical difficulties can all preclude complete and accurate data transcription. Joseph and colleagues (2000) advocate the use of videotaping as a method of data documentation during focus group activity. Videotaping has proved successful particularly with children's focus groups (Kennedy, Kools, & Krueger, 2001). Videotaping has the advantage of providing a complete recording of an individual's statement, group interaction, and individual behavior; however, it also can be viewed as intrusive and a violation of privacy. Researchers interested in using videotaping will need to consider the positives and negatives of its use.

More recently, attention has been directed at the reliability and validity of focus group data. Kidd and Parshall (2000) state that there are three criteria of reliability: stability, equivalence, and internal consistency. *Stability* refers to the consistency of issues over time. Stability becomes an important issue when group membership changes from one meeting of the group to the next.

Equivalence is a term used to describe the consistency of the moderators or coders of the focus group (Kidd & Parshall, 2000). It is essential that, to the extent possible, the same moderator lead the discussion with one group and across groups and that one researcher play a predominant role in analysis. *Internal consistency* of coding relates to the importance of having one team member assume the major responsibility for conducting the analysis, participating in as many groups and debriefings as possible, and communicating regularly with other team members as the analysis proceeds (Kidd & Parshall, 2000, p. 302).

Validity is used by Kidd and Parshall (2000) to describe a form of content validity. In other words, how convinced is the researcher that what the participants have shared is valid information? Paying careful attention to the composition of the group and interviews across groups with similar experiences are two ways to attend to validity of the data when using focus groups.

"The history of focus groups suggests that they were not originally conceived as a stand-alone method" (Kidd & Parshall, 2000). Therefore, to enhance the findings of a study that uses focus groups, the researcher should be prepared to consider using data triangulation. (For a full description of data triangulation, the reader is referred to Chapter 15.) Although not specifically related to validity, more recently, Traulsen, Almarsdottir, and Bjornsdottir (2004) have suggested interviewing the focus group moderator as a method to add "a new and valuable dimension to group interview" (p. 714). The purposes of interviewing the moderator include (1) offering information about group interaction and behavior; (2) effectively providing feedback on the research; (3) serving as an additional data point for the final analysis; and (4) adding to the richness of the data specifically about activity/conversation that occurs when the tape or video recorder is not running (Traulsen et al., 2004). The opportunity for other members of the research team to interview the moderator has important potential in adding to the study.

Using Written Narratives

Written responses by qualitative research participants are not new as a data collection strategy. Many researchers prefer written narratives to the spoken word because such narratives permit participants to think about what they wish to share. In addition, written narratives reduce costs by eliminating transcription requirements for audiotape interviews. The disadvantage of written narratives is the lack of spontaneity in responses that may occur. The popularity of the written narrative suggests it has proved an effective means of collecting qualitative research data.

In using written narratives, it becomes extremely important to be clear about what it is researchers wish the participants to write about. Because the researcher often is not present during the actual writing, it is essential that directions be focused to obtain the desired information. Researchers may need to establish mechanisms to request clarification in the event that the written document provided is unclear.

More recently, the nursing literature includes the term *narrative analysis*. Narrative analysis has been addressed primarily as a research method. Bailey (1996) defines narrative analysis as "the systematic study of stories commonly found in ethnographic interviews" (p. 187). Eaves and Kahn (2000) further share that the "terms narrative and story are used interchangeably and refer to any spoken or written presentation that includes a recounting of events that follow each other in time . . . Narrative explains by clarifying the importance of events that have taken place based on the outcome that has resulted" (p. 29).

The terms *narrative analysis* and *narrative*, as described here, refer to a data collection strategy and are **not** interchangeable concepts. Researchers interested in narrative analysis should read the works of Polkinghorne (1988) and Riessman (1993) to gain a clear understanding of this valuable research methodology. Narrative as referenced here is a data collection strategy used *in place of* or in addition to an interview.

Using Chat Rooms

With the increasing use of computer-mediated communications, the opportunities to collect data on-line grow daily. Chat rooms on the World Wide Web allow interested parties to log on and communicate synchronously. The transmissions and responses occur in real time as opposed to being delayed. A number of chat rooms are available on the Internet. Although their use as a data collection strategy has not been fully developed or completely explored, the opportunities abound. Moloney and co-researchers (2003) point out that narrative data collected in chat rooms have to be copied and pasted when the board is inactive. Also, it is difficult to scroll back to see what has been said. These peculiarities of chat rooms may make them less attractive for use as a data collection strategy. There is also the problem with synchronous communication. It may be easier to engage individuals in electronically mediated data collection when there is not a particular time demand placed on them.

Using Participant Observation

Participant observation is a method of data collection that comes from the anthropologic tradition. Therefore, it is the method of choice in ethnography. Generally, four types of participant observation are discussed in the literature. The first is *complete observer*, in which the researcher is a full observer of participants' activities. There is no interaction between the researcher and participants.

Observer as participant is the second type of participant observation. In this situation, the predominant activity of the researcher is to observe and potentially to interview. The majority of the researcher's time is spent in observation, rather than participation. To "fit" into the setting, the researcher may engage in some activities with the participants.

Participant as observer is the third type of participant observation. In this situation, the researcher acknowledges interest in studying the group; however, the researcher is most interested in doing so by becoming part of the group. A great deal has been written about "going native." This phrase demonstrates the inherent problem in getting too involved. That is, the researcher becomes so engrossed in the groups' activities that he or she loses sight of the real reason for being with the group.

The fourth type of participant observer is called *complete participant*. Complete participation requires that the researcher conceal his or her purpose. The individual becomes a member of the group. The ethical standard accepted by all disciplines makes concealment unacceptable. It is difficult, if not impossible, to justify this method. Because of a real concern for the ethics involved in data collection, individuals should not become complete participants.

Observations can also be structured or unstructured. Structured observations are more commonly found in quantitative research studies where the researcher is looking for something specific during the observation. Unstructured observations are the technique of choice in qualitative research as a way to comprehend the actions and interactions of individuals without a predetermined script. Mulhall (2003) points out that the term *unstructured* is misleading: "Observation within the naturalistic paradigm is not unstructured in the sense that it is unsystematic or sloppy. It does not, however, follow the approach of strictly checking the list of predetermined behaviors such as would occur in a structured observation" (p. 307).

Researchers should explore fully the reasons for selecting the various approaches to participant observation before initiating a study, realizing that, based on the circumstances, they may move among the approaches. There is no requirement to use only one approach. More importantly, the use of only one approach is almost impossible given the nature of fieldwork (Atkinson & Hammersley, 1998). However, it is important for researchers to think carefully about which approach they are interested in using in a given situation.

Using Field Notes

Field notes are the notations ethnographers generally make to document observations. These notes become part of data analysis. When recording field notes, it is important that researchers document what they have heard, seen, thought, or experienced. Chapter 9 offers examples of types of field notes, with detailed descriptions of how to write them.

Qualitative researchers using approaches other than ethnography for their research can use field notes. The field notes or notations made by the researcher may describe observations, assumptions about what is being heard or observed, or personal narrative about what is experienced by the researcher during a particular encounter. These notes can be very important during data collection and analysis. For example, in a phenomenological study conducted by the author (HJSS), during the interviews, notes were used to describe the participants' expressions, changes in position, and other observations that would not be captured by voice recordings. These notes were important additions during data analysis because they provided validation for important points made by the participants and facilitated appropriate emphasis on emerging themes.

MANAGING DATA

*H*ow researchers manage data will greatly affect the ease with which they analyze the data. As addressed earlier, researchers may collect data in a number of ways. Storage and retrieval are other important considerations. MacClean, Meyer, and Estable (2004) advise that there is a significant amount of attention needed to improve the accuracy of transcripts. Specifically, they offer that to ensure the quality of transcription, researchers should spot-check the work provided by the transcriptionist. This includes completely checking a subset of all completed interviews. These authors also offer information on the use of voice recognition systems, the potential for inaccurate transcription in highly charged interviews, misinterpretation of content, effect of unfamiliar terminology, language-specific errors, and difficulties in cross-cultural or multilingual transcription. Researchers must be aware of these potential problems and institute measures to minimize them.

A large amount of qualitative data can be stored on computers using a variety of available computer applications. It is beyond the scope of this book to fully share all the qualitative data collection packages available and their uses. It is important for qualitative researchers interested in using computer software to acquire and preview qualitative data analysis software and work with various software packages to determine which will be the most useful. Working with individuals who have used particular packages offers a significant opportunity to learn about the application without hours of reading and "trial and error." However, it is important to remember that what an "expert" in the program knows and what the program can do may not be the same. Therefore, gaining as much knowledge as possible about computer programs is critical. Also, remember that your purpose and needs relative to data analysis may be different from the "expert" you utilize. In conclusion, the time to review data analysis packages is *before* you begin data collection. It can be very distracting and frustrating to try to develop an understanding of the software during the data collection and analysis phases of your research.

Morison and Moir (1998) report that there are five classifications of qualitative data analysis packages:

1. Text retrievers, such as Metamorph, Orbis, Sonar Professional
2. Text base managers, such as askSam 3.0, Folio VIEWS, MAXqda
3. Code and retrievers, such as HyperQual 2, QUALPRO, the Ethnograph
4. Code-based theory builders, such as AQUAD 5.03, ATLAS/ti, HyperRESEARCH 2.6, QRS N6
5. Conceptual network builders, such as Inspiration 7.5, MECA, SemNet

Each class of programs has the ability to offer its user different types of information. The researcher must carefully match the program's capabilities with the goals of data analysis.

Richards and Richards (1994) note that if data are in text format and are part of a word processing document, computer analysis offers several features. These features include the following:

1. The ability to handle multiple documents on-screen in separate windows, which will facilitate viewing text that is similar throughout the document and will allow "cut and paste" editing
2. The ability to format files
3. The ability to include pictures, graphs, or charts to illustrate ideas
4. The ability to add video or audio data
5. Good text-searching abilities

Table 3.1 • Computerized Qualitative Data Management Programs	
Computer Program	*Source*
ATLAS/ti 5.0	SCOLARI, Sage Publications, Inc.
	1 Oliver's Yard
	55 City Road
	London EC1Y 1SP
	+44 (0) 20-7324-8500
	info@scolari.co.uk
	http://www.scolari.co.uk
Ethnograph (Version 5)	Qualis Research Associates
	P.O. Box 460728
	Denver, CO 80246
	(303) 388-1701
	Qualis@Qualisresearch.com
	http://www.Qualisresearch.com
Hyper Research 2.6	Research Ware, Inc.
	P.O. Box 1258
	Randolph, MA 02368-1258
	U.S. (888) 497-3737, or Out of US (781) 961-3909
	researchwr@aol.com
	http://www.researchware.com/
QRS N6 (NUD*IST)	SCOLARI, Sage Publications, Inc.
	1 Oliver's Yard
	55 City Road
	London EC1Y 1SP
	+44 (0) 20-7324-8500
	info@scolari.co.uk
	http://www.scolari.co.uk

6. Publish and subscribe facility, which allows for text to be changed in one document and automatically updated in a linked document
7. The ability to link documents using hypertext, which permits readers to easily move from document to document and creates a unique ability to annotate text using hypertext links; these links facilitate memo writing about identified information.

These features are available in computer applications that would not be accessible in the more traditional storage formats such as handwritten files.

Table 3.1 offers an overview of commonly used computer packages. "The CAQDAS (Computer Assisted Qualitative Data Analysis) World Wide Web Page (http://www.soc.surrey.ac.uk/caqdas/) makes available to the research community a selection of demonstration versions of qualitative data analysis packages for download" (Lewins, 1996, p. 300 and preview).

The CAQDAS Networking Project also offers "Internet resources, a support line, training courses and academic seminars" (Morison & Moir, 1998, p. 116). The network's goal is to encourage debate and discussion in addition to training and support for social and behavioral scientists interested in use of data analysis packages (Morison & Moir, 1998).

Qualitative researchers will need to practice working with these packages and, in some cases, use computer consultants to navigate the various program features. However, ultimately, the rewards of using a qualitative data analysis package will outweigh the time spent in learning about the various packages.

PERFORMING DATA ANALYSIS

When researchers have collected all their data, it is then necessary to begin analysis. Neophyte qualitative researchers are faced with the inevitability of a certain ambiguity when beginning data analysis. Qualitative data analysis requires the investigator to use mental processes to draw conclusions. In particular, the researcher will need to use "sensory impressions, intuition, images, experiences and cognitive comparisons in categorizing the findings and discerning patterns" (Hall, 2003, p. 495). These are not skills that the neophyte is generally comfortable with. The amount of data collected and the style in which researchers have stored the data will either facilitate or impede data analysis. Analysis of qualitative research is a hands-on process. Thorne (2000) states, "unquestionably, data analysis is the most complex and mysterious of all of the phases of a qualitative project" (p. 68). Researchers must become deeply immersed in the data (sometimes referred to as "dwelling" with the data). This process requires researchers to commit fully to a structured analytic process to gain an understanding of what the data convey. It requires a significant degree of dedication to reading, intuiting, analyzing, synthesizing, and reporting the discoveries. It is difficult to fully explain this process because "it is dynamic, intuitive and creative process of thinking and theorizing" (Basit, 2003, p. 143).

Data analysis in qualitative research actually begins when data collection begins. As researchers conduct interviews or observations, they maintain and constantly review records to discover additional questions they need to ask or to offer descriptions of their findings. Usually these questions or descriptions are embedded in observations and interviews. Qualitative researchers must "listen" carefully to what they have seen, heard, and experienced to discover meaning. The cyclic nature of questioning and verifying is an important aspect of data collection and analysis. In addition to the analysis that occurs throughout the study, an extended period of immersion occurs at the conclusion of data collection. During this period of dwelling, investigators question all prior conclusions in the context of the whole based on what they have discovered. Generally, this period of data analysis consumes a considerable amount of time. Researchers will spend weeks or months with their data based on the amount of information available for analysis.

The actual process of data analysis usually takes the form of clustering similar data. In many qualitative approaches, these clustered ideas are labeled *themes*. Themes are structural meaning units of data. DeSantis and Ugarriza (2000) tell us that themes emerge from the data; they are not superimposed on them. Further, they share that "a theme is an abstract entity that brings meaning identity to a recurrent experience and its variant manifestations. As such, a theme captures and unifies the nature or basis of the experience into a meaningful whole" (p. 400). For example, in a study completed by Beck (2004), participants spoke about birth trauma. In this study, Beck offers the following two statements:

> When you returned to my labor room and I was vomiting and shaking and no longer handling the contractions, you never reassured me or explained what was happening.
>
> Lying indecently and asking why the curtain behind me was open and could they close it. I felt exposed to the outside world! (p. 31)

Beck concludes based on these two statements that in the first instance the woman was feeling uninformed and lacked reassurance. In the second instance she felt that the mother was stripped of her dignity as her privacy was not respected. Her analysis of these comments leads Beck to name the theme, "To care for me: Was that too much to ask?"

Once researchers have explicated all themes relevant to a study, they report them in a way that is meaningful to the intended audience. In a phenomenological study, the researcher will relate the themes to one another to develop an *exhaustive description* of the experience being investigated.

Thorne (2000) shares that in each approach to qualitative data analysis, there is a different purpose for and different process used to draw conclusions. In grounded theory, the process for analyzing data is labeled *constant comparative method*. Using this process, the researcher compares each new piece of data with data previously analyzed. Questions are asked each time relative to the similarities or differences between each compared piece of data. The ultimate goal is the development of a theory about why a particular phenomenon exists as it does. What is the basic social-psychological process that is occurring? For a full description of the process, the reader is directed to Glaser and Strauss (1967).

In phenomenology, the process of interpretation may vary based on the philosophic tradition used. Regardless of the specific tradition, they all support "immersing oneself in data, engaging with data reflectively, and generating a rich description that will enlighten a reader as to the deeper essential structures underlying the human experience" (Thorne, 2000, p. 69).

For ethnographers, the focus of data analysis is to offer a description of a culture based on participant observation, interviews, and artifacts. "Ethnographic analysis uses an iterative process in which cultural ideas that arise during active involvement 'in the field' are transformed, translated or represented in written document" (Thorne, 2000, p. 69). The researcher asks questions, analyzes the answers, develops more questions, and analyzes the answers in a repeating pattern until a full picture of the culture emerges.

Regardless of the methodological approach used, the goal of data analysis is to illuminate the experiences of those who have lived them by sharing the richness of lived experiences and cultures. The researcher has the responsibility of describing and analyzing what is presented in the raw data to bring to life particular phenomena. It is only through rich description that we will come to know the experiences of others. As Krasner (2001) states, "Stories illuminate meaning, meaning stimulates interpretation, and interpretation can change outcome" (p. 72).

DEMONSTRATING TRUSTWORTHINESS

*M*uch debate is ongoing regarding rigor or goodness in qualitative research. The debate has mostly moved beyond the positivist convention of reliability and validity. This section of the chapter takes a conservative position regarding the ongoing debate and offers a set of criteria that has been meaningful to qualitative researchers for the past 10 to 15 years. However, taking the conservative position for the sake of sharing the *fundamentals* of qualitative research does not negate the need for nor the importance of the debate surrounding rigor. It is the authors' position that rigor in qualitative research is most important in demonstrating to the respective publics who read qualitative research that it is a respectable approach to science. On the other hand, there is an important need to constantly question the predominant paradigm's structure and function. Dualist thinking does not advance nursing knowledge, nor does it add substantially to what we know about the people we care for or the lives they lead. Advocacy for being open to alternative ways of knowing is essential. Emden and Sandelowski (1999) offer as an important criterion for addressing rigor in qualitative research a "criterion of uncertainty" (p. 5). This criterion provides for "an open acknowledgement that claims about research outcomes are at best tentative and that there may indeed be no way of showing otherwise" (p. 5).

At the outset, it is important to state that "no one set of criteria can be expected to 'fit the bill' for every research study" (Emden & Sandelowski, 1999, p. 6). Further, it is important to recognize that, ultimately, our decisions regarding the rigor in a research study amount to a judgment call (p. 6). With these two assumptions in mind, rigor in qualitative research is demonstrated through researchers' attention to and confirmation of information discovery. The goal of rigor in qualitative research is to accurately represent study participants' experiences. There are different terms to describe the processes that contribute to rigor in qualitative research. Guba (1981) and Guba and Lincoln (1994) have identified the following terms that describe operational techniques supporting the rigor of the work: *credibility, dependability, confirmability*, and *transferability*.

Credibility includes activities that increase the probability that credible findings will be produced (Lincoln & Guba, 1985). One of the best ways to establish credibility is through prolonged engagement with the subject matter. Another way to confirm the credibility of findings is to see whether the participants recognize the findings of the study to be true to their experiences (Yonge & Stewin, 1988). The act of returning to the informants to see whether they recognize the findings is frequently referred to as *member checking*. Creswell (2003) offers that member checking should be used "to determine the accuracy of the qualitative findings through taking the final report or specific descriptions or themes back to participants and determining whether these participants feel that they are accurate" (p. 196).

Dependability is a criterion met once researchers have demonstrated the credibility of the findings. The question to ask, then, is this: how dependable are these results? Sharts-Hopko (2002) submits that triangulation of methods has the potential to contribute to the dependability of the findings. Similar to validity in quantitative research, in which there can be no validity without reliability, the same holds true for dependability: there can be no dependability without credibility (Lincoln & Guba, 1985).

Confirmability is a process criterion. The way researchers document the confirmability of the findings is to leave an *audit trail*, which is a recording of activities over time that another individual can follow. This process can be compared to a fiscal audit (Lincoln & Guba, 1985). The objective is to illustrate as clearly as possible the evidence and thought processes that led to the conclusions. This particular criterion can be problematic, however, if you subscribe to Morse's (1989) ideas regarding the related matter of saturation. It is the position of Morse that another researcher may not agree with the conclusions developed by the original researcher. Sandelowski (1998a) argues that only the researcher who has collected the data and been immersed in them can confirm the findings.

Transferability refers to the probability that the study findings have meaning to others in similar situations. Transferability has also been labeled "fittingness." The expectation for determining whether the findings fit or are transferable rests with potential users of the findings and not with the researchers (Greene, 1990; Lincoln & Guba, 1985; Sandelowski, 1986). As Lincoln and Guba (1985) have stated,

> It is . . . not the naturalist's task to provide an *index of transferability*; it is his or her responsibility to provide the *database* that makes transferability judgment possible on the part of potential appliers. (p. 316)

These four criteria for judging the rigor of qualitative research are important; they define for external audiences the attention qualitative researchers render to their work.

PRESENTING THE DATA

"*T*here is no one style for reporting the findings of a qualitative research study" (Sandelowski, 1998b, p. 376). Researchers interested in sharing their results must take several things into consideration. First, who is the audience? Second, what is the purpose of the report? Third, for whom am I writing the report? Although presented linearly, the questions offered do not need to be answered linearly. The most important question, which is overarching, is this: how do I most effectively communicate the findings of my study to make them useful for others?

Sandelowski (1998b) offers some important parameters in developing the research report. These include determining focus of the narrative; balancing description, analysis, and interpretation; emphasizing character, scene, or plot; deciding whose voice will be heard; and learning how to effectively use metaphor.

Determining the focus of the study is essential. The researcher must consider carefully what needs to be told. Qualitative research studies create voluminous amounts of data. The researcher needs to decide based on the purpose of his or her study what will be told. For instance, if the purpose of the study is to discover the meaning of health to those who lived in lower Manhattan in the months following the destruction of the World Trade Center, then the purpose is to tell the story of those who experienced living there. The research report should include a rich description of what the meaning of health was for those individuals given the living conditions following the collapse of the Towers.

The way in which one tells the story is guided by the purpose of the study. If the researcher is conducting a descriptive phenomenological study, then the focus is on the description, with less attention to analysis and interpretation. This is not to suggest that the raw data are presented without analysis. Rather, the researcher will have the responsibility of digesting the narrative and distilling it into a meaningful representation of a phenomenon based on those whose experiences are shared.

If, however, the purpose of the research study is to develop a theory about recovery in the aftermath of a major crisis, then the narrative will give rise to analysis and interpretation leading ultimately to the new theory. The descriptions of individuals' recoveries will not be what are highlighted in the report. The descriptions will be the groundwork from which the theory will be derived. The focus will be analysis, interpretation, and reformulation of the data that lead to the creation of the theory.

Sandelowski (1998b) suggests that qualitative researchers also should consider "whether the stories they want to tell are best told by emphasizing, and consciously using devices to showcase, character, scene or plot" (p. 37). For example, if the researcher has studied the history of a college of nursing over 25 years, the researcher can approach the study report in a number of ways. One way is to look at an individual. Let's say the same dean presided over the college for that period of time. The researcher can look at the institution through the eyes of the dean or can analyze the findings within the context of the dean's influence over the college's growth and development. The researcher might also look at the institution in terms of its politics. For instance, if the institution was a publicly funded entity in a state with representation whose primary agenda in the state was improving the health of the populace, then the college can be described based on the effect the politics had in its growth and development. There is no one way to tell the story. The researcher should consider carefully the emphasis of the report.

Deciding whose voice will be heard is a decision that needs careful consideration. Power structures frequently overshadow choice of research topic, data collection, sampling, and analysis. Often, researchers do not even consider how what they share is cloaked in power relationships. Although the researcher needs to stay attuned to the issues of power constantly, it is enormously important when telling the story. Whose voice will be heard and how it will be shared are extremely important. For example, if the researcher has studied the culture of a trauma unit in a major city for the purpose of sharing what life is like for the health professionals and clients who use the unit, the question should be asked, Whose voice will be predominate and why? If the researcher tells the story primarily from the health professionals' points of view, is there a slant on the research report that is different than if it is told from the clients' perspectives? Power is an important factor in research. It is a particularly important factor to consider in qualitative research, which has as one of its underlying principles the commitment to convey the experiences of those studied.

Sandelowski (1998b) offers the importance of metaphor and its use in reporting qualitative research. She shares that frequently when metaphor is used in research reports, it is used incorrectly or incompletely. Metaphor is a powerful tool in helping the reader to fully grasp what the researcher is trying to convey. Therefore, it needs to be selected carefully. Those who choose to use it must realize that it is only a tool or device to help the reader understand the data. It is a directional tool and not an outcome. Hall (2003) also speaks about the value of using graphic representations to enhance sharing the richness of data.

SUMMARY

*D*ata analysis can be described as the heart of qualitative inquiry. It is the point in the research process when researchers have the opportunity to put into words their conceptualizations of the shared experiences. Through the dynamic processes of intuiting, synthesizing, analyzing, and conceptualizing, the researcher distills and then illuminates the experiences or cultures that have been part of the inquiry. Qualitative data analysis requires an openness to possibilities. It necessitates patience with abstraction and a willingness to discover the wholeness of what is shared. Qualitative data analysis entails listening carefully to narrative and sharing description and understanding of what has been said, always maintaining the highest degree of integrity.

The focus of this chapter has been on data collection, management, and analysis. The novice qualitative researcher is advised to pursue a mentor to learn good techniques and to avoid the pitfalls of data collection, management, and analysis. Beck (2003) offers that the most common data analysis problem for neophytes is premature or delayed closure. For the advanced beginner reading published studies with others and analyzing the data collection methods, data management strategies and reporting of the analysis will be helpful in further developing analysis skills. In this chapter, we have offered information on collecting data using interviews, observation, focus groups, chat rooms, and narratives. This information should be helpful in identifying the most appropriate way to collect data for your study. In the methodological chapters that follow, we offer specific information on data collection strategies that are most appropriate for the specific approach.

In the data management section, the information is focused primarily on computer programs that can help you analyze large amounts of data. There is considerable debate about the usefulness of computer programs given the dynamic nature of the analysis process. It is important, however, that you have the information so that you can make an informed decision based on what you want to achieve. Finally, we offer information on the complexity of data analysis and how very difficult it is to fully describe a process that is creative and dynamic. It is our intention to offer a foundation from which to develop data analysis skills. The integrity of qualitative research findings will be judged on the ability of researchers to tell the story of participants with truthfulness and an attention to context and power.

References

Atkinson, P., & Hammersley, M. (1998). Ethnography and participant observation. In N. K. Denzin & Y. S. Lincoln (Eds.), *Strategies of qualitative inquiry* (pp. 110-136). Thousand Oaks, CA: Sage.

Bailey, P. H. (1996). Assuring quality in narrative analysis. *Western Journal of Nursing Research, 18*(2), 186-195.

Basit, T. N. (2003). Manual or electronic? The role of coding in qualitative data analysis. *Educational Research, 45*(2), 143-154.

Beck, C. T. (2003). Initiation into qualitative data analysis. *Journal of Nursing Education, 42*(5), 231-234.

Beck, C. T. (2004). Birth trauma: In the eye of the beholder. *Nursing Research, 53*(1), 28-35.

Bianco, M. B., & Carr-Chellman, A. A. (2002). Exploring qualitative methodologies in on-line learning environments. *Quarterly Review of Distance Education, 3*(3), 251-260.

Carey, M. A. (1994). The group effect in focus groups: Planning, implementing, and interpreting focus group research. In J. M. Morse (Ed.), *Critical issues in qualitative research methods* (pp. 225-241). Thousand Oaks, CA: Sage.

Carey, M. A., & Smith, M. W. (1994). Capturing the group effect in focus groups: A special concern for analysis. *Qualitative Health Research, 4*(1), 123-127.

Carolan, M. (2003). Reflexivity: A personal journey during data collection. *Researcher, 10*(3), 7-14.

Creswell, J. W. (2003). *Research design: Qualitative, quantitative, and mixed methods/approaches* (2nd ed.). Thousand Oaks, CA: Sage.

DeSantis, L., & Ugarriza, D. N. (2000). The concept of theme as used in qualitative research. *Western Journal of Nursing Research, 22*(3), 351-377.

Dilley, P. (2004). Interviews and the philosophy of qualitative research. *Journal of Higher Education, 75*(1), 127-132.

Docherty, S., & Sandelowski, M. (1999). Focus on qualitative methods: Interviewing children. *Research in Nursing and Health Care, 22*, 177-185.

Eaves, Y. D., & Kahn, D. L. (2000). Coming to terms with perceived danger. *Journal of Holistic Nursing, 18*(1), 27-45.

Emden, C., & Sandelowski, M. (1999). The good, the bad and relative, part two: Goodness and the criterion problem in qualitative research. *International Journal of Professional Nursing Practice, 5*(1), 2-7.

Fontana, A., & Frey, J. H. (1994). Interviewing: The art and science. In N. K. Denzin & Y. S. Lincoln (Eds.), *Handbook of qualitative research* (pp. 361-376). Thousand Oaks, CA: Sage.

Glaser, B. G., & Strauss, A. (1967). *The discovery of grounded theory*. Chicago: Aldine.

Greene, J. C. (1990). Three views on nature and role of knowledge in social science. In E. Guba (Ed.), *The paradigm dialogue* (pp. 227-245). Newbury Park, CA: Sage.

Guba, E. G. (1981). Criteria for assessing the trustworthiness of naturalistic inquiries. *Educational Communication and Technology Journal, 29*, 75-92.

Guba, E. G., & Lincoln Y. S. (1994). Competing paradigms in qualitative research. In N. K. Denzin & Y. S. Lincoln (Eds.), *Handbook of qualitative research* (pp. 105-117). Thousand Oaks, CA: Sage.

Hall, J. M. (2003). Analyzing women's roles through graphic representation of narratives. *Western Journal of Nursing Research, 25*(5), 492-507.

Hudson, P. (2003). Focus group interviews: A guide for palliative care researchers and clinicians. *International Journal of Palliative Nursing, 9*(5), 202-207.

Joseph, D. H., Griffin, M., & Sullivan, E. D. (2000). Videotaped focus groups: Transforming a therapeutic strategy into a research tool. *Nursing Forum, 35*(1), 15-20.

Kennedy, C., Kools, S., & Krueger, R. (2001). Methodological considerations in children's focus groups. *Nursing Research, 50*(3), 184-187.

Kidd, P. S., & Parshall, M. B. (2000). Getting the focus and the group: Enhancing analytical rigor in focus group research. *Qualitative Health Research, 10*(3), 293-309.

Krasner, D. L. (2001). Qualitative research: A different paradigm—part 1. *Journal of Wound, Ostomy and Continence Nurses Society, 28*(2), 70-72.

Lewins, A. (1996). The CAQDAS Networking Project: Multilevel support for the qualitative research community. *Qualitative Health Research, 6*(2), 298-303.

Lincoln, Y. S., & Guba, E. (1985). *Naturalistic inquiry.* Beverly Hills, CA: Sage.

Lucasey, B. (2000). Qualitative research and focus group methodology. *Orthopedic Nursing, 19*(1), 53-55.

MacLean, L. M., Meyer, M., & Estable, A. (2004). Improving accuracy of transcripts in qualitative research. *Qualitative Health Research, 14*(1), 113-123.

MacDougall, C., & Baum, F. (1997). The devil's advocate: A strategy to avoid groupthink and stimulate discussion in focus groups. *Qualitative Health Research, 7*(4), 532-541.

Maggs-Rapport, F. (2000). Combining methodological approaches in research: Ethnography and interpretive phenomenology. *Journal of Advanced Nursing, 31*(1), 219-225.

McDougall, P. (2000). In-depth interviewing: The key issues of reliability and validity. *Community Practitioner, 73*(8), 722-724.

Moloney, J. F., Dietrich, A. S., Strickland, O. L., & Myerburg, S. (2003). Using Internet discussion boards as virtual focus groups. *Advances in Nursing Science, 26*(4), 274-286.

Morison, M., & Moir, J. (1998). The role of computer software in the analysis of qualitative data: Efficient clerk, research assistant or Trojan horse? *Journal of Advanced Nursing, 28*(1), 106-116.

Morse, J. M. (1989). Strategies for sampling. In J. M. Morse (Ed.), *Qualitative nursing research: A contemporary dialogue* (pp. 117-131). Rockville, MD: Aspen.

Mulhall, A. (2003). In the field: Notes on observation in qualitative research. *Journal of Advanced Nursing, 41*(3), 306-313.

Perry, C., Thurston, M., & Green, K. (2004). Involvement and detachment in researching sexuality: Reflections on the process of semistructured interviewing. *Qualitative Health Research, 14*(1), 135-148.

Polkinghorne, D. E. (1988). *Narrative knowing and the human sciences.* Albany: State University of New York Press.

Primeau, L. A. (2003). Reflections on self in qualitative research: Stories of family. *American Journal of Occupational Therapy, 57*(1), 9-16.

Richards, T. J., & Richards, L. (1994). Using computers in qualitative research. In N. K. Denzin & Y. S. Lincoln (Eds.), *Handbook of qualitative research* (pp. 445-462). Thousand Oaks, CA: Sage.

Riessman, C. K. (1993). *Narrative analysis.* Newbury Park, CA: Sage.

Robinson, J. P. (2000). Phases of the qualitative research interview with institutionalized elderly individuals. *Journal of Gerontological Nursing, 26*(11), 17-23.

Sandelowski, M. (1986). The problem of rigor in qualitative research. *Advances in Nursing Science, 8*(3), 27-37.

Sandelowksi, M. (1998a). The call to experts in qualitative research. *Research in Nursing & Health, 21,* 467-471.

Sandelowski, M. (1998b). Writing a good read: Strategies for re-presenting qualitative data. *Research in Nursing and Health, 21,* 375-382.

Sharts-Hopko, N. (2002). Assessing rigor in qualitative research. *Journal of the Association of Nurses in AIDS Care, 13*(4), 84-86.

Sixsmith, J., Boneham, M., & Goldring, J. E. (2003). Accessing the community: Gaining insider perspectives from the outside. *Qualitative Health Research, 13*(4), 578-589.

Thorne, S. (2000). Data analysis in qualitative research. *Evidence-Based Nursing, 3*(3), 68-70.

Traulsen, J. M., Almarsdottir, A. B., & Bjornsdottir, I. (2004). Interviewing the moderator: An ancillary method to focus groups. *Qualitative Health Research, 14*(5), 714-725.

Yonge, O., & Stewin, L. (1988). Reliability and validity: Misnomers for qualitative research. *Canadian Journal of Nursing, 20*(2), 61-67.

Ethical Considerations in Qualitative Research

*E*thical issues related to professional nursing practice arise daily in the constant struggle to do good for the patient and to avoid harm. All that nurses do in the name of patient care is wrought with tension between these two principles. As science and technology provide avenues to intervene, unanticipated and more complex ethical dilemmas will continue to arise in our practice settings. The ethical dilemmas that emerge are grounded in the fact that direct relationships with human beings are at the heart of nurses' work. Understanding ethical principles in theory, combined with life experience in practice, prepares the nurse to make sound ethical and moral decisions on a daily basis. This knowledge and experience can be transferred to an understanding of ethical issues relevant to the research process.

Ethical issues and standards must be critically considered in both quantitative and qualitative research. Nurse researchers have a professional responsibility to design research that upholds sound ethical principles and protects human rights. Ethical issues related to informed consent, participant–researcher relationships, gaining access, confidentiality, anonymity, sample size, and data analysis are addressed in this chapter. The ethical issues considered are relevant to each of the qualitative research approaches presented in the text and should be considered within the context of the method selected for a particular investigation. The protection of participants must remain at the forefront of all research studies; however, the nature of qualitative methods requires that the researcher remain alert to the possibility of unanticipated ethical dilemmas.

There has been ongoing discussion in the nursing literature regarding the ethical variances that have arisen in qualitative investigations. Clearly, guidelines established for quantitative research investigations require an expanded scope of discussion when applied to qualitative research endeavors

Table 4.1 • The "Ethics Checklist": A Guide for Critiquing the Ethical Aspects of a Qualitative Research Study	
Topic	*Guiding Questions*
Phenomenon of interest	1. Is the research study relevant, important, and most appropriately investigated through a qualitative design? Explain.
	2. Are there any aspects of the research or phenomenon of interest that appear to be misleading either in terms of the true purpose or misleading to participants? Explain.
	3. Is the research primarily being conducted for personal gain on the part of the researcher, or is there evidence that the research will somehow contribute to the greater good? What are the benefits to the participants or society as a whole?
Review of the literature	1. Has all the available literature been reviewed?
	2. Are all citations accurate in terms of referencing and quoting?
	3. Is the basis for inclusion of the articles referred to explicit?
Research design participants	1. How did the researcher protect the physical and psychological well-being of the participants?
	2. Is there evidence that informed or process consent was obtained and freely given?
	3. How were vulnerable populations recruited and protected from physical or emotional harm?
	4. Did an Institutional Review Board approve the research?
Sampling	1. How was the confidentiality of participants protected?
	2. Is there any evidence of coercion or deception?
Data generation	1. If more than one researcher collected data, were they adequately prepared?
	2. Is there evidence of falsified or fabricated data?
	3. Is there intentional use of data collection methods to obtain biased data?
	4. Was data collection covert? If so, does the researcher explain why?
	5. Have the participants been misled with regard to the nature of the research?
	6. What mechanisms did the researcher employ to ensure authenticity and trustworthiness of data? (e.g.,. audit trail, reflexive journaling)

Table 4.1 • *(Continued)*	
Topic	*Guiding Questions*
Data analysis	1. Was data analysis conducted by more than one person?
	2. Is there evidence of data manipulation to achieve intended findings?
	3. Is there evidence of missing data that may have been lost or destroyed?
Conclusions and recommendations	1. Is there evidence of intentional false or misleading conclusions and recommendations?
	2. Is confidentiality violated given the presentation of the findings?

Adapted from Firby, P. (1995). Critiquing the ethical aspects of a study. *Nurse Researcher*, 3(1), 35–41.

(Cutliffe & Ramcharan, 2002; Demi & Warren, 1995; Forbat & Henderson, 2003; Haggman-Laitila, 1999; Orb, Eisenhauer, & Wynaden, 2001; Robley, 1995). Standards for ethical conduct in the qualitative realm will continue to require in-depth examination. Although qualitative designs have improved guidelines regarding the unique concerns that emerge in this type of research, what has become increasingly clear is that the ethical aspects of the research process will always require ongoing critique and evaluation. Given this understanding, this chapter addresses ethical issues that require critical consideration in any qualitative research endeavor. Table 4.1 provides qualitative researchers with an "ethics checklist" to use as a guide when critiquing the ethical aspects of a research study.

HISTORICAL BACKGROUND

*C*odes of ethics have been established for the conduct of research in response to human rights violations that have occurred. Sadly, the human atrocities that occurred in the name of research did not happen that long ago. Ethical concerns have high visibility today because of flagrant abuses of subjects that have occurred. As a result of this abuse, some examples of which are highlighted below, varying groups have developed codes of ethics.

- ***The Nazi Medical Experiments*** (1930s–1940s) implemented by the Third Reich in Europe are one atrocious example of the violation of basic human rights with research participants. Programs of research included sterilization, euthanasia, and medical experiments that were inhumane and generated no useful scientific knowledge. Participants were exposed to permanent physical harm or death and were not allowed to refuse participation (Levine, 1986).

- *The Tuskegee Syphilis Study* (1932-1972) occurred in the United States and was sponsored by the U.S. Public Health Service. The study was conducted to determine the course of syphilis in adult black men. Some participants were unaware that they were participating in a study, and many were uninformed as to the purpose and procedures of the research. Medical treatment for syphilis was deliberately withheld, even after penicillin was determined to be an effective treatment (Levine, 1986).

- *The Jewish Chronic Disease Hospital* (1960s) conducted a study to determine patients' rejection response to live cancer cells. Elderly patients at the Jewish Chronic Disease Hospital in Brooklyn were injected with live cancer cells. The project was conducted without informed consent and without institutional review (Levine, 1986).

- *The Willowbrook Study* (1950s-1970s) deliberately infected mentally handicapped children with the hepatitis B virus. Admission to the hospital was contingent on parental consent for the children to participate in the study. However, the consent was not informed, and parents were never told of the dangerous consequences of the study (Levine, 1986).

- *The Johns Hopkins Crisis* (2001) is one of the most recent examples leading to concerns regarding research. This study involved the use of healthy volunteers to study the pathophysiology of asthma. The third subject to receive the drug hexamethonium as part of the research protocol died as a result of progressive hypotension and multiorgan failure. The study was criticized because the consent document did not indicate that the inhaled hexamethonium was experimental and did not have U.S. Food and Drug Administration (FDA) approval (Steinbrook, 2002).

Although these examples emerged from quantitative studies that employed a specific intervention, the message is clear. Guidelines are essential, but they do not always answer all the ethical or moral questions that may arise in any research study, whether the design is quantitative or qualitative. It is the responsibility of the researcher to constantly examine and question the ethical components of their work. Participants must be protected, and the researcher must remain sensitive to emerging actual or potential ethical concerns.

Early quantitative investigations paved the way for ethical codes and guidelines. Qualitative researchers are bound by the same codes and must maintain an ongoing dialogue regarding ethical dilemmas encountered during their investigations so that all researchers can benefit from the experience of others. Despite the most vigilant attempts to ensure ethical conduct during a qualitative investigation, new and important considerations are always emerging. Researchers must be willing to share their experiences. For example, Boman and Jevne (2000) report on an experience of being charged with an ethical violation in the conduct of a qualitative investigation. The article centers on a frank discussion of a qualitative research endeavor in which the identity of a study participant was disclosed (Boman & Jevne, 2000). There is much to be learned from this open and honest sharing of the researchers' experience. Similarly, Lawton (2001) discusses ethical concerns related to informed consent and role conflict that emerged during a participant observation study of dying patients. Lawton (2001) and Boman and Jevne (2000) provide relevant examples from personal experience that will serve to enhance the ethical integrity of future studies. Their open and frank discussions leave all researchers in a better position to address ethical issues that present during the conduct of a qualitative investigation.

CODES OF ETHICS

Various codes of ethics have been developed over the past five decades in response to violations of moral principles and human rights in the conduct of research. The *Nuremberg Code* was developed following the Nazi experiments of the 1930s and 1940s and remains one of the first internationally recognized efforts to establish ethical standards. The code concerns itself with the adequate protection of human subjects, the rights of participants to withdraw from a research study, and the importance of conducting research only by qualified individuals. Other international standards include the *Declaration of Helsinki*, developed in 1964 by the World Medical Association and Finland. This document is similar to the Nuremberg Code but further differentiates between research that has a therapeutic value for participants and that which does not.

In the United States, the National Commission for the Protection of Human Subjects of Biomedical and Behavioral Research, known as the *Belmont Report*, served as a model for many of the guidelines adopted by specific disciplines. The Belmont Report identified three ethical principles relevant to the conduct of research involving human subjects: the principle of respect for persons, beneficence, and justice. The regulations are available on-line (http://ohsr.od.nih.gov/guidelines/45cfr46.html).

The profession of nursing has developed a *Code of Ethics* that provides guidelines related to practice issues and research (American Nurses Association, 2001). Silva (1995) provides an explicit account of the roles and responsibilities of nurses in the conduct, dissemination, and implementation of nursing research in a document entitled *Ethical Guidelines in the Conduct, Dissemination, and Implementation of Nursing Research*.

ETHICAL ISSUES SPECIFIC TO QUALITATIVE RESEARCH DESIGN

D istinct and conceivably unanticipated ethical issues emanate from the unpredictable nature of qualitative research. As Robley (1995) noted, "ethical considerations relevant to quantitative research impact qualitative investigations in unique and more fragile ways" (p. 45). The ethical dilemmas inherent in issues surrounding informed consent, anonymity and confidentiality, data generation, treatment, publication, and participant-researcher relationships are reviewed in light of the unique issues that emerge in the design and conduct of qualitative investigations. Ethical standards for qualitative investigations must evolve from a sense that the research is dynamic and that the process, by its application, may result in unanticipated ethical concerns. The researcher must remain open to the possibility of new, and, to date, unexamined ethical concerns related to qualitative research. Further, the evolving standards must be grounded in the ethical principles of autonomy, beneficence, and justice.

Researchers must observe certain basic principles when conducting any form of research that involves human subjects. First, participants must not be harmed, thereby supporting the principle of *beneficence*. In any qualitative investigation, if researchers sense that the interview is causing issues to surface that may result in emotional trauma to participants, they must protect the welfare of the participants, perhaps by ending the interview or providing follow-up counseling and referrals. Researchers must obtain informed consent, and informant participation must be voluntary, thereby supporting the principle of *autonomy*. Furthermore, researchers must assure participants that confidentiality and anonymity will be upheld and that participants will be treated with dignity and respect. The principles of *beneficence* and *justice* are upheld in this regard (Beauchamp & Childress, 2001). The three ethical principles of autonomy, beneficence, and justice provide the organizing framework for a meaningful dialogue regarding ethical issues that pertain to qualitative investigations.

INFORMED CONSENT

I nformed consent is a topic of regular discussion in health care settings. There is an expectation that, in the clinical setting, when clients sign a consent form, they are fully aware of both the health benefits and the actual or potential risks to their health (hence, the term *informed consent*). Informed consent in research holds similar meaning, with added inherent dimensions.

Informed consent is a prerequisite for all research involving identifiable subjects. Any dialogue referencing informed consent must be grounded in the ethical principle of autonomy that encompasses the notion of being a self-governing person with decision-making capacity. Polit & Beck (2004) defined informed consent as follows: "Informed consent means that participants have adequate information regarding the research; are capable of comprehending the information; and have the power of free choice, enabling them to consent voluntarily to participate in the research or decline participation" (p. 151). The researcher is obligated to provide the participant with relevant and adequate information when obtaining informed consent. At a minimum, participants should have information about the purpose and scope of the study, the types of questions that will potentially be asked, how the results will be used, and how their anonymity will be protected (Richards & Schwartz, 2002). The emergent design of a qualitative investigation, however, presents qualitative researchers with ethical considerations that have the potential to violate the basic premise of informed consent.

Of particular concern is the notion that participants will have adequate information regarding the research study. Although a participant may consent to a study on the life experience of open heart surgery, new issues may emerge within the context of the interview for which the participant and perhaps even the researcher were unprepared. Research with vulnerable populations or topics that deal with sensitive subjects may change the direction of the research or reveal information that is not related to the original purpose of the study.

"As a minimum, it [informed consent] requires that prospective human subjects are given true and sufficient information to help them decide whether they wish to be research participants" (Behi & Nolan, 1995, p. 713). The open, emerging nature of qualitative research methods in most cases makes informed consent impossible because neither researchers nor participants can predict exactly how data will present themselves either through interview or participant observation (Holloway & Wheeler, 1995; Ramos, 1989; Richards & Schwartz, 2002; Robley, 1995). As Robley (1995) pointed out, "Questions of ethics arise within the context of the shifting focus of the study, the unpredictable nature of the research and the trust relationship between the researcher and the participant" (p. 45).

"The inherent unpredictability of the [qualitative] research process undermines the spirit of informed consent and endangers the assurance of confidentiality, two basic ethical safety nets in more quantitative research" (Ramos, 1989, p. 58). For example, in a study on the meaning of quality of life for individuals with type 1 (insulin-dependent) diabetes mellitus, data collection might begin with one open-ended question: "Tell me in as much detail as possible: What does it mean to have quality of life with type 1 insulin-dependent diabetes mellitus?" The researcher's probing questions to elicit a more detailed understanding can open a Pandora's box. Issues surrounding compliance or noncompliance may arise that endanger the client's health, or perhaps the client is depressed and concerned about issues related to loss, death, and dying. What may emerge is impossible to predict, but both researchers and participants must be informed and prepared to address issues that arise as data emerges.

The emergent design of qualitative research demands a different approach to informed consent. *Consensual decision making*, also called *process informed consent*, is more appropriate for the conduct of a qualitative investigation. This approach requires that researchers, at varying points in the research process, re-evaluate participants' consent to participate in the study. According to Munhall (1988), process consent encourages mutual participation: "Because qualitative research is conducted in an ever-changing field, informed consent should be an ongoing process. Over time, consent needs to be renegotiated as unexpected events or consequences occur" (p. 156). Information about how the researcher enters the field, participants' time commitment, and what will become of the findings are all important components to process consent (Munhall, 1988). Participants must know from the beginning of, and be reminded throughout, the investigation that they have the right to withdraw from the research study at any time. A process consent offers the opportunity to change the original consent as the study emerges and change becomes necessary. "Common sense plays a large part in renegotiating informed consent. If our focus should change, we need to ask participants for permission to change the first agreement. Continually informing and asking permission establishes the needed trust to go on further in an ethical manner" (Munhall, 1988, p. 157).

It is essential that researchers and participants discuss and clarify their understanding of the investigation (Alty & Rodham, 1998; Raudonis, 1992). As Alty and Rodham (1998) have emphasized, "At the best of times, it is difficult to know if the person you are talking to really has the same understanding of the topic as you do, indeed, if the researcher has an accurate understanding of what the subject is expressing" (p. 277).

Participant observation is an important approach to data collection in qualitative investigations. This method of data collection is useful in learning about the social practices of participants, the manner in which they relate to each other, and how they interpret their world (Merrell & Williams, 1994; Punch, 1994; Moore & Savage, 2002; Savage, 2000). *Covert participant observation*, which results when participants are unaware they are being observed, presents another ethical concern for qualitative researchers. Covert participant observation is sometimes a necessary component to data generation in some qualitative investigations. The rationale from the researcher's perspective would be to ensure that collected data are true and accurate. This type of data generation is grounded in the idea that, when the participants are aware they are being observed, their behavior will change. For example, Clarke (1996) discussed the use of covert participant observation in a secure forensic unit and the ethical issues that emerged from this method of data generation. Clarke emphasized the need to obtain an "uncontaminated picture of the unit" (p. 37).

A researcher's integrity can become damaged if the researcher uses deception to generate data. Some researchers claim that deception in the form of covert observations—or not completely describing the aims of the study or its procedures—is sometimes necessary to get reliable and valid data (Douglas, 1979; Gans, 1962). Punch (1994) agreed that field-related deception might be necessary, provided the interests of the subjects are protected. Others have argued that the need for covert research is exaggerated (Bulmer, 1982). The use of covert participant observation must be given serious consideration in the conduct of a qualitative investigation. Researchers must consider available alternative solutions for data generation, provided those solutions will maintain the integrity of the study.

Confidentiality and Anonymity

The principle of beneficence, doing good and preventing harm, applies to providing confidentiality and anonymity for research study participants. According to Polit and Beck (2004), "A promise of confidentiality is a pledge that any information participants provide will not be publicly reported in a manner that identifies them and will not be made accessible to others" (p. 150), and "anonymity occurs when even the researcher cannot link a participant to [his/her] data" (p. 149).

The very nature of data collection in a qualitative investigation makes anonymity impossible. The personal, one-to-one interaction during the interview process allows researchers to know the participants in ways that are not possible and unnecessary in quantitative designs. Qualitative research methods such as participant observation and one-to-one interviews make it "impossible to maintain anonymity at all stages; in other words, when using these methods, becoming cognizant of the source of data is unavoidable" (Behi & Nolan, 1995, p. 713).

Small sample size and thick descriptions provided in the presentation of the findings can present problems in maintaining confidentiality (Behi & Nolan, 1995; Boman & Jevne, 2000; Holloway & Wheeler, 1995; Lincoln & Guba, 1987; Ramos, 1989; Robley, 1995). Davis (1991) discussed thick descriptions as follows: "We learn from our experiences and we need to present the fruits of that learning in a full-bodied way that invites our audience to share that experience with us, and also to judge the legitimacy of our results" (p. 13). Robley (1995) emphasized that thick descriptions are extremely important to the meaning of the research and offered a solution supported by the works of Cowles (1988), Davis (1991), and Lincoln and Guba (1987): "If the narrative requires it, retain it and return to the respondent for permission, verification, and justification" (Robley, 1995, p. 48).

Often, if the research has been conducted close to home and the sample is familiar to others, the details given in the thick slices of data used to support and verify themes may reveal research participants' identities. The researcher must make every effort to ensure that confidentiality is a promise kept. "Guaranteeing confidentiality implies that the research subject's data will be used in such a way that no-one else but the researcher knows the source" (Behi & Nolan, 1995, p. 713). As Robley (1995) has pointed out, "Guarding against disclosure that may create unacceptable risks for the respondents is accomplished in part by respecting the need for withdrawal of revealing material during the interview process, and in part through the process of member checking and negotiated outcomes" (p. 46). In some instances, circulation of the research may need to be restricted to protect participants' identity (Orb et al., 2001).

Orb and colleagues (2001) note that confidentiality and anonymity can be breached by legal requirements, such as when researchers' data are subpoenaed for legal purposes (p. 95). Audit trails, commonly used to establish the confirmability of research findings, require that other researchers read the raw data. Participants need to know that this may occur within the context of data analysis. Haggerty and Hawkins (2000) discussed the limits of confidentiality within the context of the legal and ethical issues that arose in research they conducted on partner abuse. They emphasize the importance of balancing the rights of participants and furthering knowledge that has the potential to improve health care delivery. Balancing the right to privacy and confidentiality for their participants with legally mandated reporting regarding child abuse, homicidality, and suicidality are addressed.

The process of publication may also result in a breach in confidentiality or anonymity. Permission to use direct quotes must be acquired, and the researcher must be sure that examples of raw data do not reveal the participant's identity. It is imperative that, within the process of gaining consent, the participants know how the results will be used and whether they will be published (Orb et al., 2001). Finally, data may exist in a variety of formats such as written demographic data, taped interviews, videotapes, and photos. All of these formats have the potential to identify participants; they must be stored securely and, at the completion of the study, disposed of properly.

Ethical Considerations Related to the Researcher–Participant Relationship

The principle of justice concerns fair treatment and the right to privacy and anonymity. The data generation strategies associated with a qualitative investigation include such approaches as one-to-one interviews, focus groups, and participant observation. The private and intimate nature of this relationship imposes unique constraints and raises distinct ethical issues for investigators using qualitative methods. The researcher is the tool for data collection and, as such, comes to know participants in a personal way. The boundaries of the relationship may become blurred as the research progresses, and role confusion may lead to ethical concerns for the investigation. As Ramos (1989) explained, "The respondent and the investigator interact verbally, and their relationship can range from one of civil cooperation to camaraderie in problem-solving to the abiding trust and dependency of the therapeutic alliance" (p. 59).

"Nurses are legally, culturally, and historically bound to nurture and protect the health and welfare of their patients" (Ramos, 1989, p. 57). Therefore, when participants confuse the researcher's role with that of a counselor, therapist, or nurse as caregiver and unrelated issues of concern emerge, the protection of the participants' welfare must always take precedence over the research. Researchers must not move from the role of instrument in the investigation to that of counselor or therapist. "Research in nursing constitutes a delicate balance between the principles of rigorous investigation and a nurturing concern for patient welfare" (Ramos, 1989, p. 57). Investigators can attempt to guide the interview and must maintain focus on the topic under investigation. The interview is not a therapeutic intervention, and the researcher should avoid asking questions that might result in participants offering more information than they had originally consented to. Following the closure of the interview, researchers should recap for the participants issues of concern that emerged during the interview and should also provide follow-up.

Researchers must also consider the selection of participants for a qualitative research study from an ethical standpoint. "An ethical basis for selection would also involve attention to the inclusion of those whose voices need to be heard: women, minorities, children, the illiterate, and those with less personal or professional status. Social responsibility calls for attention to diversity" (Robley, 1995, p. 46).

SENSITIVE ISSUES ARISING IN THE CONDUCT OF QUALITATIVE RESEARCH

*T*he interview may be one of the few opportunities participants have to discuss the issue at hand, and the topic may well be a sensitive one. Alty and Rodham (1998) have given perspective to sensitive issues:

> The ouch! factor is a term that describes certain experiences encountered in the process of conducting qualitative research. These experiences include those ranging from a short sharp shock to the

researcher to those situations and experiences that can develop into a chronic ache if not addressed early. (p. 275)

Sensitive issues also may arise in research conducted with vulnerable populations such as dying people (Raudonis, 1992); children and adolescents (Faux, Walsh, & Deatrick, 1988); families (Demi & Warren, 1995); lesbians and gay men (Platzer & James, 1997); those involved in HIV research in poor nations (Mabunda, 2001); and individuals with intellectual disabilities (Llewellyn, 1995). Certain topics such as the "sudden violent death of a loved one, controversial involvement in political activity, a crumbling relationship, legal incarceration, and a life-threatening illness" (Cowles, 1988, p. 163) are extremely sensitive and place participants in a vulnerable situation as the researcher asks the probing questions to elicit the necessary data. Given the intensity of the interaction between researcher and participant, the researcher also may be in a vulnerable position. As Robley (1995) has observed,

> Subjectivity and collaboration makes the researcher vulnerable. Emotionally immersed in the lived experience of others, continually sensitive to the potentially injurious nature of language, and experiencing the rights of passage as an interviewer/observer—all require an inner strength that can be enhanced by self care. The researcher can use the ethics committee as a guide and support throughout the process. [He or she] can use debriefing to explore personal responses and weigh risk/benefits. Personal education in ethics and consultation with experts when it is believed that the nurse researcher is being hurt is advocated. (p. 48)

Similarly, James and Platzer (1999) discuss the risk for harm to both researcher and participant in a qualitative study with lesbians and gay men and their experiences with health care. Their account of the complex emotional and ethical issues that can arise in research with vulnerable groups emphasizes the need for researchers to pay attention to things that cause them discomfort and unease in the process of their research.

Do not stray from the focus of the investigation. Recognize that participants may need to talk, but make clear that the researcher will address the issue after the interview. "All research (particularly that which focuses on sensitive issues) may stir up emotions of such intensity that failure to provide an opportunity for the respondent to talk may be perceived as irresponsible" (Alty & Rodham, 1998, p. 279). Allowing time for feedback and discussion of participants' feelings brings with it the possibility that the researcher will hear too much, but it must be done. After each interview, ask participants if they need follow-up. Provide a contact for additional help (Alty & Rodham, 1998; Holloway & Wheeler, 1995; Richards & Swartz, 2002).

GATHERING, INTERPRETING, AND REPORTING QUALITATIVE DATA

G athering, interpreting, and reporting qualitative research findings require that researchers spend time planning how data will be collected and then reading and rereading verbatim transcriptions of interviews and field notes. Procedures such as bracketing (defined in Chapter 2) are required if researchers are to have any confidence in the final data analysis. Researchers must keep any presuppositions and personal biases separate or set aside throughout the entire investigation. Having a second researcher review data and verify categories can also serve as a validity check. According to Ramos (1989),

> The investigator, even with the validation of inferences afforded by the relationship with the respondent, imposes his or her logic and values onto the communicated reality of the respondent. He or she imposes his or her subjective reality upon the interpretation of meaning-data from the respondent. The researcher cannot extract correct meanings unilaterally. Without the validation afforded by member checking, a leap in logic could occur, and a serious misinterpretation of sensitive information can occur. (p. 60)

Returning final descriptions to participants so that they may validate that the interpretation of the interview or observation is authentic and true further adds to final data analysis. This procedure can assist researchers in verifying that there were no serious misinterpretations or omissions of critical information. Respondent validation does, however, have limitations. The repeated contact with participants may be impractical and present undo burden on participants (Richards & Schwartz, 2002).

Haggman-Laitila (1999) expands on the discussion of authenticity of data and overcoming the researcher's personal views. Haggman-Laitila bases a discussion of data collection and analysis on the assumption that the researcher cannot detach from his or her own view in phenomenological research. The researcher is able to understand the experiences of an individual only through the researcher's own view. The research process is a balanced cooperative relationship between the subjects and the researcher (p. 13). Given this assumption, Haggman-Laitila offers practical guidelines for the purpose of data gathering and interpretation in a qualitative investigation.

During the process of data gathering, Haggman-Laitila (1999) suggests that researchers plan key interview questions in advance, keep interviews open and discussion-like, verify interpretations by asking more questions and allowing additions and corrections, avoid rhetorical or leading questions, and keep a diary or videotape to facilitate recognition of the researchers' own views during the data analysis process. During data analysis, the researcher must look for additional questions raised in the data, write down questions that emerge during the reading of the data, compare researcher and participant views, re-examine all experiences, and be sure that the presentation of findings is based on the views expressed by the participants. Smith (1999) illustrates the importance of considering the researcher's reflections through the use of a reflexive journal. Smith used the journaling process in his study of the lived experience of suffering among six problem drinkers. The information reported in the reflexive journal added to the contextual richness of the study.

HUMAN SUBJECTS AND INTERNET RESEARCH

*T*he Internet is a comprehensive electronic database of material that represents the opinions and concerns of those individuals who utilize this resource. Qualitative analysis of material communicated on the Internet can describe needs, values, concerns, and preference of consumers and professionals relevant to health and health care. Although the Internet provides innovative access to human interactions, such research raises new issues in research ethics.

Within the context of ethics and Internet research, questions emerge regarding what may be public versus private information, whether informed consent has been obtained, and the extent to which the subjects can be identified. Im and Chee (2002) discuss issues related to the protection of human subjects in Internet research that emerged in a study exploring gender and ethnic diversity in cancer pain experiences. Issues raised in their study include concerns regarding anonymity and confidentiality, security, full disclosure, and fair treatment. The authors focus on mechanisms employed to address ethical concerns that emerged in the study. As more and more research is conducted through the Internet, ethical codes will need to be examined to ensure they address the issues that emerge in this type of research. Traditional tenets of informed consent and public and private information must be questioned when researchers use electronic databases for their research.

SUMMARY

*A*lthough the ethical principles governing qualitative and quantitative research are similar, the complex, personal, and intense nature of qualitative research requires a fresh perspective regarding the research process. The dynamic nature of qualitative methodologies presents unique concerns regarding informed consent. Treating consent as an ongoing process rather than an isolated event allows participants to re-evaluate their participation in a particular study should the focus change. Qualitative data collection strategies prevent participant anonymity. Maintaining the focus of the research and clarifying the purpose can prevent the development of close, intimate relationships between participants and the researcher from turning into what may be interpreted as therapeutic encounters. Presentation of the findings with thick descriptions and slices of raw data may complicate issues of confidentiality. When writing the analysis, the researcher should take care to prevent the identity of participants from being revealed through the incorporation of examples of raw data. Internet research presents new and emerging concerns regarding anonymity and confidentiality. Additionally, researchers must consider and address the vulnerability of certain populations. These issues are important in the ongoing development and use of qualitative research methods. Finally, it is important to remember that although established ethical guidelines may give some direction, the ethical and moral picture of qualitative research is much more complicated. Even though an ethical review board may have approved a research study, problems may still arise. "We should not simply assume that because research has been accepted by a committee it is morally justifiable in its methods" (Firby, 1995, p. 36). Ethical guidelines for qualitative research will continue to emerge, and researchers must consider those guidelines from a different perspective than those associated with quantitative designs.

References

Alty, A., & Rodham, K. (1998). The ouch! factor: Problems in conducting sensitive research. *Qualitative Health Research, 8*(2), 275–282.

American Nurses Association. (2001). *Code for nurses with interpretive statements.* Kansas City, MO: Author.

Beauchamp, T. L., & Childress, J. F. (2001). *Principles of biomedical ethics* (5th ed.). Oxford, UK: Oxford University Press.

Behi, R., & Nolan, M. (1995). Ethical issues in research. *British Journal of Nursing, 4*(12), 712–716.

Boman, J., & Jevne, R. (2000). Ethical evaluation in qualitative research. *Qualitative Health Research, 10*(4), 547–554.

Bulmer, M. (Ed.). (1982). *Social research ethics.* New York: Macmillan.

Clarke, L. (1996). Covert participant observation in a secure forensic unit. *Nursing Times, 92*(48), 37–40.

Cowles, K. V. (1988). Issues in qualitative research on sensitive topics. *Western Journal of Nursing Research, 10*(2), 163–179.

Cutliffe, J. R., & Ramcharan, P. (2002). Leveling the playing field? Exploring the merits of the ethics-as-process approach for judging qualitative research proposals. *Qualitative Health Research, 12*(7), 1000–1010.

Davis, D. S. (1991). Rich cases: The ethics of thick description. *Hastings Center Report, 21*(4), 12–16.

Demi, A. S., & Warren, N. A. (1995). Issues in conducting research with vulnerable families. *Western Journal of Nursing Research, 17*(2), 188-202.

Douglas, J. D. (1979). Living morality versus bureaucratic fiat. In C. B. Klockers & F. W. O. Connor (Eds.), *Deviance and decency: The ethics of research with human subjects* (pp. 13-33). Beverly Hills, CA: Sage.

Faux, S. A., Walsh, M., & Deatrick, J. A. (1988). Intensive interviewing with adolescents. *Western Journal of Nursing Research, 10*(2), 180-194.

Firby, P. (1995). Critiquing the ethical aspects of a study. *Nurse Researcher, 3*(1), 35-41.

Forbat, L., & Henderson, J. (2003). "Stuck in the middle with you": The ethics and process of qualitative research with two people in an intimate relationship. *Qualitative Health Research, 13*(10), 1453-1462.

Gans, H. J. (1962). *The urban villagers: Group and class in the life of Italian-Americans.* New York: Free Press.

Haggerty, L. A., & Hawkins, J. (2000). Informed consent and the limits of confidentiality. *Western Journal of Nursing Research, 22*(4), 508-515.

Haggman-Laitila, A. (1999). The authenticity and ethics of phenomenological research: How to overcome the researcher's own views. *Nursing Ethics, 6*(1), 12-22.

Holloway, I., & Wheeler, S. (1995). Ethical issues in qualitative nursing research. *Nursing Ethics, 2*(3), 223-232.

Im, E. & Chee, W. (2002). Issues in protection of human subjects in Internet research. *Nursing Research, 51*(4), 266-269.

James, T., & Platzer, H. (1999). Ethical considerations in qualitative research with vulnerable groups: Exploring lesbians' and gay men's experiences of health care—a personal perspective. *Nursing Ethics, 6*(1), 73-81.

Lawton, J. (2001). Gaining and maintaining consent: Ethical concerns raised in a study of dying patients. *Qualitative Health Research, 11*(5), 693-705.

Levine, R. (Ed.). (1986). *Ethics and regulation of clinical research* (2nd ed.). Baltimore-Munich: Urban & Schwarzenberg.

Lincoln, Y. S., & Guba, E. (1987). Ethics: The failure of positivist science. *Review of Higher Education, 12*, 221-240.

Llewellyn, G. (1995). Qualitative research with people with intellectual disability. *Occupational Therapy International, 2*, 108-127.

Mabunda, G. (2001). Ethical issues in HIV research in poor countries. *Journal of Nursing Scholarship, 33*(2), 111-114.

Merrell, J., & Williams, A. (1994). Participant observation and informed consent: Relationships and tactical decision-making in nursing research. *Nursing Ethics, 1*(3), 163-172.

Moore, L., & Savage, J. (2002). Participant observation, informed consent and ethical approval. *Nurse Researcher, 9*(4), 58-70.

Munhall, P. (1988). Ethical considerations in qualitative research. *Western Journal of Nursing Research, 10*(2), 150-162.

Orb, A., Eisenhauer, L., & Wynaden, D. (2001). Ethics in qualitative research. *Journal of Nursing Scholarship, 33*(1), 93-98.

Platzer, H., & James, T. (1997). Methodological issues conducting sensitive research on lesbian and gay men's experience of nursing care. *Journal of Advanced Nursing, 25*, 626-633.

Polit, D. F., & Beck, C. T. (2004). *Nursing research: Methods, appraisal, and utilization* (7th ed.). Philadelphia: Lippincott Williams & Wilkins.

Punch, M. (1994). Politics and ethics in qualitative research. In N. K. Denzin & Y. S. Lincoln (Eds.), *Handbook of qualitative research* (pp. 86-97). Thousand Oaks, CA: Sage.

Ramos, M. C. (1989). Some ethical implications of qualitative research. *Research in Nursing and Health, 12,* 57-63.

Raudonis, B. A. (1992). Ethical considerations in qualitative research with hospice patients. *Qualitative Health Research, 2*(2), 238-249.

Richards, H. M., & Schwartz, L. J. (2002). Ethics of qualitative research: Are there special issues for health services research? *Family Practice, 19*(2), 135-139.

Robley, L. R. (1995). The ethics of qualitative nursing research. *Journal of Professional Nursing, 11*(1), 45-48.

Savage, J. (2000). Participative observation: Standing in the shoes of others? *Qualitative Health Research, 10*(3), 324-339.

Silva, M. (1995). *Ethical guidelines in the conduct, dissemination, and implementation of nursing research.* Washington, DC: American Nurses Publishing.

Smith, B. A. (1999). Ethical and methodological benefits of using a reflexive journal in hermeneutic-phenomenologic research. *Journal of Nursing Scholarship, 31*(4), 359-363.

Steinbrook, R. (2002). Protecting research subjects: The Crisis at John Hopkins. *New England Journal of Medicine, 346,* 716.

CHAPTER 5

Phenomenology as Method

*P*henomenology has been and continues to be an integral field of inquiry that cuts across philosophic, sociologic, and psychological disciplines. This rigorous, critical, systematic method of investigation is a recognized qualitative research approach applicable to the study of phenomena important to the discipline of nursing. Phenomenological inquiry brings to language perceptions of human experience with all types of phenomena. As several authors have noted, phenomenology, both as philosophy and research approach, allows nursing to explore and describe phenomena important to the discipline (Arrigo & Cody, 2004; Beck, 1994; Caelli, 2000, 2001; Todres & Wheeler, 2001; Van der Zalm & Bergum, 2000). Because professional nursing practice is enmeshed in people's life experiences, phenomenology as a research approach is well suited to the investigation of phenomena important to nursing.

Phenomenological inquiry as a philosophy and developing science continues to undergo interpretation and explication in terms of its pragmatic use as a nursing research method. This chapter addresses the variety of methodological interpretations detailed within the discipline of phenomenological inquiry. Phenomenology as philosophy and as method is discussed, along with fundamental differences between descriptive and interpretive phenomenology. Highlights of specific elements and interpretations of phenomenology as a research approach provide readers with a beginning understanding of common phenomenological language and themes. This chapter also addresses methodological concerns specific to conducting a phenomenological investigation.

Introductory concepts for researchers interested in conducting a phenomenological investigation are presented in the content that follows. The reader should keep in mind that there is no quick step-by-step method to phenomenological inquiry. The methodology is philosophically complex, and the analytic processes required to participate in the method require scientific discipline. Researchers interested in conducting a phenomenological investigation must read original philosophically based work and identify a mentor with expertise in the discipline to acquire an in-depth understanding of phenomenology both as a philosophy and as a research approach.

PHENOMENOLOGY DEFINED

P *henomenology* is a science whose purpose is to describe particular phenomena, or the appearance of things, as lived experience. Cohen (1987) has pointed out that phenomenology was first described as the study of phenomena or things by Immanuel Kant in 1764. Merleau-Ponty (1962), in the preface to his text *Phenomenology of Perception*, asked the question, What is phenomenology? His description reflects the flow of phenomenological thinking, but Merleau-Ponty never offered a definitive answer or step-by-step approach to what phenomenology actually entailed. Essentially, not much has changed. Merleau-Ponty offered the following description:

> Phenomenology is the study of essences; and according to it, all problems amount to finding definitions of essences: the essence of perception, or the essence of consciousness, for example. But phenomenology is also a philosophy, which puts essences back into existence, and does not expect to arrive at an understanding of man and the world from any starting point other than that of their "facticity." It is a transcendental philosophy which places in abeyance the assertions arising out of the natural attitude, the better to understand them: but it is also a philosophy for which the world is always "already there" before reflection begins—as an inalienable presence; and all its efforts are concentrated upon re-achieving a direct and primitive contact with the world, and endowing that contact with a philosophical status. It is the search for a philosophy which shall be a "rigorous science," but it also offers an account of space, time and the world as we "live" them. It tries to give a direct description of our experience as it is, without taking account of its psychological origin and the causal explanations which the scientist, the historian or the sociologist may be able to provide. (p. vii)

The historian Herbert Spiegelberg (1975) explained phenomenology as a movement rather than a uniform method or set of doctrines. The account provided by Spiegelberg emphasizes the fluid nature of phenomenology and the fact that a list of steps to the approach would not reflect the philosophic depth of the discipline. Spiegelberg defined phenomenology as "the name for a philosophical movement whose primary objective is the direct investigation and description of phenomena as consciously experienced, without theories about their causal explanation and as free as possible from unexamined preconceptions and presuppositions" (p. 3).

Spiegelberg (1975) and Merleau-Ponty (1962) described phenomenology as both a philosophy and a method. Phenomenology was further explained by Wagner (1983) as a way of viewing ourselves, others, and everything else whom or with which we come in contact in life. "Phenomenology is a system of interpretation that helps us perceive and conceive ourselves, our contacts and interchanges with others, and everything else in the realm of our experiences in a variety of ways, including to describe a method as well as a philosophy or way of thinking" (Wagner, 1983, p. 8).

Omery (1983) addressed the question, What is the phenomenological method? Although researchers have interpreted this question in a variety of ways, the approach is inductive and descriptive in its design. Phenomenological method is "the trick of making things whose meanings seem clear, meaningless, and then, discovering what they mean" (Blumensteil, 1973, p. 189).

Lived experience of the world of everyday life is the central focus of phenomenological inquiry. Schutz (1970) described the world of everyday life as the "total sphere of experiences of an individual which is circumscribed by the objects, persons, and events encountered in the pursuit of the pragmatic objectives of living" (p. 320). In other words, it is the lived experience that presents to the individual what is true or real in his or her life. Furthermore, it is this lived experience that gives meaning to each individual's perception of a particular phenomenon and is influenced by everything internal and external to the individual. Perception is important in phenomenological philosophy and method, as explained by Merleau-Ponty (1956):

> Perception is not a science of the world, nor even an act, a deliberate taking up of a position. It is the basis from which every act issues and it is presupposed by them. The world is not an object the law of whose constitution I possess. It is the natural milieu and the field of all my thoughts and of all my explicit perceptions. Truth does not "dwell" only in the "interior man" for there is no interior man. Man is before himself in the world and it is in the world that he knows himself. When I turn upon myself from the dogmatism of common sense or the dogmatism of science, I find, not the dwelling place of intrinsic truth, but a subject committed to the world. (p. 62)

Phenomenology is as much a way of thinking or perceiving as it is a method. The goal of phenomenology is to describe lived experience. To further clarify both the philosophy and method of phenomenology, it is helpful to gain a sense of how the movement developed historically. An overview of the roots of phenomenology as a philosophy and science follows.

PHENOMENOLOGICAL ROOTS

*T*he phenomenological movement began around the first decade of the 20th century. This philosophic movement consisted of three phases: (1) preparatory; (2) German; and (3) French. The following text describes common themes of phenomenology within the context of these three phases.

Preparatory Phase

The Preparatory phase was dominated by Franz Brentano (1838–1917) and Carl Stumpf (1848–1936). Stumpf was Brentano's first prominent student and, through his work, demonstrated the scientific rigor of phenomenology. Clarification of the concept of intentionality was the primary focus during this time (Spiegelberg, 1965). *Intentionality* means that consciousness is always consciousness of something. Merleau-Ponty (1956) explained "interior perception is impossible without exterior perception, that the world as the connection of phenomena is anticipated in the consciousness of my unity and is the way for me to realize myself in consciousness" (p. 67). Therefore, one does not hear without hearing something or believe without believing something (Cohen, 1987).

German Phase

Edmund Husserl (1857–1938) and Martin Heidegger (1889–1976) were the prominent leaders during the German, or second, phase of the phenomenological movement. Husserl (1931, 1965) believed that philosophy should become a rigorous science that would restore contact with deeper human concerns and that phenomenology should become the foundation for all philosophy and science. According to Spiegelberg (1965), Heidegger followed so closely in the steps of Husserl that his work is probably a direct outcome of Husserl's. The concepts of essences, intuiting, and phenomenological reduction were developed during the German phase (Spiegelberg, 1965).

Essences are elements related to the ideal or true meaning of something, that is, those concepts that give common understanding to the phenomenon under investigation. Essences emerge in both isolation and in relationship to one another. According to Natanson (1973), "Essences are unities of meaning intended by different individuals in the same acts or by the same individuals in different acts" (p. 14). Essences, therefore, represent the basic units of common understanding of any phenomenon. For example, Schwarz (2003) explored how nurses experience and respond to patients' requests for assistance in dying. Schwarz (2003) describes the continuum of interventions provided by the nurses in her phenomenological study that includes "refusal, providing palliative care that might secondarily hasten dying, respecting and not interfering with patients' or families' plans to hasten dying, and providing varying types and degrees of direct AID" (p. 377). In a study examining patient experiences living with rheumatoid arthritis, Iaquinta and Larrabee (2003) describe the essences of this experience as "grieving while growing, persuading self and others of RA's authenticity, cultivating resilience, confronting negative feelings, navigating the healthcare system, and masterminding new lifeways" (p. 282).

Intuiting is an eidetic comprehension or accurate interpretation of what is meant in the description of the phenomenon under investigation. The intuitive process in phenomenological research results in a common understanding about the phenomenon under investigation. Intuiting in the phenomenological sense requires that researchers imaginatively vary the data until a common understanding about the phenomenon emerges. Through imaginative variation, researchers begin to wonder about the phenomenon under investigation in relationship to the various descriptions generated. To further illustrate, in a study on commitment to nursing (Rinaldi, 1989), the essences of commitment gleaned from the data were varied in as many ways as possible and compared with participants' descriptions. From this imaginative variation, a relationship between the essences of commitment and to whom or what the nurse was committed emerged. For example, the nurse may be committed to clients, colleagues, the employing institution, the profession, or self. To whom or what the nurse is committed is then examined in relationship to the essences of commitment. Researchers might vary the essences of commitment within the descriptions of the person to whom or the thing to which the nurse is committed. Some essences may apply when the issue is commitment to clients, and other essences if the issue is commitment to the institution. In a study on the lived experience of caring for a child with cystic fibrosis, the intuitive process resulted in emergence of phenomena unique to caring for a child with a chronic illness at the time of diagnosis. The essential elements of the experience included Falling Apart, Pulling Together, and Moving Beyond (Carpenter & Narsavage, 2004).

Phenomenological reduction is a return to original awareness regarding the phenomenon under investigation. Husserl specified how to describe, with scientific exactness, the life of consciousness in its original encounter with the world through phenomenological reduction. Husserl (1931, 1965) challenged individuals to go "back to the things themselves" to recover this original awareness. Husserl's reference "to the things" meant "a fresh approach to concretely experienced phenomena, as free as possible from conceptual presuppositions and an attempt to describe them as faithfully as possible" (Spiegelberg, 1975, p. 10).

Phenomenological reduction begins with a suspension of beliefs, assumptions, and biases about the phenomenon under investigation. Isolation of pure phenomenon, versus what is already known about a particular phenomenon, is the goal of the reductive procedure. The only way to really see the world clearly is to remain as free as possible from preconceived ideas or notions. Complete reduction may never be possible because of the intimate relationship individuals have with the world (Merleau-Ponty, 1956).

As part of the reductive process, phenomenological researchers must first identify any preconceived notions or ideas about the phenomenon under investigation. Having identified these ideas, the researchers must bracket or separate out of consciousness what they know or believe about the topic under investigation. *Bracketing* requires researchers to remain neutral with respect to belief or disbelief in the existence of the phenomenon. Bracketing begins the reductive process and, like that process, must continue throughout the investigation. Essentially, researchers set aside previous knowledge or personal beliefs about the phenomenon under investigation to prevent this information from interfering with the recovery of a pure description of the phenomenon. Bracketing must be constant and ongoing if descriptions are to achieve their purest form. Haggman-Laitila (1999) holds the position that the researcher cannot detach from his or her own view and offers practical aspects to help in overcoming the researcher's views during data gathering and analysis. Chapter 4 offers an overview of strategies to address this very issue within the context of ethical standards.

French Phase

Gabriel Marcel (1889–1973), Jean-Paul Sartre (1905–1980), and Maurice Merleau-Ponty (1905–1980) were the predominant leaders of the French, or third phase, of the phenomenological movement. The primary concepts developed during this phase were embodiment and being-in-the-world. These concepts refer to the belief that all acts are constructed on foundations of perception or original awareness of some phenomenon. Lived experience, given in the perceived world, must be described (Merleau-Ponty, 1956). Munhall (1989) explained these key concepts, originally described by Merleau-Ponty, as follows:

> Embodiment explains that through consciousness one is aware of being-in-the-world and it is through the body that one gains access to this world. One feels, thinks, tastes, touches, hears, and is conscious

through the opportunities the body offers. There is talk sometimes about expanding the mind or expanding waistlines. The expansion is within the body, within the consciousness. It is important to understand that at any point in time and for each individual a particular perspective and/or consciousness exists. It is based on the individual's history, knowledge of the world, and perhaps openness to the world. Nursing's focus on the individual and the "meaning" events may have for an individual, is this recognition that experience is individually interpreted. (p. 24)

The philosophic underpinnings of phenomenology are complex. Given this understanding, one can appreciate why the methodological applications remain dynamic and evolving. Different philosophers may have different interpretations of phenomenology as both a philosophy and method. The dynamic nature and evolving interpretations provide phenomenological researchers with a variety of options from which to choose when embarking on an investigation of this nature. The content that follows presents these options, in a very pragmatic format, along with other issues related to actually conducting a phenomenological investigation.

At this particular juncture, the following words of caution are offered: Imperative to gaining an in-depth understanding of the method and philosophy of phenomenology is a return to the original works. Readers should take the time to read the works of Husserl, Heidegger, Merleau-Ponty, Spiegelberg, Ricoeur, Gadamer, and others to ensure a solid foundation and understanding of the philosophy behind the method. It is also advised that beginning researchers connect with a mentor who can guide their development in the area of phenomenology. Paley (1997) suggested that "a problematic feature of the way in which phenomenology has been imported into nursing is that sources tend to be second-hand and several 'tiers' in the literature are apparent" (p. 187). Paley's work addresses how original concepts can become distorted when interpreted second-hand and emphasizes the point made earlier: researchers who are embarking on a phenomenological investigation must return to the original works, secure a mentor with expertise in the discipline, and recognize that there is no simplistic step-by-step approach to phenomenological inquiry.

FUNDAMENTAL CHARACTERISTICS OF THE PHENOMENOLOGICAL METHOD

*P*henomenology as a research method is a rigorous, critical, systematic investigation of phenomena. "The purpose of phenomenological inquiry is to explicate the structure or essence of the lived experience of a phenomenon in the search for the unity of meaning which is the identification of the essence of a phenomenon, and its accurate description through the everyday lived experience" (Rose, Beeby, & Parker, 1995, p. 1124).

Several procedural interpretations of phenomenological method are available as guidelines to this research approach (Colaizzi, 1978; Giorgi, 1985; Paterson & Zderad, 1976; Spiegelberg, 1965, 1975; Streubert, 1991; van Kaam, 1984; van Manen, 1990). Because there is more than one legitimate way to proceed with a phenomenological investigation, the researcher must be familiar with the philosophic underpinnings and ground the study in the approach that would offer the most rigorous and accurate interpretations of the phenomenon under investigation. Appropriateness of the method to the phenomenon of interest should guide the method choice. Clearly, phenomenology is grounded in a variety of philosophic positions and procedural interpretations. The philosophic underpinnings of phenomenology are critical to the discipline. The guidelines in provide meaningful direction for method application and highlight various procedural interpretations. Once again the reader is encouraged to return to the original works to ensure a comprehensive understanding of the philosophic positions associated with the method. Chapter 6 provides a critical discussion of method application along with selected examples of research that apply the approaches described in Table 5.1.

Six Core Steps

Spiegelberg (1965, 1975) identified a core of steps or elements central to phenomenological investigations. These six steps are (1) descriptive phenomenology; (2) phenomenology of essences; (3) phenomenology of appearances; (4) constitutive phenomenology; (5) reductive phenomenology; and (6) hermeneutic phenomenology (Spiegelberg, 1975). A discussion of each of the six elements follows. As Spiegelberg (1965) has explained, the purpose of this discussion is to "present this method as a series of steps, of which the later will usually presuppose the earlier ones, yet not be necessarily entailed by them" (p. 655). As such, phenomenology as a movement is described. A combination of one or more of the elements identified as central to the movement can be found in the plethora of published phenomenological investigations.

DESCRIPTIVE PHENOMENOLOGY

Descriptive phenomenology involves "direct exploration, analysis, and description of particular phenomena, as free as possible from unexamined presuppositions, aiming at maximum intuitive presentation" (Spiegelberg, 1975, p. 57). Descriptive phenomenology stimulates our perception of lived

TABLE 5.1 • Methodological Interpretations	
Author(s)	*Procedural Steps*
Colaizzi (1978)	1. Describe the phenomenon of interest.
	2. Collect participants' descriptions of the phenomenon.
	3. Read all participants' descriptions of the phenomenon.
	4. Return the original transcripts and extract significant statements.
	5. Try to spell out the meaning of each significant statement.
	6. Organize the aggregate formalized meanings into clusters of themes.
	7. Write an exhaustive description.
	8. Return to the participants for validation of the description.
	9. If new data are revealed during the validation, incorporate them into an exhaustive description.
Giorgi (1985)	1. Read the entire description of the experience to get a sense of the whole.
	2. Reread the description.
	3. Identify the transition units of the experience.
	4. Clarify and elaborate the meaning by relating constituents to each other and to the whole.
	5. Reflect on the constituents in the concrete language of the participant.
	6. Transform concrete language into the language or concepts of science.
	7. Integrate and synthesize the insight into a descriptive structure of the meaning of the experience.
Paterson & Zderad (1976)	1. Compare and study instances of the phenomenon wherever descriptions of it may be found (putting descriptions in a logbook).
	2. Imaginatively vary the phenomenon.
	3. Explain through negation.
	4. Explain through analogy and metaphor.
	5. Classify the phenomenon.
van Kaam (1984)	1. Obtain a core of common experiences.
	2. List and prepare a rough preliminary grouping of every expression presented by participants.
	3. Reduce and eliminate. Test each expression for two requirements:

TABLE 5.1 • *(Continued)*	
Author(s)	*Procedural Steps*
	a. Does it contain a moment of the experience that might eventually be a necessary and sufficient constituent of the experience?
	b. If so, is it possible to abstract this moment and to label it, without violating the formulation presented by the participant?
	4. Eliminate expressions not meeting these two requirements.
	5. Tentatively identify the descriptive constituents; bring together all common relevant constituents in a cluster labeled with the more abstract formula expressing the common theme.
	6. Finally, identify the descriptive constituents by application; this operation consists of checking the tentatively identified constituents against random cases of the sample to see whether they fulfill the following conditions. Each constituent must:
	a. be expressed explicitly in the description,
	b. be expressed explicitly or implicitly in some or the large majority of descriptions,
	c. be compatible with the description in which it is not expressed.
	7. If a description is found incompatible with a constituent, the description must be proved not to be an expression of the experience under study, but of some other experience that intrudes on it.
van Manen (1990)	1. Turn to the nature of lived experience by orienting to the phenomenon, formulating the phenomenological question, and explicating assumptions and preunderstandings.
	2. Engage in existential investigation, which involves exploring the phenomenon: generating data, using personal experience as a starting point, tracing etymologic sources, searching idiomatic phrases, obtaining experiential descriptions from participants, locating experiential descriptions in the literature, and consulting phenomenological literature, art, and so forth.
	3. Engage in phenomenological reflection, which involves conducting thematic analysis, uncovering thematic aspects in life-world descriptions, isolating thematic statements, composing linguistic transformations, and gleaning thematic descriptions from artistic sources.

TABLE 5.1 • *(Continued)*	
Author(s)	*Procedural Steps*
	4. Engage in phenomenological writing, which includes attending to the speaking of language, varying the examples, writing, and rewriting.
Streubert (1991)	1. Explicate a personal description of the phenomenon of interest.
	2. Bracket the researcher's presuppositions.
	3. Interview participants in unfamiliar settings.
	4. Carefully read the interview transcripts to obtain a general sense of the experience.
	5. Review the transcripts to uncover essences.
	6. Apprehend essential relationships.
	7. Develop formalized descriptions of the phenomenon.
	8. Return to participants to validate descriptions.
	9. Review the relevant literature.
	10. Distribute the findings to the nursing community.

experience while emphasizing the richness, breadth, and depth of those experiences (Spiegelberg, 1975, p. 70). Spiegelberg (1965, 1975) identified a three-step process for descriptive phenomenology: (1) intuiting; (2) analyzing; and (3) describing.

Intuiting

The first step, *intuiting*, requires the researcher to become totally immersed in the phenomenon under investigation and is the step in the process whereby the researcher begins to know about the phenomenon as described by the participants. The researcher avoids all criticism, evaluation, or opinion and pays strict attention to the phenomenon under investigation as it is being described (Spiegelberg, 1965, 1975).

The step of intuiting the phenomenon in a study of quality of life would involve the "researcher as instrument" in the interview process. The researcher becomes the tool for data collection and listens to individual descriptions of quality of life through the interview process. The researcher then studies the data as they are transcribed and reviews repeatedly what the participants have described as the meaning of quality of life.

Analyzing

The second step is *phenomenological analyzing*, which involves identifying the essence of the phenomenon under investigation based on data obtained and how the data are presented. As the researcher distinguishes the phenomenon with regard to elements or constituents, he or she explores the relationships and connections with adjacent phenomena (Spiegelberg, 1965, 1975).

As the researcher listens to descriptions of quality of life and dwells with the data, common themes or essences will begin to emerge. Dwelling with the data essentially involves complete immersion in the generated data to fully engage in this analytic process. The researcher must dwell with the data for as long as necessary to ensure a pure and accurate description.

Describing

The third step is *phenomenological describing*. The aim of the describing operation is to communicate and bring to written and verbal description distinct, critical elements of the phenomenon. The description is based on a classification or grouping of the phenomenon. The researcher must avoid attempting to describe a phenomenon prematurely. Premature description is a common methodological error associated with this type of research (Spiegelberg, 1965, 1975). Description is an integral part of intuiting and analyzing. Although addressed separately, intuiting and analyzing are often occurring simultaneously.

In a study on quality of life, phenomenological describing would involve classifying all critical elements or essences that are common to the lived experience of quality of life and describing these essences in detail. Critical elements or essences are described singularly and then within the context of their relationship to one another. A discussion of this relationship follows.

PHENOMENOLOGY OF ESSENCES

Phenomenology of essences involves probing through the data to search for common themes or essences and establishing patterns of relationships shared by particular phenomena. *Free imaginative variation*, used to apprehend essential relationships between essences, involves careful study of concrete examples supplied by the participants' experiences and systematic variation of these examples in the imagination. In this way, it becomes possible to gain insights into the essential structures and relationships among phenomena. Probing for essences provides a sense for what is essential and what is accidental in the phenomenological description (Spiegelberg, 1975). The researcher follows through with the steps of intuiting, analyzing, and describing in this second core step (Spiegelberg, 1965, 1975). According to Spiegelberg (1975), "Phenomenology in its descriptive stage can stimulate our perceptiveness for the richness of our experience in breadth and in depth" (p. 70).

PHENOMENOLOGY OF APPEARANCES

Phenomenology of appearances involves giving attention to the ways in which phenomena appear. In watching the ways in which phenomena appear, the researcher pays particular attention to the different ways in which an object presents itself. Phenomenology of appearances focuses attention on the phenomenon as it unfolds through dwelling with the data. Phenomenology of appearances "can heighten the sense for the inexhaustibility of the perspectives through which our world is given" (Spiegelberg, 1975, p. 70).

CONSTITUTIVE PHENOMENOLOGY

Constitutive phenomenology is studying phenomena as they become established or "constituted" in our consciousness. Constitutive phenomenology "means the process in which the phenomena 'take shape' in our consciousness, as we advance from first impressions to a full 'picture' of their structure" (Spiegelberg, 1975, p. 66). According to Spiegelberg (1975), constitutive phenomenology "can develop the sense for the dynamic adventure in our relationship with the world" (p. 70).

REDUCTIVE PHENOMENOLOGY

Reductive phenomenology, although addressed as a separate process, occurs concurrently throughout a phenomenological investigation. The researcher continually addresses personal biases, assumptions, and presuppositions or sets aside these beliefs to obtain the purest description of the phenomenon under investigation. Suspending judgment can make us more aware of the precariousness of all our claims to knowledge, "a ground for epistemological humility" (Spiegelberg, 1975, p. 70).

This step is critical for the preservation of objectivity in the phenomenological method. For example, in a study investigating the meaning of quality of life for individuals with type 1 (insulin-dependent) diabetes mellitus, the investigator begins the study with the reductive process. The researcher identifies all presuppositions, biases, or assumptions he or she holds about what quality of life means or what it is like to have diabetes. This process involves a critical self-examination of personal beliefs and an acknowledgment of understandings that the researcher has gained from experience. The researcher takes all he or she knows about the phenomenon and brackets it or sets it aside in an effort to keep what is already known separate from the lived experience as described by the participants.

Phenomenological reduction is critical if the researcher is to achieve pure description. The reductive process is also the basis for postponing any review of the literature until the researcher has analyzed the data. The researcher must always keep separate from the participants' descriptions what he or she knows or believes about the phenomenon under investigation. Therefore, postponing the literature review until data analysis is complete facilitates phenomenological reduction.

INTERPRETIVE NURSING RESEARCH
AND HERMENEUTIC PHILOSOPHY

Interpretive frameworks within phenomenology are used to search out the relationships and meanings that knowledge and context have for each other (Lincoln & Guba, 1985). Increasingly, published nursing research is grounded in the philosophic theory of hermeneutics, and several authors have discussed the philosophic underpinnings of this particular research approach, offering clarity and direction for others (Crist & Tanner, 2003; Geanellos, 2000; Todres & Wheeler, 2001; Van der Zalm & Bergum, 2000). A phenomenological-hermeneutic approach is essentially a philosophy of the nature of understanding a particular phenomenon and the scientific interpretation of phenomena appearing in text or written word. Hermeneutics as an interpretive approach is based on the work of Ricoeur (1976), Heidegger (1927/1962), and Gadamer (1976). The methodology allows for increasingly sensitive awareness of humans and their ways of being-in-the-world (Dreyfus, 1991). Allen and Jenson (1990) emphasized that,

> The value of knowledge in nursing is, in part, determined by its relevance to and significance for an understanding of the human experience. In order to obtain that understanding, nursing requires modes of inquiry that offer the freedom to explore the richness of this experience. Hermeneutics offers such a mode of inquiry. With this interpretive strategy, a means is provided for arriving at a deeper understanding of human existence through attention to the nature of language and meaning. (p. 241)

Hermeneutic phenomenology is a "special kind of phenomenological interpretation, designed to unveil otherwise concealed meanings in the phenomena" (Spiegelberg, 1975, p. 57). Gadamer (1976) elaborated by noting that hermeneutics bridges the gap between what is familiar in our worlds and what is unfamiliar: "Its field of application is comprised of all those situations in which we encounter meanings that are not immediately understandable but require interpretive effort" (p. xii). As in all research, congruence between the philosophic foundations of the study and the methodological processes of the research are critical. The basic elements of hermeneutic philosophy and interpretive inquiry are addressed in the following narrative within the context of the work of Ricoeur (1976), Heidegger (1927/1962), and Gadamer (1976).

Paul Ricoeur's interpretive approach is one way in which nurse researchers can apply hermeneutic philosophy to a qualitative investigation. Ricoeur (1976) describes the interpretive process as a series of analytic steps and acknowledged the "interrelationship between epistemology (interpretation) and ontology (interpreter)" (Geanellos, 2000, p. 112). Crist and Tanner (2003) also describe the interpretive process of hermeneutic phenomenology. They note that although it is not required, having a team of researchers that can debate, brainstorm, and discuss interpretations adds depth and insight to the content area of the inquiry (Crist & Tanner, 2003). A major difference between hermeneutic phenomenology and other interpretations of phenomenological research methods is the fact that the method does not require researchers to bracket their own preconceptions or theories during the process (Lowes & Prowse, 2001). Analysis is essentially the hermeneutic circle, which proceeds from a naïve understanding to an explicit understanding that emerges from explanation of data interpretation

As described by Allen and Jenson (1990),

> The hermeneutical circle of interpretation moves forward and backward, starting at the present. It is never closed or final. Through rigorous interaction and understanding, the phenomenon is uncovered. The interpretive process that underlies meaning arises out of interactions, working outward and back from self to event and event to self. (p. 245)

There are three main steps to the process of hermeneutic phenomenology:

1. First, during the *naïve reading*, the researcher reads the text as a whole to become familiar with the text and begins to formulate thoughts about its meaning for further analysis. Lindholm, Uden, and Rastam (1999) in a study on nursing management note that during this particular component of data analysis, they "read all the interviews individually to gain a sense of the whole text. Their impressions of the text were then documented and discussed. The naïve reading directed attention to the phenomenon of power" (p. 103).

2. *Structural analysis* follows as the second step and involves identifying patterns of meaningful connection. This step is often referred to as an *interpretive reading*. To illustrate, Lindholm, Uden, and Rastam (1999) noted that the researchers met to compare and discuss the texts. They describe this step in the following manner: "The text was divided into meaning units, which were transformed with the contents intact. Arising from every transformed meaning unit a number of labels were created, to discover common themes. During the analysis there was continuous movement between the whole and the parts of the text" (p. 103).

3. Third, *interpretation of the whole* follows and involves reflecting on the initial reading along with the interpretive reading to ensure a comprehensive understanding of the findings. Several readings are usually required. Lindholm, Uden, and Rastam (1999) performed a separate interpretation of their data during this step and described themes and subthemes within the data.

Ricoeur (1981) has addressed the difference between text and discourse, referring to these differences as distancing. The four principles of distancing are (1) the transcription itself and the meaning of the written word; (2) the relationship between what has been written and the intent of the person who wrote the text; (3) the meaning of the text beyond its original intent as well as the author's original intent; and (4) the new interpreted meaning of the written word and the audience. The process of hermeneutic interpretive phenomenology is not linear. "Within the circular process, narratives are examined simultaneously with the emerging interpretation, never losing sight of each informant's particular story and context" (Crist & Tanner, 2003, p. 203). Christ and Tanner describe five phases of hermeneutic phenomenology. Their interpretation provides detailed steps for those new researchers engaging in hermeneutic interpretive research. Crist and Tanner emphasize that the phases of inquiry in interpretive research frequently overlap due to the nature of the circular process of examining narratives. The phases include the following:

1. *Early Focus and Lines of Inquiry:* This phase involves critical evaluation of the investigators' interview and observation techniques and identification of missing or unclear data. New research questions emerge and direct future sampling (Crist & Tanner, 2003, p. 203).
2. *Central Concerns, Exemplars, and Paradigm Cases:* During this second phase, the researchers identify themes or meanings. Development of the interpretations occurs through writing and rewriting central of concerns. Transcript review of summaries begins (Crist & Tanner, 2003, p. 204).
3. *Shared Meanings:* Connections between meanings found within and across stories are made (Crist & Tanner, 2003, p. 204).
4. *Final Interpretations:* Development of in-depth interpretations, central concern summaries, and interpretive summaries is undertaken (Crist & Tanner, 2003, p. 204).
5. *Dissemination of the Interpretation:* Refinement of manuscripts and development of audit trail are accomplished (Crist and Tanner, p. 204, 2003).

Allen and Jenson (1990) illustrated the application of hermeneutic inquiry in their exploration of what it means to have eye problems and to be visually impaired. Their example emphasizes the applicability of hermeneutics in the description and explanation of human phenomena. According to Allen and Jenson (1990),

> The task ... of modern hermeneutics is to describe and explain human phenomena (such as health and illness). The purpose of hermeneutical description and explanation is to achieve understanding through interpretation of the phenomena under study. It is the written description of the phenomena (text) that is the object of interpretation. (p. 242)

Interpretive phenomenology is a valuable method for the study of phenomena relevant to nursing education, research, and practice. Several investigations have used interpretive phenomenology in areas such as educational innovation (Diekelmann, 2001); caring for dying patients with air hunger (Tarzian, 2000); and examining the experience of isolation in blood and marrow transplantation (Cohen, Ley, & Tarzian, 2001). Applying any interpretation of phenomenological research methodology to a particular investigation will require a careful examination of the researcher's role, generation and treatment of data, and ethical issues connected with a phenomenological investigation. A discussion of these topics as they relate to the selection of phenomenology as a research method follows.

SELECTION OF PHENOMENOLOGY AS METHOD

*H*ow do researchers decide to use the phenomenological method for the investigation of phenomena important to nursing? This is a complex decision that should be grounded in the understanding that the approach selected must be the best one to answer the questions relevant to the study. Nursing's philosophic beliefs about humans and the holistic nature of professional nursing will provide direction and guidance as well.

Nursing encourages detailed attention to the care of people as humans and grounds its practice in a holistic belief system that nurses care for mind, body, and spirit. Holistic care and avoidance of reductionism are at the center of professional nursing practice. The holistic approach to nursing is rooted in the nursing experience and is not imposed artificially from without. Just as caring for only part of the client is inconsistent with nursing practice, so, too, is the study of humans by breaking them down into parts. The following example illustrates the nature of holistic nursing practice. When caring for a client who has had a mastectomy, the nurse addresses not only body image but also the effect the surgery may have on family, work, and psychological well-being. The nurse might ask, "How are you feeling about your surgery?" or "What kinds of changes in your life do you anticipate as a result of your mastectomy?" These questions elicit more about the client as a person, with a life and feelings, as opposed to a question such as, Do you want to look at the scar? An approach that deals only with the removed body part narrows the understanding of the overall impact of this life-altering event and can potentially result in misdirected care.

Because phenomenological inquiry requires that the integrated whole be explored, it is a suitable method for the investigation of phenomena important to nursing practice, education, and administration. Spiegelberg (1965) remarked that phenomenological method investigates subjective phenomena in the belief that essential truths about reality are grounded in lived experience. What is important is the experience as it is presented, not what anyone thinks or says about it. Therefore, investigation of phenomena important to nursing requires that researchers study lived experience as it is presented in the everyday world of nursing practice, education, and administration. Human experience is the central tenet, and how human beings experience phenomena important to nursing practice directs phenomenological investigations.

A holistic perspective and the study of experience as lived serve as the foundation for phenomenological inquiry. A positive response to the following questions will help researchers clarify whether phenomenological method is the most appropriate approach for the investigation. First, researchers should ask, Is there a need for further clarity on the chosen phenomenon? Evidence leading researchers to conclude that phenomena need further clarity may be that there is little if anything published on a subject, or perhaps what is published needs to be described in more depth. Second, researchers should consider the question, Will the shared lived experience be the best data source for the phenomenon under investigation? Because the primary method of data collection is the voice of the people experiencing a particular phenomenon, researchers must determine that this approach will provide the richest and most descriptive data. Third, as in all research, investigators should ask, What are the available resources, the time frame for the completion of the research, the audience to which the research will be presented, and my own personal style and ability to engage in the method in a rigorous manner while accepting the inherent ambiguity?

Topics appropriate to phenomenological research method include those central to humans' life experiences. Examples include happiness, fear, being there, commitment, being a chairperson, being a head nurse, or the meaning of stress for nursing students in the clinical setting. Health-related topics suitable for phenomenological investigation might include a myriad of topics such as the meaning of pain, living with chronic illness, and end-of-life issues. Chapter 6 offers readers a selective sample of published research using phenomenological research methodology in the areas of practice, education, and administration.

ELEMENTS AND INTERPRETATIONS OF THE METHOD

Researcher's Role

As lived experience becomes the description of a particular phenomenon, the investigator takes on specific responsibilities in transforming the information. Reinharz (1983) articulated five steps that occur in phenomenological transformation as the investigator makes public what essentially was private knowledge. The first transformation occurs as people's experiences are transformed into language. During this step, the researcher, through verbal interaction, creates an opportunity for the lived experience to be shared (Reinharz, 1983). In the example of research on quality of life for individuals with type 1 diabetes mellitus, the researcher would create an opportunity for individuals living with this chronic illness to share their experiences related to the meaning of quality of life.

The second transformation occurs as the researcher transforms what is seen and heard into an understanding of the original experience. Because one person can never experience what another person has experienced in exactly the same manner, researchers must rely on the data participants have shared about a particular experience and from those develop their own transformation (Reinharz, 1983). In this instance, the researcher studying quality of life takes what participants have said and produces a description that lends understanding to the participants' original experiences.

Third, the researcher transforms what is understood about the phenomenon under investigation into conceptual categories that are the essences of the original experience (Reinharz, 1983). Data analysis of interviews addressing the meaning of quality of life would involve clarifying the essences of the phenomenon. For example, the data may reveal that quality of life for an individual with type 1 diabetes mellitus may center on freedom from restrictions in daily activities, independence, and prevention of long-term complications.

Fourth, the researcher transforms those essences into a written document that captures what the researcher has thought about the experience and reflects the participants' descriptions or actions. In all transformations, information may be lost or gained; therefore, it is important to have participants review the final description to ensure that the material is correctly stated and nothing has been added or deleted (Reinharz, 1983).

Fifth, the researcher transforms the written document into an understanding that can function to clarify all preceding steps (Reinharz, 1983). The intent of this written document, often referred to as the exhaustive description, is to synthesize and capture the meaning of the experience into written form without distorting or losing the richness of the data. In other words, the exhaustive description of quality of life would reveal the richness of the experience identified from the very beginning of the investigation as perceived by individuals with type 1 diabetes mellitus.

In addition to the five transformational steps outlined by Reinharz (1983), the investigator must possess certain qualities that will permit access to data that participants possess. The abilities to communicate clearly and to help participants feel comfortable expressing their experiences are essential qualities in a phenomenological researcher. The researcher is the instrument for data collection and must function effectively to facilitate data collection. The researcher must recognize that personal characteristics such as manner of speaking, gender, age, and other personality traits may interfere with data retrieval. For this reason, researchers must ask whether they are the appropriate people to access a given person's or group's experiences (Reinharz, 1983).

Data Generation

Purposive sampling is used most commonly in phenomenological inquiry. This method of sampling selects individuals for study participation based on their particular knowledge of a phenomenon for the purpose of sharing that knowledge. "The logic and power of purposeful sampling lies in selecting information-rich cases for study in depth. Information-rich cases are those from which one can learn a great deal about issues of central importance to the purpose of the research, thus the term purposeful sampling" (Patton, 1990, p. 169).

Sample selection provides the participants for the investigation. Researchers should contact participants, once they have agreed to participate, before the interview to prepare them for the actual meeting and to answer any preliminary questions. At the time of the first interview, the researcher may obtain informed consent and permission to tape-record, if using this data-gathering instrument. Piloting interview skills and having a more experienced phenomenological researcher listen to the tape of an interview can assist in the development of interviewing skills. According to Benoliel (1988), an "effective observer-interviewer needs to bring knowledge, sensitivity, and flexibility into a situation. Interviewing is not an interpersonal exchange controlled by the interviewer but rather a transaction that is reciprocal in nature and involves an exchange of social rewards" (p. 211).

Researchers should help participants describe lived experience without leading the discussion. Open-ended, clarifying questions such as the following facilitate this process: What comes to mind when you hear the word *commitment*? What comes to mind when you think about quality of life? Open-ended interviewing allows researchers to follow participants' lead, to ask clarifying questions, and to facilitate the expression of the participants' lived experience. Interviews usually end when participants believe they have exhausted their descriptions. If interviews are not feasible, researchers may ask participants to write an extensive description of some phenomenon by responding to a pre-established question or questions. The concern with written responses versus tape-recorded interviews is that descriptions may not reveal the depth and detail that can be achieved through interviews. During the interview, researchers can help participants explain things in more detail by asking questions. This valuable opportunity is eliminated when participants write their descriptions.

The interview allows entrance into another person's world and is an excellent source of data. Complete concentration and rigorous participation in the interview process improve the accuracy, trustworthiness, and authenticity of the data. However, researchers must remember to remain centered on the data, listen attentively, avoid interrogating participants, and treat participants with respect and sincere interest in the shared experience.

Data generation or collection continues until the researcher believes saturation has been achieved, that is, when no new themes or essences have emerged from the participants and the data are repeating. Therefore, predetermination of the number of participants for a given study is impossible. Data collection must continue until the researcher is assured saturation has been achieved.

Morse (1989) stated that saturation is a myth. She proposed that, given another group of informants on the same subject at another time, new data may be revealed. Therefore, investigators will be able to reach saturation only with a particular group of informants and only during specific times. "The long term challenge for the phenomenologist interested in generating theory is to interview several samples from a variety of backgrounds, age ranges and cultural environments to maximize the likelihood of discovering the essences of phenomena across groups" (Streubert, 1991, p. 121).

Ethical Considerations

The personal nature of phenomenological research results in several ethical considerations for researchers. Informed consent differs in a qualitative study as opposed to a quantitative investigation. There is no way to know exactly what might transpire during an interview. Researchers must consider issues of privacy. When preparing a final manuscript, researchers must determine how to present the data so that they are accurate yet do not reveal participants' identities. For an in-depth discussion of ethical issues in qualitative research, see Chapter 4.

Data Treatment

Researchers may handle treatment of the data in a variety of ways. Use of open-ended interviewing techniques, tape recordings, and verbatim transcriptions will increase the accuracy of data collection. High-quality tape-recording equipment is essential. Researchers will make handwritten notes. Adding handwritten notes to verbally transcribed accounts helps to achieve the most comprehensive and accurate description. A second interview may be needed, giving researchers an opportunity to expand, verify, and add descriptions of the phenomenon under investigation and assist participants in clarifying and expounding on inadequate descriptions. In addition, often participants will have additional thoughts about the phenomenon under study after the initial interview. Following an interview, researchers should immediately listen to the tape, checking that the interview made sense and verifying the need for a follow-up interview. Also, researchers should make extensive, detailed notes immediately after the interview in case the tape recording has failed.

When data collection begins, so, too, does data analysis. From the moment researchers begin listening to descriptions of a particular phenomenon, analysis is occurring. These processes are inseparable. Therefore, the importance of the reductive process cannot be overemphasized. Separating one's beliefs and assumptions from the raw data occurs throughout the investigation. Journaling helps in continuing the reductive process. Researchers' use of a journal can facilitate phenomenological reduction. Writing down any ideas, feelings, or responses that emerge during data collection supports reductive phenomenology. Drew (1989) has offered the added perspective that journaling that addresses a researcher's own experience can be "considered data and examined within the context of the study for the part it has played in the study's results" (p. 431).

Following data collection and verbatim transcription, researchers should listen to the tapes while reading the transcriptions for accuracy. This step will help to familiarize them with the data and begin immersing them in the phenomenon under investigation.

Data Analysis

Data analysis requires that researchers dwell with or become immersed in the data. The purpose of data analysis, according to Banonis (1989), is to preserve the uniqueness of each participant's lived experience while permitting an understanding of the phenomenon under investigation. This begins with listening to participants' verbal descriptions and is followed by reading and rereading the verbatim transcriptions or written responses. As researchers become immersed in the data, they may identify and extract significant statements. They can then transcribe these statements onto index cards or record them in a data management file for ease of ordering later in the process. Apprehending or capturing the essential relationships among the statements and preparing an exhaustive description of the phenomenon constitute the final phase. Through free imaginative variation, researchers make connections between statements obtained in the interview process. It is critical to identify how statements or central themes emerged and are connected to one another if the final description is to be comprehensive and exhaustive.

Microcomputers and word processing software can make data storage and retrieval more efficient. Examining available software packages for qualitative data analysis may be an appropriate option, depending on researchers' personal preferences. See Chapter 3 for an in-depth discussion of data generation and management strategies including available software for data storage, retrieval, and analysis.

Review of the Literature

The review of the literature generally follows data analysis. The rationale for postponing the literature review is related to the goal of achieving a pure description of the phenomenon under investigation. The fewer ideas or preconceived notions researchers have about the phenomenon under investigation, the less likely their biases will influence the research. A cursory review of the literature may be done to ensure the necessity of the study and the appropriateness of method selection. Once data analysis is complete, researchers review the literature to place the findings within the context of what is already known about the topic.

Trustworthiness and Authenticity of Data

The issue of trustworthiness in qualitative research has been a concern for researchers engaging in these methods and is discussed at length in the literature (Beck, 1993; Krefting, 1991; Yonge & Stewin, 1988). The issue of rigor in qualitative research is important to the practice of good science.

The trustworthiness of the questions put to study participants depends on the extent to which they tap the participants' experiences apart from the participants' theoretical knowledge of the topic (Colaizzi, 1978). Consistent use of the method and of bracketing prior knowledge helps to ensure pure description of data. To ensure trustworthiness of data analysis, researchers return to each participant and ask if the exhaustive description reflects the participant's experiences. When the findings are recognized to be true by the participants, the trustworthiness of the data is further established. If elements are noted to be unclear or misinterpreted, the researchers must return to the analysis and revise the description.

Requesting negative descriptions of the phenomenon under investigation is helpful in establishing authenticity and trustworthiness of the data. For example, in the study investigating the meaning of quality of life in individuals with type 1 diabetes mellitus, the researcher may ask, "Can you describe a situation in which you would feel that you did not have quality of life?" This question gives an opportunity to compare and contrast data.

Finally, the audit trail is critical to establishing authenticity and trustworthiness of the data. This process allows the reader to clearly follow the line of thinking that the researcher used during data analysis. Clear connections between how the research moved from raw data to interpreted meanings are made through detailed examples. Rigor in qualitative research is a critical component to the process. Data analysis occurs through complex mental processes, critical thinking, and analysis. Researchers must prepare their final descriptions in such a way that the line of thinking and interpretation that occurred is clear to the reader and true to the data.

SUMMARY

*P*henomenology is an integral field of inquiry to nursing, as well as philosophy, sociology, and psychology. As a research method, phenomenology is a rigorous scientific process whose purpose is to bring to language human experiences. The phenomenological movement has been influenced by the works of Husserl, Brentano, Stumpf, Merleau-Ponty, and others. Hermeneutic phenomenology offers a different approach to qualitative understanding through the interpretive process of the written and spoken word. Concepts central to the method include intentionality, essences, intuiting, reduction, bracketing, embodiment, and being-in-the-world.

Phenomenology as a method of research offers nursing an opportunity to describe and clarify phenomena important to practice, education, and research. Researchers selecting this approach for the investigation of phenomena should base their decision on suitability and a need for further clarification of the selected phenomenon. Specific consideration must be given to the issues of researcher as instrument, data generation, data treatment and authenticity, and trustworthiness of data. Investigations that use this approach contribute to nursing's knowledge base and can provide direction for future investigations.

The relevance of phenomenology as a research method for nursing is clear. Within the qualitative paradigm, this method supports "new initiatives for nursing care where the subject matter is often not amenable to other investigative and experimental methods" (Jasper, 1994, p. 313). Nursing maintains a unique appreciation for caring, commitment, and holism. Phenomena related to nursing can be explored and analyzed by phenomenological methods that have as their goal the description of lived experience.

References

Allen, M. N., & Jenson, L. (1990). Hermeneutical inquiry, meaning and scope. *Western Journal of Nursing Research, 12*(2), 241-253.

Arrigo, B., & Cody, W. K. (2004). A dialogue on existential-phenomenological thought in psychology and in nursing. *Nursing Science Quarterly, 17*(1), 6-11.

Banonis, B. C. (1989). The lived experience of recovering from addiction: A phenomenological investigation. *Nursing Science Quarterly, 2*(1), 37-42.

Beck, C. T. (1993). Qualitative research: The evaluation of its credibility, fittingness, and auditability. *Western Journal of Nursing Research, 15*(2), 263-265.

Beck, C. T. (1994). Phenomenology: Its use in nursing research. *International Journal of Nursing Studies, 31*(6), 499-510.

Benoliel, J. Q. (1988). Commentaries on special issue. *Western Journal of Nursing Research, 10*(2), 210-213.

Blumensteil, A. (1973). A sociology of good times. In G. Psathas (Ed.), *Phenomenological sociology: Issues and applications.* New York: Wiley.

Caelli, K. (2000). The changing face of phenomenological research: Traditional and American phenomenology in nursing. *Qualitative Health Research, 10*(3), 366-377.

Caelli, K. (2001). Engaging with phenomenology: Is it more of a challenge than it needs to be? *Qualitative Health Research, 11*(2), 273-281.

Carpenter, D. R., & Narsavage, G. (2004). One breath at a time: Living with cystic fibrosis. *Journal of Pediatric Nursing, 19*(1), 25-31.

Cohen, M. Z. (1987). A historical overview of the phenomenological movement. *Image, 19*(1), 31-34.

Cohen, M. Z., Ley, C., & Tarzian, A. J. (2001). Isolation in blood and marrow transplantation. *Journal of Nursing Scholarship, 23*(6), 592-609.

Colaizzi, P. F. (1978). Psychological research as the phenomenologist views it. In R. Valle & M. King (Eds.), *Existential phenomenological alternative for psychology* (pp. 48-71). New York: Oxford University Press.

Crist, J. D., & Tanner, C. A. (2003). Interpretation/analysis methods in hermeneutic phenomenology. *Nursing Research, 52*(3), 202-205.

Diekelmann, N. (2001). Narrative pedagogy: Heideggerian hermeneutical analysis of lived experiences of students, teachers, and clinicians. *Advances in Nursing Science, 23*(3), 53-71.

Drew, N. (1989). The interviewer's experience as data in phenomenological research. *Western Journal of Nursing Research, 11*(4), 431-439.

Dreyfus, H. L. (1991). *Being-in-the-world: A commentary on Heidegger's being and time.* Division I. Cambridge, MA: MIT Press.

Gadamer, H. G. (1976). *Philosophical hermeneutics* (D. E. Linge, Trans. & Ed.). Los Angeles: University of California Press.

Geanellos, R. (2000). Exploring Ricoeur's hermeneutic theory of interpretation as a method of analyzing research texts. *Nursing Inquiry, 7*(2), 112-119.

Giorgi, A. (1985). *Phenomenology and psychological research.* Pittsburgh, PA: Duquesne University Press.

Haggman-Laitila, A. (1999). The authenticity and ethics of phenomenological research: How to overcome the researcher's own views. *Nursing Ethics, 6*(1), 12-22.

Heidegger, M. (1962). *Being and time.* New York: Harper & Row. (Original work published 1927.)

Husserl, E. (1931). *Ideas: General introduction to pure phenomenology* (W. R. Boyce Gibson, Trans.). New York: Collier.

Husserl, E. (1965). *Phenomenology and the crisis of philosophy* (Q. Laver, Trans.). New York: Harper & Row.

Iaquinta, M. L., & Larrabee, J. H. (2003). Phenomenological lived experience of patients with rheumatoid arthritis. *Journal of Nursing Care Quality, 19*(3), 280-289.

Jasper, M.A. (1994). Issues in phenomenology for researchers of nursing. *Journal of Advanced Nursing, 19,* 309-314.

Krefting, L. (1991). Rigor in qualitative research: The assessment of trustworthiness. *American Journal of Occupational Therapy, 45*(3), 214-222.

Lincoln, Y. S., & Guba, E. G. (1985). *Naturalistic inquiry.* Beverly Hills, CA: Sage.

Lindholm, M., Uden, G., & Rastam, R. (1999). Management from four different perspectives. *Journal of Nursing Management, 7,* 101-111.

Lowes, L., & Prowse, M.A (2001). Standing outside the interview process? The illusions of objectivity in phenomenological data generation. *International Journal of Advanced Nursing, 31,* 219-255.

Merleau-Ponty, M. (1956). What is phenomenology? *Cross Currents, 6,* 59-70.

Merleau-Ponty, M. (1962). *Phenomenology of perception* (C. Smith, Trans.). New York: Humanities Press.

Morse, J. M. (1989). *Qualitative nursing research: A contemporary dialogue.* Rockville, MD: Aspen.

Munhall, P. (1989). Philosophical ponderings on qualitative research. *Nursing Science Quarterly, 2*(1), 20-28.

Natanson, M. (1973). *Edmund Husserl: Philosopher of infinite tasks.* Evanston, IL: Northwestern University Press.

Omery, A. (1983). Phenomenology: A method for nursing research. *Advances in Nursing Science, 5*(2), 49-63.

Paley, J. (1997). Husserl, phenomenology and nursing. *Journal of Advanced Nursing, 26,* 187-193.

Paterson, G. J., & Zderad, L. T. (1976). *Humanistic nursing.* New York: Wiley.

Patton, M. Q. (1990). *Qualitative evaluation and research methods* (2nd ed.). Newbury Park, CA: Sage.

Reinharz, S. (1983). Phenomenology as a dynamic process. *Phenomenology and Pedagogy, 1*(1), 77-79.

Ricoeur, P. (1976). *Interpretation theory: Discourse and the surplus of meaning.* Fort Worth, TX: Texas Christian University Press.

Ricoeur, P. (1981). *Hermeneutics and the social sciences* (J. Thompson, Trans. & Ed.). New York: Cambridge University Press.

Rinaldi, D. M. (1989). The lived experience of commitment to nursing. Dissertation Abstracts International (University Microfilms No. 1707).

Rose, P., Beeby, J., & Parker, D. (1995). Academic rigour in the lived experience of researchers using phenomenological methods in nursing. *Journal of Advanced Nursing, 21,* 1123-1129.

Schutz, A. (1970). *On phenomenology and social relations.* Chicago: University of Chicago Press.

Schwarz, J. K. (2003). Understanding and responding to patients' requests for assistance in dying. *Journal of Nursing Scholarship, 35*(4), 377-384.

Spiegelberg, H. (1965). *The phenomenological movement: A historical introduction* (2nd ed., Vol. 1-2). Dordrecht, The Netherlands: Martinus Nijhoff.

Spiegelberg, H. (1975). *Doing phenomenology.* Dordrecht, The Netherlands: Martinus Nijhoff.

Streubert, H. J. (1991). Phenomenological research as a theoretic initiative in community health nursing. *Public Health Nursing, 8*(2), 119-123.

Tarzian, A. J. (2000). Caring for dying patients who have air hunger. *Journal of Nursing Scholarship, 32*(2), 137-143.

Todres, L., & Wheeler, S. (2001). The complexity of phenomenology, hermeneutics and existentialism as a philosophical perspective for nursing research. *International Journal of Nursing Studies, 38,* 1-8.

Van der Zalm, J. E., & Bergum, V. (2000). Hermeneutic phenomenology: Providing living knowledge for nursing practice. *Journal of Advanced Nursing, 31*(1), 211-218.

van Kaam, A. (1984). *Existential foundation of psychology.* New York: Doubleday.

van Manen, M. (1990). *Researching the lived experience.* Buffalo: State University of New York.

Wagner, H. R. (1983). *Phenomenology of consciousness and sociology of the life and world: An introductory study.* Edmonton, Alberta: University of Alberta Press.

Yonge, O., & Stewin, L. (1988). Reliability and validity: Misnomers for qualitative research. *Canadian Journal of Nursing Research, 20*(2), 61-67.

CHAPTER 6

Phenomenology in Practice, Education, and Administration

*T*he acceptance of qualitative methods as legitimate approaches to the discovery of knowledge continues to grow as an increasing number of nurse researchers apply these methods to investigations that have as their phenomena of interest people's life experiences. Very often in nursing we are faced with practice, education, and administrative experiences that seem to present patterns that are familiar to us. To validate our perceptions, research must be conducted to explore and describe phenomena fully and accurately. This process, in turn, leads to improved understanding and ultimately better outcomes in all domains of nursing. Hudacek's (2000) work, *Making a Difference: Stories from the Point of Care,* which is published in book form, uses phenomenological principles to analyze nurse stories. Her work has implications for nursing practice, education, and administration. As evidenced by published works, phenomenology as one approach to qualitative investigations has made a significant contribution to the substantive body of nursing knowledge. Qualitative methods allow exploration of the life experiences of human beings in ways that respect and acknowledge the importance of all knowledge to be gained through subjective experiences and the importance of accepting different ways of knowing.

This chapter provides an overview and critique of three phenomenological investigations, published as journal articles, in the areas of nursing practice, education, and administration. An article by Judith Kennedy Schwarz (2003), "Understanding and Responding to Patients' Requests for Assistance in Dying," is reprinted at the end of the chapter. It is provided as a sample of a phenomenological investigation and is critiqued to offer the reader an example of the process used to assess the quality of a phenomenological investigation. The practice, education, and administrative studies presented in this chapter were reviewed according to the criteria found in Box 6.1. These guidelines offer readers of qualitative investigations a guide to recognizing the essential methodological points of a published report. The guidelines allow readers to examine how the research has contributed to the scientific base of nursing knowledge. This chapter also provides readers with selected examples of published research using the phenomenological method. These examples are presented in Table 6.1.

Box 6.1

Qualitative Critique Criteria

Focus/Topic

1. What is the focus or the topic of the study? What is it that the researcher is studying? Is the topic researchable? Is it focused enough to be meaningful but not too limited so as to be trivial?
2. Why is the researcher using a qualitative design? Would the study be more appropriately conducted in the quantitative paradigm?
3. What is the philosophical tradition or qualitative paradigm upon which the study is based?

Purpose

1. What is the purpose of the study? Is it clear?

Significance

1. What is the relevance of the study to what is already known about the topic?
2. How will the results be useful to nursing and/or health care?

Method

1. Given the topic of the study and the researcher's stated purpose, how does the selected research method help to achieve the stated purpose?
2. What methodological components/strategies (?) has the researcher identified to conduct the study?
3. Based on the material presented, how does the researcher demonstrate that he or she has followed the method?
4. If the researcher used any form of triangulation, explain how he or she maintained the integrity of the study.

Sampling

1. How were participants selected?
2. Explain how the selection process supports a qualitative sampling paradigm.
3. Are the participants in the study the appropriate people to inform the research? Explain.

Box 6.1 *(Continued)*

Data Collection

1. How does the data collection method reported support discovery, description, or understanding?
2. What data collection strategies does the researcher use?
3. Does the researcher clearly state how human subjects were protected?
4. How was data saturation achieved?
5. Are the data collection strategies appropriate to achieve the purpose of the study? Explain.

Data Analysis

1. How were data analyzed?
2. Based on the analysis reported, can the reader follow the researcher's stated processes?

Findings/Trustworthiness

1. How do the reported findings demonstrate the participants' realities?
2. How does the researcher relate the findings of the study to what is already known?
3. How does the researcher demonstrate that the findings are meaningful to the participants?

Conclusions/Implications/Recommendations

1. How does the researcher provide a context for use of the findings?
2. Are the conclusions drawn from the study appropriate? Explain.
3. What are the recommendations for future research?
4. Are the recommendations, conclusions, and implications clearly related to the findings? Explain.

APPLICATION TO PRACTICE

*M*any nursing interventions performed in clinical settings lend themselves to quantitative measurement. Examples include measurement of blood pressure, central venous pressure, or urine-specific gravity. However, nurses enmeshed in practice settings are well aware that much of what is done for patients is subjective and based on how nurses come to know their patients and the patients' life experiences. For example, caring, reassurance, and quality of life are phenomena central to nursing practice, but they do not necessarily lend themselves to quantitative measurement. Even areas of practice that are studied primarily from a quantitative perspective can be enriched when examined from a qualitative lens. Therefore, phenomena unique to the practice of professional nursing need investigative approaches suitable to their unique nature. Phenomenology as a qualitative research method has been used to explore a variety of practice-related experiences and facilitates understanding

Text continued on page 111.

Table 6.1 • Selective Sampling of Phenomenological Research Studies

Author(s)	Date	Domain	Phenomenon Of Interest	Sample	Data Generation	Findings
Ohman, Soderberg, & Lundman	2003	Practice	The meaning of living with a serious chronic illness	10 men and 10 women	Semi-structured interviews, tape-recorded and transcribed verbatim	Three major themes were identified: Experiencing the body as a hindrance; Being alone in illness; and Struggling for normalcy.
Secrest, Norwood, & Keatley	2003	Education	Baccalaureate student nurses' perspectives of what it means to be professional	69 baccalaureate nursing students at different educational levels	Written narratives collected in a classroom setting	The student experience of professionalism was grounded in a world of self and others with the emergence of three interrelated themes: Ground-belonging; Knowing; and Affirmation.
Schwarz	2003	Practice	How nurses experience and respond to patients' requests for assistance in dying	10 self-selected nurses	Personal interview, tape-recorded and transcribed verbatim. All but one participant was interviewed twice. One interview was conducted by telephone.	Four major themes were described: Being open to hear and hearing; Interpreting and responding to the meaning; Responding to persistent requests for assistance in dying; Reflections. A continuum of

						Findings (continued)
						interventions was described and included refusal, providing palliative care that might secondarily hasten dying, respecting and not interfering with patients' or families' plans to hasten dying, and providing varying types and degrees of direct assistance in dying. Few nurses agreed or refused to help a patient die. Most struggled alone and in silence with feelings of conflict, guilt, and moral distress.
Carpenter & Narsavage	2004	Practice	The lived experience of parents caring for a child newly diagnosed with cystic fibrosis	Eleven families caring for children newly diagnosed with cystic fibrosis	One focus group, tape-recorded and transcribed verbatim. Detailed written narratives from study participants	Three major themes emerged that were fluid in nature. They included Falling apart; Pulling together; and Moving beyond. Sub-themes were evident within each of the major themes described. Families

Table 6.1 • (Continued)

Author(s)	Date	Domain	Phenomenon of Interest	Sample	Data Generation	Findings
						reported moving back and forth among the three main areas of adjustment depending on the health of the child or other life events that occurred.
Cheung & Hocking	2004	Practice	Spousal carers' experience of caring for their partner with multiple sclerosis	Ten spousal carers of people with multiple sclerosis	Unstructured, in-depth interviews, tape-recorded and transcribed verbatim	The constitutive pattern of weaving through a web of paradoxes emerged from the data. Experiences of loss and gain and feelings of vulnerability and strength were reported.
Hinck	2004	Practice	The lived experience of oldest-old adults aged 85–98 years	19 adults— 13 women and 6 men	In-depth interviews, audiotaped and transcribed verbatim	Description of how historical, cultural, and environmental contexts shaped everyday thoughts, activities, and what was meaningful to the participants

| Iaquinta & Larrabee | 2004 | Practice | The lived experience of rheumatoid arthritis | 6 individuals with rheumatoid arthritis (RA) | Personal interview, tape-recorded and transcribed verbatim | Six major themes emerged and included: Grieving while growing; Persuading self and others of RA's authenticity; Cultivating resilience; Confronting negative feelings; Navigating the health care system; and Masterminding new life ways. |
| McNeill | 2004 | Practice | Experiences of fathers who have a child with juvenile rheumatoid arthritis (JRA) | 22 fathers | Semi-structured interviews, tape-recorded and transcribed verbatim | A substantive theory of fathers' experience of caring for a child with JRA. Fathers were profoundly affected. JRA served as a catalyst for meaningful involvement, and a multitude of emotions were expressed. Efforts to remain strong for others created high levels of stress. |

Table 6.1 • (Continued)						
Author(s)	Date	Domain	Phenomenon of Interest	Sample	Data Generation	Findings
Ohman & Soderberg	2004	Practice	The meaning of close relatives' experiences of living with a person with serious chronic illness	14 close relatives (10 women and 4 men)	40 to 60-minute interviews, tape-recorded and transcribed verbatim	Three major themes were identified: A shrinking life, Forced to take responsibility, and Struggling to keep going.
Thomas-MacLean	2004	Practice	Women's experiences of embodiment after breast cancer	12 women	In-depth interviews, tape-recorded and transcribed verbatim	Five themes emerged: Issues of control; suffering; Encountering medicine, Visible loss, and Leaving active treatment.

Text continued from page 105.

of subjective interactive experiences (Cheung & Hocking, 2004; Iaquinta & Larrabee, 2003; McNeill, 2004; Thomas-MacLean, 2004). Examples of published research related to the practice domain can be found in Table 6.1.

Nurses are in a special position to influence patient care. They not only are responsible for the patient as an individual in the health care setting but also frequently make observations about the effects of illness on family members and other related aspects of the illness experience. They are in a prime position to identify issues related to nursing practice that need to be understood and described more fully. One example of a phenomenological research study as applied to the practice setting is "Understanding and Responding to Patients' Requests for Assistance in Dying" by Schwarz (2003). In this study, the authors share how they used qualitative data to provide a fuller understanding of how nurses experience and respond to patients' requests for assistance in dying.

The purpose of the study by Schwarz (2003) was "to explore how nurses understand the meaning of being asked by a decisionally capable person for assistance in dying and given that understanding, how they determine what their response ought to be" (p. 377). The purpose was clearly articulated in the abstract and early in the article. Schwarz has made explicit the importance of the research at the outset of this comprehensive and well-articulated phenomenological investigation. It is clear to the reader that a problem exists that lends itself to a qualitative approach.

Schwarz (2003) emphasized the need for a qualitative research design, noting that "American nurses increasingly report being asked by dying patients or their family members for assistance in dying" (p. 377). Through narrative review of published research and detailed discussion of the need to understand lived experience from the caregiver perspective, the author has supplied the reader with sound rationale for the research approach as well as the study's significance. The qualitative approach applied by this author provides an added and important dimension to understanding the lived experience of caring for terminally ill patients who request assistance in dying.

Schwarz (2003) described in detail the methodological strategies used to conduct her study. The author's detailed description clearly demonstrates how the method was followed throughout the study. For purposes of this investigation, the researcher used interpretive phenomenology as described by van Manen (1990). Although the philosophical underpinnings of phenomenological method were not specifically addressed, the author did discuss in detail the method used for this investigation. The methodology was appropriate for this phenomenological study, and the method application is clearly articulated by the researchers.

Sampling was purposeful and is clearly addressed by Schwarz (2003). "Nurses were invited to participate if they believed a competent patient had asked them for help in dying and were willing to talk about the experience" (p. 378). The author notes that the study was reviewed and approved by an Institutional Review Board. Based on this statement, the reader can make the assumption that protection of human subjects was addressed. Schwarz (2004) adds more detail to the discussion of ethical issues relevant to her research and connects this to the nature of her topic and vulnerability of her participants. This adds significantly to the integrity of the study.

Baseline open-ended interviews were conducted. Her narrative clarifies the approach to data collection, which is appropriate to phenomenological methodology. Schwarz (2003) offers the following:

> Most interviews occurred in participants' homes and lasted approximately 2 hours. One nurse who practiced on the West Coast was interviewed by telephone, and with one exception, participants were interviewed at least twice. Each was asked, "Tell me about a time when a patient asked you for help in dying" and were prompted to fully describe the experience. The second discussion occurred 2 weeks later to clarify details and meanings. (p. 379)

Data analysis is described in detail and follows the rigorous research methodology described by van Manan (1990). The reader can follow the data analysis process. This adds to the authenticity and trustworthiness of the findings. Schwarz (2003) notes,

> Analysis of these data was on-going throughout data collection, transcription, and repeated readings of the text. Analysis proceeded from an initial overview of each participant's experience to more focused reflection followed by preliminary coding of these data and identification of themes. Once individual thematic summaries were written, recurring aspects of the experience common to all participants were identified and described. An auditor reviewed interview transcripts, themes, and the organization, description, and interpretation of findings. (p. 379)

The findings demonstrate the participants' realities as they relate to the experience for nurses caring for a terminally ill patient who has requested assistance in dying. The four major themes described by Schwarz (2003) included Being Open to Hear and Hearing; Interpreting and Responding to the Meaning; Responding to Persistent Requests for Assistance in Dying; and Reflections. The findings of the study are discussed within the context of what is already known about the topic, followed by detailed recommendations for future research. Schwarz provides an excellent example of phenomenological research using van Manen's (1990) approach to data analysis. This study also offers an excellent example of some of the benefits to be achieved through qualitative research methods.

APPLICATION TO EDUCATION

*N*ursing education also lends itself to objective and subjective research interests. Test construction and critical thinking are education-related examples that are appropriate for quantitative investigation, although not exclusively. The educational domain of nursing also lends itself to qualitative investigation in areas such as educational experiences, caring and the curriculum, or the effect of evaluation on student performance in the clinical setting.

Nursing education is an important area of research that can be studied using qualitative approaches. An overview and critique of the study "I Was Actually a Nurse: The Meaning of Professionalism for Baccalaureate Nursing Students" by Secrest, Norwood, and Keatley (2003) is provided for this example of the phenomenological method applied to the educational domain of nursing.

The phenomenon of interest for this study is relevant to nursing education and had as its purpose to understand "how students experience professionalism" and "baccalaureate student nurses' perspectives of what it means to be professional" (Secrest et al., 2003, p. 77). The authors provide rationale for their study through a literature review of topics related to nursing education and professionalism for baccalaureate nursing students. The authors emphasize the importance of their study in the following statement: "Understanding how students experience professionalism is important to provide appropriate education experiences to foster this aspect of professional socialization" (p. 77).

Secrest and colleagues (2003) base their methodology on an interpretive existential-phenomenological framework. The research method is consistent with this branch of phenomenological research. Rationale for the method and philosophical underpinnings are clearly articulated. "This qualitative study was based on Pollio, Henley, and Thompson's (1997) interpretive framework, which takes an existential-phenomenological approach. The purpose of the interpretation was to recognize patterns or themes in an experience" (p. 78).

Participant selection also was described in great detail. The selection of participants supported a qualitative framework in that it was purposeful, and subjects had experience with the phenomenon under investigation. The sample was drawn from a baccalaureate program in a metropolitan university in the southeastern portion of the United States. Three classes of students taking a professional nursing issues course were invited to participate (Secrest et al., 2003).

Secrest and colleagues (2003) also address protection of human subjects and note that ethical principles were honored:

> Students provided oral and written consent, and the written consent forms were kept separate from the data. Students were told they were not obligated to participate and would not be penalized for not participating. Names did not appear on any of the written work. Demographic data were collected on a separate page and were not connected to the written descriptions. Students also were assured that the written descriptions would be typed by a secretary prior to faculty analysis so handwriting could not be identified. (p. 79)

The data collection strategies used by Secrest and colleagues (2003) support phenomenological approaches to discovery, description, and understanding. The strategies used by the researchers are detailed and appropriate to achieve the purposes of the study. Further, data analysis follows the interpretive approach described by the authors. In addition to the narrative analysis, the authors diagram for the reader the relationship of the findings, facilitating a clearer understanding of their line of thinking in the data analysis process. Saturation is not addressed.

Discussion of the findings demonstrates how the data reflected participants' realities and how the researcher related findings of the study to what is already known. Secrest and colleagues (2003) described in detail for the reader the three relational themes that resulted: belonging, knowing, and affirmation. Examples of raw data related to each relational theme are provided, allowing the reader to follow the line of thinking of the researcher and adding credibility to the study. The conclusions drawn from the study are appropriate, and recommendations for future research are made. The article makes an important contribution to the literature on professionalism and nursing education.

APPLICATION TO ADMINISTRATION

*T*he qualitative research literature addressing issues uniquely related to nursing administration is limited, possibly because many of the issues that lend themselves to qualitative education in nursing administration overlap with the practice arena. For example, studies related to professional nurse behavior and work satisfaction, successful leadership strategies, and perspectives on nurse empowerment would cross over between administration and practice. An example of this overlap is the study by Duchscher (2001), "Out in the Real World: Newly Graduated Nurses in Acute-Care Speak Out." This article describes the perceptions of five nurses regarding their work environment. Although the implications from the study relate directly to nursing practice, they can also be applied to nursing administration in that the result provides "insight into, and enhances understanding of, recruitment and retention issues for nursing administrators who serve as gatekeepers to the practice orientations and ongoing workplace environments of new nursing graduates" (p. 426). This study, reported as a phenomenological investigation, provides an example of how this particular methodology can be applied to nursing administration.

For purposes of the critique, the following study, which is purely administrative, is reviewed. The study "Management From Four Different Perspectives" by Lindholm, Uden, and Rastam (1999) is presented as one example of the application of qualitative research in the area of nursing administration. The phenomenon of interest, clearly identified in the study, focused on gaining an understanding of the process of nursing management in a developing organization. The specific rationale for using a qualitative format, as well as the philosophic underpinnings of the approach, was clearly described. Despite the fact that the Swedish health care system has a variety of management positions to which nurses have legal access, nurses have traditionally held middle management positions. Ongoing decentralization has moved nurses into senior management positions. Therefore, "Elucidating the significance of nursing management increases the possibility of developing the management area of the nursing profession and of using recently acquired knowledge to influence the development of the nursing profession" (Lindholm et al., 1999, p. 102).

The purpose of the study was to "illuminate nursing management in a developing organization from the perspectives of nurse managers, chief physicians, hospital directors and politicians, respectively" (Lindholm et al., 1999, p. 102). The authors make explicit their purpose and support it with a review of the literature.

The sample included 15 nurse managers, 11 chief physicians, and 3 politicians who were chairmen of the local health boards. "The nurse managers were all women, except for one. In the other groups all the participants were men"(Lindholm et al., 1999, p. 102).

The method used to collect data was compatible with the research purpose and adequately addressed the phenomenon of interest. Lindholm and co-researchers (1999) interviewed their participants individually. All interviews were tape-recorded and transcribed verbatim. The authors used Ricoeur's process of phenomenological hermeneutics. Detailed examples of the steps of the hermeneutic circle are provided, demonstrating for the reader how the researchers followed the stated method. Although the researchers do not make an explicit statement regarding data saturation, they do comment that the interviews were comprehensive and "provided good coverage of the issues leaving no need to increase the number of informants" (Lindholm et al., 1999, p. 102).

Data analysis followed the phenomenological hermeneutic approach inspired by Ricoeur. The author provides clear examples of the data analysis process in relationship to each step of the hermeneutic circle.

> The first step was the naïve reading of each interview to acquire a sense of the whole of the text, to gain an impression and to formulate ideas for further analysis. The second step was a structural analysis to identify meaning units, to explain, through revealing the structure and the internal dependent relations, what constitutes the static state of the text. The third step was the understanding of the interpreted whole, from reflection on the naïve reading and the structural analysis (Lindholm et al., 1999, p. 103).

The findings demonstrate the participants' realities, and the researchers relate the findings of the study to what is already known. Through the discussion of the findings, the researchers provide a context for their use and conclusions are drawn. Recommendations for future research are made and the conclusions and implications are clearly related to the findings. This work makes an important contribution to the nursing administration knowledge base.

SUMMARY

*T*he body of published phenomenological research has grown considerably since the first publication of this textbook. Clearly, the body of practice-related research is expanding, with considerable development of research in the area of education and administration. Examples of phenomenological research applied to the areas of nursing practice, education, and administration emphasize the important contribution that phenomenological research has made to nursing's substantive body of knowledge. The critiquing guidelines provide the reader with a guide to evaluating phenomenological research. Examples of phenomenological research using the method interpretations described in Chapter 5 have been highlighted to facilitate method comprehension and application.

Phenomenology as a research approach provides an avenue for investigation that allows description of lived experiences. The voice of professional nurses in practice, education, and administration can be a tremendous source of data that have yet to be fully explored. Identifying subjective phenomena unique to the domains of nursing education, practice, and administration is important to the ever-expanding body of nursing knowledge.

References

Carpenter, D. R., & Narsavage, G. (2004). One breath at a time: Living with cystic fibrosis. *Journal of Pediatric Nursing, 19*(1), 25-31.

Cheung, J., & Hocking, P. (2004). The experience of spousal carers of people with multiple sclerosis. *Qualitative Health Research, 14*(2), 153-166.

Chinn, P. (1985). Debunking myths in nursing theory and research. *Image, 17*(2), 171-179.

Hinck, S. (2004). The lived experience of oldest-old rural adults. *Qualitative Health Research, 14*(6), 779-791.

Hudacek, S. (2000). *Making a difference: Stories from the point of care.* Indianapolis, IN: Sigma Theta Tau Press.

Iaquinta, M. L., & Larrabee, J. H. (2003). Phenomenological lived experience of patients with rheumatoid arthritis. *Journal of Nursing Care Quality, 19*(3), 280-289.

Lindholm M., Uden, G., & Rastam, L. (1999). Management from four different perspectives. *Journal of Nursing Management, 7,* 101-111.

McNeill, T. (2004). Fathers' experience of parenting a child with juvenile rheumatoid arthritis. *Qualitative Health Research, 14*(4), 526-545.

Ohman, M., & Soderberg, S. (2004). The experiences of close relatives living with a person with serious chronic illness. *Qualitative Health Research, 14*(3), 296-410.

Ohman, M., Soderberg, S., & Lundman, B. (2003). Hovering between suffering and enduring: The meaning of living with serious chronic illness. *Qualitative Health Research, 13*(4), 528-542.

Pollio, H. R., Henley, R., & Thompson, C. (1997). The phenomenology of everyday life. New York: Cambridge University Press.

Schwarz, J. K. (2003). Understanding and responding to patients' requests for assistance in dying. *Journal of Nursing Scholarship, 35*(4), 377-384.

Secrest, J. A., Norwood, R. A., & Keatley, V. M. (2003). "I was actually a nurse": The meaning of professionalism for baccalaureate nursing students. *Journal of Nursing Education, 42*(2), 77-83.

Thomas-MacLean, R. (2004). Memories of treatment: The immediacy of breast cancer. *Qualitative Health Research, 14*(5), 628-643.

van Manen, M. (1990). *Researching lived experience: Human science for an action sensitive pedagogy.* Albany, NY: State University of New York.

Research Article

Understanding and Responding to Patients' Requests for Assistance in Dying

Judith Kennedy Schwarz

Purpose: To explore how nurses experience and respond to patients' requests for assistance in dying (AID).

Design and Methods: A phenomenological study of 10 self-selected nurses.

Findings: Four major themes: Being Open to Hear and Hearing; Interpreting and Responding to the Meaning; Responding to Persistent Requests for AID, and Reflections. When faced with persistent requests for AID, participants provided a continuum of interventions; refusal, providing palliative care that might secondarily hasten dying, respecting and not interfering with patients' or families' plans to hasten dying, and providing varying types and degrees of direct AID. Their responses were context-driven rather than rule-mandated, and they drew a distinction between secondarily hastening and directly causing death.

Conclusions: Few nurses in this study unequivocally agreed or refused to directly help a patient die. Most struggled alone and in silence to find a morally and legally acceptable way to help patients who persisted in requesting AID. Regardless of how they responded, many described feelings of conflict, guilt, and moral distress.

JOURNAL OF NURSING SCHOLARSHIP, 2003; 35:4, 377-384. ©2003 SIGMA THETA TAU INTERNATIONAL.

[Key words: death, palliative end-of-life care, assisted suicide]

When a nurse is asked by a decisionally capable person for assistance in dying (AID), defined in this inquiry to include either assisted suicide or voluntary active euthanasia, hearing that request often results in a profound moral dilemma. Assisted suicide includes providing the means to end life, such as a prescription for a lethal amount of drugs, the drugs themselves, or other measures to a person with knowledge of that person's intentions (American Nurses Association [ANA], 1994; Brody, 1992). Voluntary active euthanasia is a deliberate act that causes death at the voluntary request of a person incapable of causing his or her own death (Brody, 1992).

Judith Kennedy Schwarz, RN, PhD, *Delta Zeta*, Consultant, New York University, New York. Correspondence to Dr. Schwarz, 450 West End Ave., New York, NY 10024. E-mail: Judschwarz@rcn.com

Accepted for publication March 6, 2003.

American nurses increasingly report being asked by dying patients or their family members for AID, and several recent studies have shown the frequency of their responses to such requests (Asch, 1996; Ferrell, Virani, Grant, Coyne, & Uman, 2000; Leiser, Mitchell, Hahn, Slome, & Abrams, 1998; Matzo & Emanuel, 1997). Little is known about how nurses understand what patients are asking them to do, or about the process used to determine their responses to such requests. The purpose of this study was to explore how nurses understand the meaning of being asked by a decisionally capable person for AID and given that understanding, how they determine what their response ought to be.

Background

Public support for the idea of physician-assisted suicide for those who are terminally ill and suffering continues to grow in America. The most recent Harris poll reported that the percentage of surveyed Americans who support legalization of assisted suicide is now more than 60% (Reuters Health, 2002). Many Americans consider an assisted death a positive alternative to their fears of dying an institutionalized death that is painful, undignified, and senselessly prolonged (Schwarz, 1999). Hospitalized patients continue to die in unrecognized and poorly managed pain; the study to understand progress and preferences for outcomes and risks of treatment (SUPPORT) data indicated the incidence of untreated pain among hospitalized dying patients (more than 50%), clinicians' lack of competence in pain-management, and institutional limitations on end-of-life (EOL) care (SUPPORT, 1995).

Nurses have argued that if effective symptom management were provided to dying patients who experience pain and suffering, requests for assisted dying would be virtually eliminated (Coyle, 1992; Kazanowski, 1997). Although many clinicians assert that uncontrolled pain is a major risk factor for suicide among terminally ill patients (Block & Billings, 1994; Foley, 1995), recent studies have shown that the relationship between severe pain and a desire for a hastened death is more complex than straightforward (Breitbart & Rosenfeld, 1999). The few studies to explore why terminally ill patients ask clinicians for AID have indicated that physical pain is not the principal reason for such requests, but just one among other more frequently cited concerns, such as fears about loss of personal dignity and control, increasing dependency, and becoming a burden on family members (Meier, et al. 1998; Sullivan, Hedberg, & Fleming, 2000).

People who are incurably ill or dying might look forward to death and have occasional thoughts about suicide (Foley, 1995; Quill, Meier, Block, & Billings, 1998), or long for an end to the dying process (Coyle, 1992). In contrast to fleeting thoughts about hastening death, some people make serious and repeated requests for AID (Quill et al., 1998). Sometimes the clinician asked to provide AID is a nurse, and some nurses do assist patients in dying, although nurse-assisted dying is illegal and contrary to the ANA code of ethics (ANA, 2001) and professional guidelines (ANA, 1991; 1994).

Five descriptive studies have indicated American nurses' clinical experiences and responses to patients or family members who requested nurses' AID (Asch, 1996; Ferrell et al., 2000; Leiser et al., 1998; Matzo & Emanuel, 1997; Volker, 2001). Asch surveyed 1,600 critical care nurses (73% return rate) about their experiences with AID; 16% indicated participation in assisted suicide or euthanasia. Leiser and colleagues (1998) surveyed 428 nurses who worked in facilities that served AIDS patients in San Francisco and received 215 responses; 15% reported assisting in suicides. Matzo and Emanuel (1997) received 440 surveys (74% return rate) from New England oncology nurses; 1% acknowledged assisting in suicide and 4.5% reported assisted patient-requested euthanasia. Of those 440 nurses, 110 wrote comments on their completed questionnaires indicating that nurses wanted to discuss this issue.

In the largest study to date, Ferrell and colleagues (2000) reported results of a survey completed by 2,333 oncology nurses. Respondents reported support for legalization of assisted suicide (30%) and euthanasia (23%) and the frequency of patients' requests for AID: 23% had been asked for a lethal prescription and 22% had been asked for a lethal injection. Three percent of respondents reported helping patients obtain prescriptions and 3% reported administering lethal medication. Volker (2001) used naturalistic descriptive analysis of 48 stories anonymously submitted by 40 nurses identified as direct care providers or clinical nurse specialist members of the Oncology Nursing Society. Respondents submitted stories about the experience of being asked for AID by terminally ill cancer patients.

Many of these researchers have acknowledged uncertainty in determining the true prevalence and actual meaning of these data, in part because respondents who acknowledged AID may have instead provided symptom relief that was perceived to secondarily hasten death. Questions in these surveys had a forced-answer format, and some respondents indicated difficulty understanding the meaning of researchers' questions about assisted suicide or euthanasia (Davis et al. 1995; Ferrell et al., 2000). No study was found to report results of interviews with nurses who responded to patients' requests for AID.

The current study was focused on nurses who believed they had been asked by patients for AID. This topic was difficult to explore; conducting research about clinical practices that participants believed were illegal or professionally condemned acts presented ethical and practical challenges.

Methods

Interpretive phenomenology was the methodologic basis for this study. The research question was, "What is the nature of the experience of being asked to help someone die?"

This report includes stories nurses told about the meaning to them of being asked by patients for AID, and analysis was based on van Manen's (1990) methodologic approach for interpretive phenomenology.

Participants

Nurses were invited to participate if they believed a competent patient had asked them for help in dying and they were willing to talk about that experience. The concept of AID was not researcher-defined; by telling their stories, participants described what AID meant to them. A self-selected group of 10 nurses participated: four nurses worked in hospice home care; three were experts in the care of people with AIDS; two worked in critical care, and one was a clinical nurse specialist (CNS) in the care of patients with spinal cord injuries. Two of the 10 nurses were male (only female pseudonyms are used), all were Caucasian, middle-aged, and well-educated (three PhDs; five MSNs), and experienced (from 6 to 35 years). Eight worked in clinical settings on the East Coast, and two practiced on the West Coast of the United States.

Ethical Considerations

The need to assure potential participants that their identity would be kept confidential was paramount because of possible disclosure of illegal or professionally unsanctioned interventions. The university institutional review board that approved this research agreed to waive the requirement that participants sign an informed consent document so no records indicated their identity. Participants verbally agreed to participate in this study after receiving written information necessary for potential participants to make an informed choice about participation. All identifying characteristics of participants, their institutional affiliations, and descriptions of patients were altered or were removed before transcription. The researcher personally transcribed the interviews and then destroyed the audiotapes.

Generation and Analysis of Text

Most interviews occurred in participants' homes and lasted approximately 2 hours. One nurse who practiced on the West Coast was interviewed by telephone, and with one exception, participants were interviewed at least twice. Each was asked, "Tell me about a time when a patient asked you for help in dying" and were prompted to fully describe the experience. The second discussion occurred 2 weeks later to clarify details and meanings. Participants were given a thematic summary of my understanding of their experience; they provided reactions, clarifications, and written comments on the summaries that were included in the analysis.

Analysis of these data was on-going throughout data collection, transcription, and repeated readings of the text. Analysis proceeded from an initial overview of each participant's experience to more focused reflection followed by preliminary coding of these data and identification of themes. Once individual thematic summaries were written, recurring aspects of the experience common to all participants were identified and described. An auditor reviewed interview transcripts, themes, and the organization, description, and interpretation of findings.

Findings

The findings of this study are presented as themes and subthemes identified from the stories of participants. The four major themes were: Being open to hear and hearing; interpreting and responding to the meaning; responding to persistent requests for AID; and reflections.

Being Open to Hear and Hearing

Each narrative began the same way—a nurse heard a person's plea for help in dying. The first theme revealed how nurses experienced hearing such a request.

Unlike the hospice nurses who heard requests for AID fairly often, the six non-hospice participants described them as upsetting, unusual, and sometimes life-altering events, Charlotte, a CNS said, "It was the most important professional experience I've ever had." Sandy said, "I'll always remember it."

Participants heard a person's plea for help in dying within the culture of their own clinical experiences, personal and professional values, and spiritual or religious beliefs. Sophie, a home hospice nurse said "Patient's open up to me.... They will say things to me that they have not said to other nurses.... I will go back to the primary nurse and say, 'You know, the patient asked if I could help him to die. Has he asked that of you?' And that nurse often said 'no.'" Many participants described long-term relationships with patients who requested AID and strong commitments to their role as patient advocates.

Interpreting and Responding to the Meaning

The second theme included steps taken to explore what patients meant by the request for AID; requests were not taken at face value. Participants described active measures used to uncover and explore hidden meanings and unmet needs. A hospice nurse said, "Things are often not as they seem. It takes detective work to find out what they mean by 'help me die.'" A critical care nurse said, "Anytime somebody says to you, 'I want to die;' you have to assess why, And if it's pain, I can take care of that."

Most nurses said requests for AID were not associated with unmanaged physical pain, but often indicated suffering such as existential or spiritual distress, weariness with the prolonged process of dying, or determination to control the circumstances of dying. Participants also found meanings other than a desire for AID. Patients frequently wanted help in achieving a "good" death—as they defined it. When patients received good EOL care, their request for a hastened death was often withdrawn. Similar findings were reported by physicians in Oregon who found that when good palliative care was provided to dying patients; almost half reconsidered their request for assisted suicide (Ganzini et al., 2000).

When Stephany promised to help her patient die, she knew he was not asking to be killed. His death from end-stage AIDS was both imminent and inevitable. What he meant when he asked her to "Help me die" was that he wanted her to ensure that his EOL wishes were honored: that he would not be connected to machines, that his pain would be well managed, and that his family would be nearby as he died. When care was focused on facilitating "good" deaths, participants acknowledged that their EOL interventions might secondarily and unintentionally hasten dying; occasionally, death might be directly or knowingly hastened.

Multiple meanings of hastening death. Participants who provided opiate analgesia to relieve symptoms of pain or suffering acknowledged the possibility of an opiate-related hastened death. As a critical care nurse said, "If a hastened death occurs secondarily as a result of giving opiates for pain, that's not a problem." Participants agreed that such instances of opiate-related hastening death were morally justified because their intentions were good; because their intent was to relieve suffering and not to cause death, additional moral reflection was deemed unnecessary.

Although they condoned opiate-related hastened death, most participants distinguished opiate-related hastening death from opiate-caused death. A critical care nurse said, "If you're dialing up the morphine [drip] too fast, and your intent is to decrease the respiratory drive, that's a different story.... Of course if you depress their respirations enough, they're obviously going to die." Two participants who were palliative care educators characterized the presumed association between appropriate use of opiates for dying patients and the likelihood that such opiate use caused death as an "over-blown myth." Brandy said, "I've never seen anyone on a morphine drip who died as a result of the morphine." Stephany said about the morphine drip that helped her patient to die peacefully, "I'm sure that it contributed to his death in that, even if it didn't kill him, it may have allowed him to let go ... to release himself and allow himself to die."

Nurses in this study accepted the possibility of opiate-related hastened death because they believed that effective pain management for dying patients was a moral imperative. They also distinguished between secondarily hastening death and intentionally or directly causing death. Participants explicitly or implicitly appealed to the principle of double effect as moral justification for assuming the risk of secondarily and unintentionally hastening death.

Use of double-effect reasoning and the meaning of intentions. The principle of double effect, formulated by Roman Catholic moral theologians in the Middle Ages, continues to be used as a guide to decisions when clinicians cannot avoid all harmful action but they must decide whether one potentially harmful action is preferable to another (Quill, Dresser, & Brock, 1997). Properly applied, the principle requires that the agent intend only the good effect and not the bad, but it does not indicate how to determine the nature of a good or bad outcome when dying patients want a hastened death. Some clinicians have challenged the usefulness of this principle in cases that involve conflicts in values. Elizabeth, a hospice nurse, was unusually candid in her description of the difficulties in its use.

> I think we manipulate it [double effect] a little; I know personally I have—when I'm medicating someone, if they're truly at the end of life, and they just want it over.... I have found myself saying, 'Oh yes, I'm increasing that dose because of respiratory distress' or 'because of the pain'. But truly, in my heart I know, I really want that suffering over for that patient, because I think that their journey has been long and hard, and enough is enough. So I consider it a form of euthanasia.

Her hospice nurse colleagues challenged her description of such interventions as a form of euthanasia: One colleague said, "Oh no! That's the principle of double effect, and your intent was to manage the symptoms, not end that patient's life." Elizabeth said, "And I think we say that to make ourselves feel it's okay. I think euthanasia has been happening for years.... Physicians have done it; I'm sure nurses have done it, and family members too." Elizabeth stated that hospice nurses "hide behind the principle of double effect" to ease their consciences as they struggled to help patients die well. She claimed that their appeal to this principle sometimes functioned as a sort of moral "rubber stamp" that short-circuited thoughtful reflection about their intentions when caring for symptomatic dying patients. As a patient's death became imminent, participants acknowledged the difficulty in knowing whether their intent was exclusively to palliate symptoms or also to hasten a suffering patient's death. Sophie continually examined her intentions when assessing the analgesia needs of dying patients. She said,

> There are times when I question, "Did that just put them over the edge?" And if I were honest with myself, I would have to say yes.... It's a very fine line, and I struggle with it quite a bit ... I have that moment of "Hummm. Is this going to put them over the edge?" And sometimes it does, but I'm controlling a symptom of dying. I'm giving the medication for a specific reason. I'm not giving it to kill that patient. So for me there is a line.... It's not black and white; it's a gray area.

Sophie felt uneasy when intervening in ways she believed hastened death, yet she said those feelings of discomfort were good to have. "If I was comfortable with it, [knowingly hastening death] that would be very dangerous because I might cross that line without even knowing it and give myself permission to make decisions that aren't mine to make."

In contrast, other participants seemed unconcerned about the distinction between opiate-hastened death and opiate-caused deaths. Casey, a hospice nurse who publicly advocated for legalization of assisted suicide, said that if a patient was suffering and wanted help in dying, her response was to "aggressively titrate" opiate drugs. Although she maintained that her "primary intent was to eliminate suffering," she acknowledged; "I know that this has led to death on a number of occasions." She considered herself legally and morally blameless for any hastened death that resulted from achieving her goal of eliminating patient suffering.

Other participants explicitly or implicitly referred to the principle of double effect as justification for their use of other EOL interventions that they experienced as secondarily hastening dying, such as withdrawing feeding tubes or other treatments that prolonged dying, giving dying patients "permission" to die, or answering patients' questions about how they could hasten their own dying with information about stopping eating and drinking. Elizabeth said, "We all hesitate to acknowledge that we hasten death, but I think indeed we do. When we tell someone it's okay to withhold or withdraw their nutrition, that hastens the dying process ... but that's not a bad thing." Such instances of secondarily hastening death were viewed as morally acceptable and professionally appropriate EOL care.

Responding to Persistent Requests for AID

For most participants persistent requests for AID were uncommon. When they occurred participants paused to consider how far they would travel on their journey with dying patients, and where they recognized or drew a line on their commitment to help patients die well.

Finding a moral line. Most participants described a moral line that limited their responses to persistent requests for AID. That point was based on strongly held personal values, moral or spiritual beliefs, their sense of professional responsibility or duty, and fears of legal or professional liability. Some thought their beliefs were clear until they tried to explain that decisions depend upon patient context. For example, Rose, a hospice nurse whose early religious training and education occurred within Roman Catholic tradition, found those beliefs consistent with hospice practice that prohibits clinicians from intervening to intentionally hasten the dying process. Yet she was proud of the one time that she had helped hasten a suffering patient's death in response to his family's plea for her help.

The patient was dying from metastasized cancer and had stopped taking all fluids and food 10 days earlier, in an effort to hasten his own death. She called the hospice physician and said, "The family is saying that he really wants to go; we have morphine suppositories and thorazine pills in the house. What can we do?" Rose repeated the physician's suggestions out loud for the family to hear. "You can give one every hour or every half hour—alternating morphine with thorazine. It will make him quite sleepy and of course pain free." Though she was not present when her patient died, she knew that the family helped him to die. She approved of their actions, and characterized her own involvement as "absolutely the right thing to do." Although she crossed her hospice's line by helping hasten this patient's death, she experienced no moral or personal conflict from doing so. She never discussed with her physician colleague their collusion in the patient's death; even when clinicians agreed that hastening a patient's death was "absolutely the right thing to do," they did not acknowledge or discuss such experiences.

Although Elizabeth said that intentionally intervening to hasten a patient's death is wrong, she acknowledged occasionally doing so when suffering patients were near the end of life. Although those occasions were not experienced as moral conflicts, she described a different incident when she believed she crossed her moral line. Her patient was dying from AIDS and was in terrible pain; he kept screaming and saying that he wanted to die. She phoned the hospice physician for help and he said, "Just do what you have to do to get him comfortable and I'll write the orders later." She continued trying to ease his distress, but all her efforts failed. "I had done everything that I could—I didn't know what else to do, so I took the timer off the [morphine] pump ... and I just kept pumping the boluses until he stopped screaming." He died 12 hours later. Despite assurances from hospice colleagues that she had not caused his death, she believed her actions were morally wrong because she directly intervened to hasten his death. She remains haunted by her memories of that experience, conflicted and distressed about her role in that patient's death.

The closer participants' responses were to their predetermined moral line, the more uncomfortable they became. Often the source of their discomfort was conflict between their desire to do the right thing and fears about the consequences of doing so. Sandy, a nurse with over 38 years of experience with dying patients, said unequivocally that people ought to have the right to be helped to die, and it was wrong for society to intervene and dictate whether people could end their lives. Yet, when a neighborhood friend who was dying from AIDS asked her to help him die she realized, "The two things that scared . . . me were my Catholic upbringing—it's a mortal sin to help someone commit suicide—and the other was my license." She said to her neighbor, "I can't do it for you, but I'll help you in what little way I can." She told her neighbor's companion to buy *Final Exit*, and guided them through its directions. She was not present when he died, and she did not feel proud of her role in her neighbor's death. She wondered whether she "should have been more able to assist in some way."

In contrast Jones, an ANP who cared for persons with AIDS, experienced no conflict between her theoretical support for a persons' right to make important life choices and her willingness to act upon those convictions by providing those who requested AID with the means to end their lives. She believed that decisionally capable people ought to be permitted to determine whether the benefits of continued life outweighed the burdens. Her respect for individual autonomy included the right to determine the circumstance and time of death and essentially outranked all competing values.

Sophie also experienced no conflict between the theoretical location of her moral line and the clinical decisions she made when faced with persistent requests for AID. Because of her religious beliefs, on numerous occasions when she "got right up to the edge," she always stopped. She never crossed her line because she believed "I do not have the right to intervene and decide when a person's life should end ... I'm not The Boss." Brandy, a critical care nurse, also knew why she would not cross her line when an elderly patient in the ICU requested that she "help him out." He knew he was dying, he was ready, his family was exhausted, and he wanted the dying process over. Although she sympathized with his wishes, "There was no question in my mind, I was not going to give him enough [morphine] to push him over the edge. He was not in pain, and I really didn't know this man. In no way would I jeopardize myself professionally."

In contrast, Charlotte spent months trying to determine the right response to the dilemma she experienced when her 17-year-old patient requested that his ventilator be removed so he could die. When he realized that he would never "get better" and would always be paralyzed below his chin, he wanted to be allowed to die. She believed he had a "right to die" and advocated for his ethical right to have his wishes respected, but she was unable to persuade other members of the health care team or his parents of his right to have the life-sustaining treatment stopped. Because of his fractured neck he could not exercise his right to self-determination without help; he was dependent upon those whose moral and professional duty to care conflicted with his right to die. "There wasn't any way that the kid could die. He couldn't kill himself and we weren't going to help him."

Those events occurred more than 25 years ago, before legal case law recognized an adult patient's right to refuse unwanted life-sustaining treatment; aside from his quadriplegia, David was a healthy young man who was neither terminally ill nor dying. At that time in America, removing a ventilator from a young person in David's condition was considered tantamount to murder. When David said to her, "You've got to help me. You are the only hope I have left," her initial reaction was, "The morally courageous thing to do would be to help him." Her second response was to consider the consequences if she did. Regretfully, she told him, "I can't help you because I really want to be a nurse. And I'm afraid that I wouldn't ever get to be a nurse again for anybody if I helped you." And then they both cried. He lived for 7 more years; 26 years later, Charlotte remains uncertain whether she did the right thing by not helping David to die as he wanted.

When determining how to respond to persistent requests for AID, participants considered their spiritual or religious beliefs, fears about "getting caught," and their moral obligations to particular patients. They did not consider or consult their profession's code of ethics or written position statements on EOL care. Jones purposefully avoided consulting these guidelines because, "I thought it would terrify me. It would make me lose heart. It's like not knowing the nurse practice act—if you don't know the act and disobey it, that's bad. But it's really bad if you know it and disobey it." Participants kept their experiences secret; most did not discuss patients' requests or their responses with nurse colleagues, they did not consult or collaborate with other clinicians, and they did not subsequently talk with physicians about their shared experience of collusion to facilitate a hastened death.

Participants described a continuum of responses they provided to persistent requests for AID that included refusal, not interfering with patient or family plans to hasten or cause death, and providing varying degrees and kinds of assistance. Whether they passively "stood by" or actively intervened with assistance that patients or family members used to cause death, nurses were concerned about "who ought to control dying."

Conflicts in control over dying. To directly intervene to cause death is the ultimate act of controlling dying; participants strongly resisted assuming control or responsibility for another's death. They instead worked to empower patients to control and manage their own dying, recognizing that seriously ill and dying people are highly vulnerable and unempowered. To be empowered, patients must have relevant and accurate information to make informed choices about their EOL experiences.

Sandy informed her neighbor about the instructions in *Final Exit*, and Jones told her patient how he could end his life with an overdose of insulin. Jones knew Robert well; she had cared for him for months as he suffered from end-stage AIDS; he also had diabetes. His previous suicide attempt was unsuccessful, despite the many drugs he had available because of what Jones described as his "knowledge deficit." She believed that access to this information was a question of fairness. Though she provided Robert with the information, he controlled the decision about its use. "He really made the decision; all I did was choose to give him the information that, if he had been educated enough, he could have found on his own."

Rose noted that many of her hospice patients were truly ambivalent about wanting a hastened death. "Some patients begged 'Please, please, please help me to die!' and with their next breath said, 'Give me some water,' or 'Give me something to eat.'" Sometimes, when they persisted in asking, "How can I end this?" she replied,

> If you want to die, don't drink. Water is life, you can't live without water—you simply cannot—it would be a matter of days. And you can see it click! You can see it register in their eyes like, "Oh ya. Of course that's true." Then they'd say, "Oh no. I couldn't do that to my family."

Because Rose believed, "Every death happens as it is supposed to" she readily accepted this patient's decision to not hasten dying. Rose presented EOL options to her patients and their families, but she removed herself from controlling which option they chose. These nurses believed that if patients were decisionally capable, had received good EOL care, and still wanted to end their lives "They have the right to do that. They have the right to do whatever they choose." However, most did not believe that patients had a right to their help in dying.

Another way some hospice nurse participants avoided feeling responsible for a patient's death was to purposefully distance themselves from plans made by patients or families to hasten or cause death. Family members sometimes asked hospice nurses, "What would happen if [we] gave an increased amount of opiate or other drugs more often than ordered?" Hospice nurses in this study implicitly gave family members permission to do what they thought right for their loved ones, but stipulated that they did not want to know the family's plans, and promised not to document the conversation or to reveal the plan. When family members asked Rose about doses of drugs, she replied that she didn't know, but added,

> "You have the medication, there's stuff in the house. If you want to give more, that's up to you." I always gave people the choice and I never knew precisely what they did. She described this support as a "human-to-human response. If this were my loved one, I would want to know what I could do to help accelerate the dying process. Its fine-tuning EOL care.

Sophie also gave families permission to do what they thought right for their dying loved ones and said, "'What you do after I leave is what you do after I leave.' I have a lot of respect for people in their own homes. The family has rights that I don't have."

These nurses were clear about the line they drew, families could do what they thought best for their loved one, but the nurses would neither assist nor intervene to stop them. They covertly provided permission then actively looked away; they wanted their patients to die well, but they did not want to be morally responsible for death.

Providing Direct AID. Two nurses explicitly acknowledged providing direct AID; each had well thought out reasons for doing so. When Paula helped people to commit suicide in Oregon, she limited her assistance to those who met the criteria specified in Oregon's Death With Dignity Act; they had to be competent and terminally ill and resolute in their desire. She emphasized the importance of ensuring that the request was not because of inadequate palliative care, and she often recommended hospice care, and provided opportunities to reconsider the decision. When those criteria were met, she mixed and gave the lethal medication to those who had to be able to ingest the lethal mixture on their own. Although she believed her assistance was lawful, what was more important was her certainty that she was doing the right thing. She believed that people ought to be able to end their lives when and under circumstances they chose. "I think that's as much a human right as anything." Paula knew the ANA opposed nurse-assisted suicide, but maintained that, "We need to balance the scales and speak up for the other side;" she spoke for those who shared her convictions that terminally ill people had a right to be assisted in suicide. Casey shared those convictions in support of assisted suicide, but was more circumspect than was Paula in describing her own role in assisting patients to die. She said she knew that hospice and other nurses who care for dying patients are assisting in suicides and providing active euthanasia.

Jones actively helped two terminally ill people obtain the means to end life. She obtained a prescription for a lethal amount of drugs for another patient with AIDS, and helped an elderly friend who feared a pain-filled cancer death, by providing her with lethal drugs. In neither case did Jones think that suicide was the right choice, yet she firmly believed the decision was theirs and not hers to make. Neither patient committed suicide; one died from her disease and the other lived with his disease and retained the means to end his life.

The final theme, Reflections, included participants' thoughts about their experiences, what they wished they had done, and what they thought they might do in the future. Most acknowledged an ambivalent mix of emotions when they considered their responses to a request for AID. Regardless of what they actually did, nurses who believed their actions were instrumental in helping a person die experienced feelings of guilt and moral distress. All participants except Casey and Paula opposed further legalization of assisted suicide or active euthanasia because of fears about the potential for abuse and that clinicians might too readily accept a patient's fleeting wish to die.

Discussion

A covert "underground" practice exists in the United States of providing assistance to people who wish to die well and wisely (Leiser et al., 1998), thus tension often is felt between what is legally permitted and what is morally required. Tuten (2001) noted that, "We teach what is right but practice what is legal. And we are disturbed when what is right is not legal and what is legal is not right" (p. 64).

Participants' stories gave compelling evidence of the difficulty in knowing intentions when (a) their identified goal of care was to manage EOL suffering, and (b) facilitating peaceful dying resulted in a hastened death, often secondarily and unintentionally, and occasionally knowingly. Participants kept silent about their experiences, some because they believed they had crossed a moral line, and others feared professional or legal sanction. Those who believed themselves directly or indirectly responsible for a person's death described feelings of guilt and moral conflict. Sophie almost decided to stop practicing as a hospice nurse after colleagues "jokingly" referred to her as the "angel of death." When nursing interventions result in feelings of guilt and unresolved moral distress, nurses are at increased risk for professional burnout and leaving the profession; those who remain at the bedside of dying patients might cope with their stress by becoming emotionally detached and distancing themselves from patients and colleagues (Cameron, 1997).

Although familiar with basic ethical principles important to good EOL care, such as the central role of respect for people, and the principle of double effect, participants did not refer to the code of ethics or the profession's position statements on AID, instead their responses were context-driven rather than rule-mandated. These findings also showed that some nurses appealed to the principle of double effect in name only, and thereby avoided the work of thoughtful moral reflection that is necessary if this construct is to be appropriately applied to EOL decisions.

Conclusions

Few nurses in this study unequivocally agreed or refused to participate in helping patients die. Most struggled alone and in silence to find another way to respond by providing good EOL care and remaining present when patients and families suffered.

The question of what constitutes "doing harm" to dying patients who request AID remained unresolved. When the goal of care was to help patients die well, these nurses experienced difficulty identifying a reliable moral line that distinguished among palliative interventions that allowed, hastened, or caused death. They described unspoken understandings and covert agreements with family members, and collusion with physician colleagues. When acts of collusion and secrecy become routine, they undermine the important role of collaboration and consultation in good hospice and palliative EOL care. These findings indicate a need to further explore how nurses understand the meaning of intentions when providing palliative care to dying patients.

References

American Nurses Association. (1991). Position statement on the promotion of comfort and relief of pain in dying patients. Washington, DC: Author.

American Nurses Association. (1994). Position statement on assisted suicide. Washington, DC: Author.

American Nurses Association. (2001). Code of ethics for nurses with interpretive statements. Washington, DC: Author.

Asch, D.A. (1996). The role of critical care nurses in euthanasia and assisted suicide. New England Journal of Medicine, 334, 1374–1401.

Block, S.D., & Billing, J.A. (1994). Patient requests to hasten death: Evaluation and management in terminal care. Archives of Internal Medicine, 154, 2039–2047.

Breitbart, W., & Rosenfeld, B.D. (1999). Physician-assisted suicide: The influence of psychosocial issues. Cancer Control, 6, 146–161.

Brody, H. (1992). Assisted dying—A compassionate response to a medical failure. The New England Journal of Medicine, 327, 1384–1388.

Brody, H. (1998). Double effect: Does it have a proper use in palliative care? Journal of Palliative Medicine, 1, 329–332.

Cavanaugh, T.A. (1996). The ethics of death-hastening or death-causing palliative analgesic administration to the terminally ill. Journal of Pain and Symptom Management, 12, 248–254.

Cameron, M.E. (1997). Legal and ethical issues: Ethical distress in nursing. Journal of Professional Nursing, 13, 280.

Coyle, N. (1992). The euthanasia and physician-assisted suicide debate: Issues for nursing. Oncology Nursing Forum, 19(Suppl. 7), 41–46.

Davis, A.J., Phillips, L., Drought, T.S., Sellin, S., Ronsman, K., & Hershberger, K.A. (1995). Nurses' attitudes toward active euthanasia. Nursing Outlook, 43, 174–179.

Ferrell, B., Virani, R., Grant, M., Coyne, P., & Uman, G. (2000). Beyond the Supreme Court decision: Nursing perspectives on end-of-life care. Oncology Nursing Forum, 27, 445–455.

Field, D., & James, N. (1993). Where and how patients die. In D. Clark (Ed.), The future of palliative care: Issues of policy and practice (pp. 6–29). Buckingham, United Kingdom: Open University Press.

Foley, K.M. (1995). Pain, physician-assisted suicide and euthanasia. The Pain Forum, 4, 163–178.

Ganzini, L., Nelson, H.D., Schmidt, T.A., Kraemer, D.F., Delorit, M.A., & Lee, M.A. (2000). Physicians' experiences with the Oregon Death with Dignity Act. New England Journal of Medicine, 342, 557–563.

Kazanowski, M. (1997, March). A commitment to palliative care: Could it impact assisted suicide? Journal of Gerontological Nursing, 36–42.

Latimer, E.J. (1991). Ethical decision-making in the care of the dying and its application to clinical care. Journal of Pain and Symptom Management, 6, 329–335.

Leiser, R.J., Mitchell, T.F., Hahn, J., Slome, L., & Abrams, D.I. (1998). Nurses' attitudes and beliefs toward assisted suicide in AIDS. Journal of the Association of Nurses in AIDS Care, 9, 26–33.

Matzo, L.M., & Emanuel, E.J. (1997). Oncology nurses' practices of assisted suicide and patient-requested euthanasia. Oncology Nursing Forum, 24, 1725–1732.

Matzo, L.M., & Schwarz, J.K. (2001). In their own words: Oncology nurses respond to patient requests for assisted suicide and euthanasia. Applied Nursing Research, 14, 64–71.

Meier, D.E., Emmons, C., Wallenstein, S., Quill, T., Morrison, R.S., & Cassel, C.K. (1998). A national survey of physician-assisted suicide and euthanasia in the United States. The New England Journal of Medicine, 338, 1193–1201.

Quill, T.E. (1998). Principle of double effect and end-of-life pain management: Additional myths and a limited rule. Journal of Palliative Medicine, 1, 333–336.

Quill, T.E., Dresser, R., & Brock, D. (1997). The rule of double effect—A critiques of its role in end-of-life decision making. New England Journal of Medicine, 337, 1768–1771.

Quill, T.E., Lo, B., & Brock, D.W. (1997). Palliative options of last resort: A comparison of voluntarily stopping eating and drinking, terminal sedation, physician-assisted suicide, and voluntary active euthanasia. Health Law and Ethics, 278, 2099–2104.

Quill, T.E., Meier, D.E., Block, S.D., & Billings, J.A. (1998). The debate over physician-assisted suicide: Empirical data and convergent views. Annals of Internal Medicine, 128, 522–558.

Reuters Health. (January 13, 2002). New survey claims majority support assisted suicide. Retrieved October 22, 2003, from http://www.priestsforlife.org/news/infonet/infonet02-01-13.htm#NewSurvey

Schwarz, J.K. (1999). Assisted dying and nursing practice. Image: Journal of Nursing Scholarship, 31, 367–373.

Study to Understand Progress and Preferences for Outcomes and Risks of Treatment (SUPPORT), Connors, A.F., Dawson, N.V., Desbiens, N.A., Fulkerson, W.J. Goldman, L., Knaus, W.A., et al. (1995). A controlled trial to improve care for seriously ill hospitalized patients. JAMA, 274, 1591–1598.

Sullivan, A.D., Hedberg, K., & Fleming, D. (2000). Legalized physician-assisted suicide in Oregon—the second year. New England Journal of Medicine, 342, 598–604.

Tuten, M. (2001). A death with dignity in Oregon. Oncology Nursing Forum, 28, 58–65.

van Manen, M. (1990). Researching lived experience: Human science for an action sensitive pedagogy. Albany, NY: State University of New York.

Volker, D.L. (2001). Perspectives on assisted dying: Oncology nurses' experiences with requests for assisted dying from terminally ill patients with cancer. Oncology Nursing Forum, 28, 39–49.

Grounded Theory as Method

Grounded theory is a qualitative research approach used to explore the social processes that present within human interactions. As a research approach, grounded theory differs from other qualitative approaches in that the primary purpose is to develop a theory about dominant social processes rather than to describe a particular phenomenon. The roots of grounded theory can be found in the interpretive tradition of symbolic interactionism, which speculates on social roles as they relate to human behavior. Through application of the approach, researchers develop explanations of key social processes or structures that are derived from or grounded in empirical data (Hutchinson, 2001). Grounded theorists assume that each group shares a specific social psychological problem that is not necessarily articulated (Hutchinson, 2001). Glaser and Strauss (1967) developed the method and published the first text addressing method issues: *The Discovery of Grounded Theory*.

Nursing used grounded theory to describe phenomena important to professional nursing as early as the 1960s and more extensively in the last decade (Beck, 1993, 2002; Benoliel, 1967; D'Abundo & Chally, 2004; Hutchinson, 1992; Meeker, 2004; Olson, 2002). Since the publication of the first edition of this textbook, grounded theory research has expanded significantly. Benoliel (1996) noted that grounded theory began to influence nursing knowledge development in the early 1960s. In her manuscript, "Grounded Theory and Nursing Knowledge," she examined how the method has contributed to nursing's body of substantive knowledge from the 1960s through the 1990s. Benoliel (1967) suggested that the major focus of the contributions to nursing knowledge over these decades was on "adaptations to illness, infertility, nurse adaptation and interventions, and status passages of vulnerable persons and groups" (p. 406). Grounded theory has continued to evolve and has become an extensively applied research approach. The methodology makes important contributions to nursing's development of a substantive body of knowledge, primarily because of its ability to develop middle-range theory, which can be tested empirically.

This chapter reviews fundamental characteristics of grounded theory and addresses methodological issues specific to engaging in this qualitative research approach. The chapter also reviews the systematic techniques and procedures of analysis essential to grounded theory investigations. Additional reading of primary sources is necessary to grasp the method in a comprehensive manner.

GROUNDED THEORY ROOTS

*A*s a qualitative research method, grounded theory has been used extensively in the discipline of sociology. Based on the symbolic interactionist perspective of human behavior, the development of this qualitative research approach has been credited to Barney Glaser and Anselm Strauss, two sociologists at the University of California in San Francisco. Grounded theory as a method of qualitative research is a form of field research. Field research refers to qualitative research approaches that explore and describe phenomena in naturalistic settings such as hospitals, outpatient clinics, and nursing homes. The basic assumption of this qualitative research approach is that people make sense and order of their social worlds. Essentially, common perceptions are shared within particular social groups, and theoretical constructs are described through grounded theory methodology (McCann & Clark, 2003a).

Grounded theory explores basic social processes. Symbolic interactionism theory, described by George Herbert Mead (1964) and Herbert Blumer (1969), provides the theoretical underpinnings of grounded theory method. In symbolic interactionism theory, it is believed that people behave and interact based on how they interpret or give meaning to specific symbols in their lives, such as style of dress or verbal and nonverbal expressions. For example, the nurse's cap, which is seen less frequently, was a style of dress that gave meaning to patients, which is apparent from statements such as, "How do I know you are my nurse if you do not wear your cap?" or "I liked it better when nurses wore caps—they looked more professional." Language can also have different meanings for different people. A common statement made by many nurses is, "I'm working on the floor today." Individuals familiar with the health care environment are likely to interpret that statement to mean that the nurse has been assigned to a specific unit in the hospital where he or she is providing nursing care to clients. Someone who is unfamiliar with the hospital setting or is from a different culture may interpret this statement differently. To them, "I'm working on the floor today" may mean cleaning or repairing the floor. Stern, Allen, and Moxley (1982) emphasized, it is also through the meaning and value of which these symbols have for us that we try to interpret our world and the actors who interact with us. In this way, we try to read minds, and to act accordingly. Learning the meaning and value of interactional symbols is everyone's lifetime study, and no easy task. (p. 203)

The study and exploration of the social processes present within human interactions in grounded theory are linked directly to symbolic interactionism.

Nurse researchers have widely recognized the significance of grounded theory as a method to investigate phenomena important to nursing and have used this approach extensively. Benoliel (1996), a pioneer in the use of grounded theory method for nursing research, examined the roots of grounded theory in nursing and its development over the past several decades. She identified the knowledge generation that occurred during this period as the Decade of Discovery, 1960-1970, followed by the Decade of Development, 1970-1980; the Decade of Diffusion, 1980-1990; and the Decade of Diversification, 1990 to present.

During the Decade of Discovery (1960-1970), grounded theory emerged as a major research method within the field of sociology. As the method entered the Decade of Development (1970-1980), seminars for the continued development of grounded theorists emerged, as well as funding for postdoctoral research training programs (Benoliel, 1996). The Decade of Diffusion (1980-1990) resulted in even further expansion of the research method, and nursing became visible as a group of researchers who could explain and implement grounded theory method. Nursing journals gave more attention to grounded theory, and university centers evolved that focused on grounded theory research in nursing (Benoliel, 1996). The Decade of Diversification (1990 to present) has resulted in the dissemination of the knowledge gained through grounded theory research.

Methodological issues raised by more recent attempts to refine the process of generating grounded theory continue to be addressed in the literature (Baker, Wuest, & Stern, 1992; Keddy, Sims, & Stern, 1996; Robrecht, 1995; Wuest, 1995). Baker and colleagues (1992) discussed method slurring between grounded theory and phenomenology, which mixed steps from both methods, and addressed the importance of being specific about method. Robrecht (1995) proposed "dimensional analysis, described by Schatzman in 1991 as a method for the generation of grounded theory" (p. 169). Within a feminist framework, the grounded theory method incorporates diversity and change (Wuest, 1995).

Unlike quantitative research, grounded theory does not begin with an existing theory but rather generates theory in a specific substantive area. The primary purpose of grounded theory research is the discovery of theory from methodical data generation. Precise procedural steps are applied to ultimately develop a grounded theory, or a theoretically complete explanation about a particular phenomenon (Benoliel, 1967; McCann & Clark, 2003a, 2003b, 2003c; Stern, 1980; Strauss & Corbin, 1990). Strauss and Corbin (1990) have explained grounded theory as follows:

> A grounded theory is one that is inductively derived from the study of the phenomenon it represents. That is, it is discovered, developed, and provisionally verified through systematic data collection and analysis of data pertaining to that phenomenon. Therefore, data collection, analysis, and theory stand in reciprocal relationship with each other. One does not begin with a theory, and then prove it. Rather, one begins with an area of study and what is relevant to that area is allowed to emerge. (p. 23)

The goal of grounded theory investigations is to discover theoretically complete explanations about particular phenomena. According to Strauss and Corbin (1990), grounded theory involves "systematic techniques and procedures of analysis that enable the researcher to develop a substantive theory that meets the criteria for doing 'good' science: significance, theory-observation compatibility, generalizability, reproducibility, precision, rigor, and verification" (p. 31).

McCann and Clark (2003b) noted that the "main criticism of grounded theory method is that the epistemological assumptions have not been clearly explicated and its links with existing social theory have been decreased" (p. 20). Further, there are essentially two accounts of grounded theory methodology: the Glaser and Strauss (1967) approach, which has been expanded by Glaser (1992); and the Strauss and Corbin approach (1990, 1998). The approaches share common characteristics but differ in their philosophical underpinnings. The common elements include theoretical sensitivity, theoretical sampling, constant comparative analysis, coding and categorizing data, literature as a data source, integration of theory, and theoretical memos (McCann & Clark, 2003b). A discussion of these common elements as they relate to grounded theory method follows.

FUNDAMENTAL CHARACTERISTICS OF GROUNDED THEORY METHOD

*T*he goal of grounded theory is the generation of theory and the refinement and further development of existing theories. Through an inductive approach, researchers use the method to generate theory that can be either formal or substantive. *Substantive theory* is that developed for a substantive, or empirical, area of inquiry (Glaser & Strauss, 1967). Examples pertinent to nursing might include taking care of oneself in a high-risk environment

(Rew, 2003) or concerns of intimate partners or patients experiencing sudden cardiac arrest after implantation of an internal defibrillator (Dougherty, Pyper, & Benoliel, 2004). *Formal theory* is developed for a formal, or conceptual, area of inquiry (Glaser & Strauss, 1967). Examples might include socialization to professional nursing or authority and power in nursing practice. Substantive and formal theories are considered to be middle-range theories in that both types fall between the working hypotheses and the all-inclusive grand theories (Glaser & Strauss, 1967). *Middle-range theories* have a narrower scope than grand theories and encompass limited concepts and aspects of the real world (Fawcett, 1995). Middle-range theories are most useful in nursing research since they can be empirically tested. Grand theories are broadest in scope, frequently lack operationally defined concepts, and are unsuitable to direct empirical testing (Fawcett, 1995). *Partial theories* are the most limited in scope and utility, comprising summary statements of isolated observation within a narrow range of phenomena. Some partial or micro theories may be developed into middle-range theories with additional research (Fawcett, 1995).

An important concept for new grounded theorists to recognize is that researchers do not begin with theory. Instead, researchers identify essential constructs from generated data, and from these data, theory emerges. Procedural steps in grounded theory are specific and occur simultaneously (see Figure 7.1 later in chapter). Because the information pertinent to the emerging theory comes directly from the data, the generated theory remains connected to or grounded in the data (Glaser & Strauss, 1967; Stern, 1980; Strauss & Corbin, 1990, 1998).

Grounded theory methodology combines both inductive and deductive research methods (Glaser & Strauss, 1967; Stern, 1980; Strauss & Corbin, 1990, 1998). From an inductive perspective, theory emerges from specific observations and generated data. The theory then can be tested empirically to develop predictions from general principles such as a deductive research method. Hutchinson (2001) addressed an important difference between verificational research and grounded theory research. Her explanation is helpful in clarifying the inductive nature of grounded theory:

> In verificational research, the researcher chooses an existing theory or conceptual framework and formulates hypotheses, which are then tested in a specific population. Verificational research is linear; the researcher delineates a problem, selects a theoretical framework, develops hypotheses, collects data, tests the hypotheses, and interprets the results. On a continuum, verificational research is more deductive, whereas grounded theory research is more inductive. Verificational research moves from a general theory to a specific situation, whereas grounded theorists aim for the development of a more inclusive, general theory through the analysis of specific social phenomena. (p. 212)

Stern (1980) differentiated grounded theory from other qualitative methodologies. There are five basic differences:

1. The conceptual framework of grounded theory is generated from the data rather than from previous studies.
2. The researcher attempts to discover dominant processes in the social scene rather than describe the unit under investigation.
3. The researcher compares all data with all other data.
4. The researcher may modify data collection according to the advancing theory; that is, the researcher drops false leads or asks more penetrating questions as needed.
5. The investigator examines data as they arrive and begins to code, categorize, conceptualize, and write the first few thoughts concerning the research report almost from the beginning of the study.

Constant comparative analysis is another fundamental characteristic that guides data generation and treatment. *Constant comparative analysis* of qualitative data combines an analytic procedure of constant comparison with an explicit coding procedure for generated data. "The aim of this method is the generation of theoretical constructs that, along with substantive codes and categories and their properties, form a theory that encompasses and explains as much behavioral variation as possible" (Hutchinson, 2001, p. 228). *Core variables* that are broad in scope interrelate concepts and hypotheses that emerge during data analysis. *Basic social psychological processes* (BSPPs) illustrate the social processes that emerge from the data analysis. A later section on the application of the grounded theory method explains these fundamental characteristics in greater detail.

GROUNDED THEORY AS A METHOD

*T*he need for more middle-range theories in nursing that can be empirically tested is one reason for using grounded theory to conduct scientific investigations of phenomena important to nursing. Stern and colleagues (1982) further articulated the factors linking grounded theory to nursing: nursing occurs in a natural rather controlled setting, and the nursing process requires "constant comparison of collected and coded data, hypothesis generation, use of the literature as data, and collection of additional data to verify or reject hypotheses" (p. 201).

Grounded theorists embarking on a new investigation should ask themselves, Have I paid enough attention to this particular phenomenon in terms of the individual's viewpoint? Have empirical research and the published literature offered what seems to be an oversimplification of the concepts relevant to the phenomenon under investigation? Is there a need for a deeper understanding of specific characteristics related to a particular phenomenon? Has the phenomenon been previously investigated? Positive answers to these or similar questions can validate for grounded theorists that the method choice is appropriate. As in any type of research, grounded theorists must consider the issues of available resources, time frame, and personal commitment to the investigation.

ELEMENTS AND INTERPRETATION OF THE METHOD

*W*hen individuals choose to conduct a grounded theory investigation, usually they have decided there is some observed social process requiring description and explanation. Application of grounded theory research techniques to the investigation of an observed social process important to nursing education, practice, or administration involves the application of several nonlinear phases. The phases are described in the following narrative as they relate to the methodological steps familiar to the research process. Development and refinement of the research question, sample selection, researcher's role, and ethical considerations in grounded theory investigations are described along with procedures for data generation, treatment, and analysis.

Research Question

The main purpose of using the grounded theory approach is to explore social processes with the goal of developing theory. The research question in a grounded theory investigation identifies the phenomenon to be studied. More specifically, the question lends focus and clarity about what the phenomenon of interest is (Strauss & Corbin, 1990, 1998). Furthermore, researchers need a research question or questions that will give them the flexibility and freedom to explore a phenomenon in depth. Also underlying this approach to qualitative research is the assumption that all of the concepts pertaining to a given phenomenon have not yet been identified, at least not in this population or place; or if so, then the relationships between the concepts are poorly understood or conceptually undeveloped (Strauss & Corbin, 1990, 1998).

The nature of grounded theory methodology requires that investigators refine the research question as they generate and analyze the study data. Because the study focus may change depending on the data generated, the original question merely lends focus to the study. A truly accurate research question is impossible to ask before beginning any grounded theory study (Hutchinson, 2001).

An example of a grounded theory question that begins an investigation and lends focus to the study is, How do nursing faculty address unsafe skill performance by nursing students? The question is broad but adds focus to the investigation by clarifying that the study will explore faculty evaluation and feedback techniques as they relate to unsafe student clinical performance. As data collection and analysis proceed, the focus of the study may change, given the emerging theory. Hypothetically, the focus of the study could change to, What is unsafe skill performance? Researchers must begin with a broad question that also provides focus. Researchers should expect that they will refine the question throughout the research process.

Sampling

Theoretical sampling is used in the data collection process for the purpose of generating theory. In theoretical sampling, the sample size is determined by generated data. The researcher simultaneously collects, codes, and analyzes data. Participants for a grounded theory investigation must be selected based on their experience with the social process under investigation. Just as it is impossible to finalize the research question before a grounded theory investigation, it is equally impossible to know how many participants will be involved. The sample size is determined by the data generated and their analysis. For example, in a grounded theory investigation on nurses' commitment to professional nursing practice, understanding the perspective of the nurse who has stayed in nursing as well as that of the nurse who has left the profession illustrates the need for theoretical sampling. Grounded theorists continue to collect data until they achieve saturation of conceptual information and no new codes emerge. The researcher can gain closure by constant questioning and re-examination of the data (Hutchinson, 2001).

Researcher's Role

Stern (1980) emphasized that, in a naturalistic setting, it is impossible to control for the presence of the researcher. Investigators bring personal experience to a study to enhance understanding of the problem. According to Stern and colleagues (1982), in the conduct of naturalistic research, investigators do not attempt to remove themselves from the study. Rather, researchers openly recognize they have a role in the investigation. Stern and colleagues (1982) further delineated the grounded theorist's role as follows:

> The grounded theory researcher works within a matrix where several processes go on at once rather than following a series of linear steps. The investigator examines data as they arrive, and begins

to code, categorize, conceptualize, and to write the first few thoughts concerning the research report almost from the beginning of the study." (p. 205)

The researcher is an integral part of the investigation and, consequently, must recognize the intimate role with the participants and include the implications of that role in the actual investigation and interpretation of the data.

Strauss and Corbin (1990, 1998) have identified skills needed for doing qualitative research: the ability "to step back and critically analyze situations, to recognize and avoid bias, to obtain valid and reliable data, and to think abstractly" (p. 18). Furthermore, "a qualitative researcher requires theoretical and social sensitivity, the ability to maintain analytical distance while at the same time drawing upon past experience and theoretical knowledge to interpret what is seen, astute powers of observation, and good interactional skills" (p. 18). To conduct a grounded theory investigation, researchers must possess excellent interpersonal and observational skills, compelling analytical abilities, and writing skills that facilitate communication in written word, with a high degree of accuracy, regarding what they have learned.

Ethical Considerations

Researchers must also consider the ethical implications of conducting a grounded theory investigation or, for that matter, any qualitative investigation. Obtaining informed consent, maintaining confidentiality, and handling sensitive information are a few examples of ethical considerations researchers must address. Because it is impossible to anticipate what sensitive issues might emerge during data collection in a grounded theory investigation, researchers must be prepared for unexpected concerns. Chapter 4 provides an extensive discussion of ethical considerations pertinent to qualitative investigations.

Steps in the Research Process

Stern (1980) described five steps in the process of grounded theory research that compose the fundamental components of the method. They are (1) the collection of empirical data; (2) concept formation; (3) concept development; (4) concept modification and integration; and (5) production of the research report.

DATA GENERATION

Researchers may collect grounded theory data from interview, observation, or documents, or from a combination of these sources (Stern, 1980). Daily journals, participant observation, formal or semi-structured interviews, and informal interviews are valid means of generating data. As concepts and categories emerge during data analysis, the required sampling of particular data sources continues until each category is saturated. No limits are set on the number of participants, interviewees, or data sources (Cutcliffe, 2000). Sampling in grounded theory research is consequently theoretical rather than purposeful (Glaser & Strauss, 1978). Participant selection and data generation sources are a function of the emerging hypothesis. Theoretical sampling is the process of data generation that requires the researcher to collect, code, and analyze data simultaneously. This process develops in response to the emerging theory and allows the research to develop richer data where needed.

Rew (2003) described her data generation techniques in her study, "A Theory of Taking Care of Oneself Grounded in Experiences of Homeless Youth."

> All interviews were tape recorded with permission from the participants. Interviews lasted an average of 30 minutes and were guided by two main tour questions: (a) What helps you remain healthy living as you do? And (b) What would you like to tell me about how you take care of yourself? Upon completion of the interview, each participant received compensation of $10, a snack bar and a beverage. The investigator also recorded field notes that detailed the youths' physical appearance and gestures during the interviews. Following each interview, the investigator's personal impressions of the participant and the participant's response were written in a journal. (p. 236)

The researcher examines and analyzes the data gathered using field techniques, observational methods, documents, and publications through a system of constant comparison until the investigation generates a number of hypotheses. As investigators develop hypotheses, they consult the literature for previously developed theories that relate to the emerging hypotheses of the study in progress. The developed theory, consisting of related factors or variables, should be suitable for testing (Hutchinson, 2001; Stern, 1980; Strauss & Corbin, 1990, 1998).

DATA TREATMENT

The choice of data treatment and collection methods is influenced primarily by researcher preference. Researchers generally tape-record interviews and transcribe them verbatim. Researchers should transcribe and type double-spaced field notes immediately. It is also helpful to leave at least a 2-inch margin on one side of the transcribed data sheets for coding purposes. The availability of computer programs for qualitative data analysis offers another option. Table 7.1 provides readers with an example of a field note and Level I coding.

DATA ANALYSIS: GENERATING THEORY

The discovery of a core variable is the goal of grounded theory. "The researcher undertakes the quest for this essential element of the theory, which illuminates the main theme of the actors in the setting, and explicates what is going on in the data" (Glaser, 1978, p. 94). The core variable serves as the foundational concept for theory generation, and "the integration and density

Table 7.1 • Sample Field Note	
Field Note	*Level I Coding*
9/10/2005	
There are 7 students, 1 faculty member, and 3 staff members to care for 35 orthopedic clients. Each student has been assigned 1 client. The students are juniors in a baccalaureate nursing program. This is their <u>1st clinical experience</u> and their 4th week on the unit. The instructor is working with a student as she prepares an intramuscular injection. <u>The student's hands are trembling.</u> The student drops the uncapped syringe on the floor, bends down, picks up the syringe to prepare to use the contaminated syringe to prepare the injection. <u>The instructor asks her what is wrong with the way she is proceeding.</u> <u>The student does not know. Tears are welling up in the student's eyes. The instructor's face is flushed, and she seems frustrated.</u> The instructor <u>explains</u> what is wrong, <u>tells</u> the student she is unprepared for the experience, and <u>asks</u> a staff member to give the injection. The staff member comments that she doesn't have time. <u>The student leaves the medication room crying. The instructor takes her to a conference room to discuss the incident.</u>	Fear Questioning Overwhelming Frustration Telling Asking Privacy

of the theory are dependent on the discovery of a significant core variable" (Hutchinson, 2001, p. 222). The core variable has six essential characteristics:

1. It recurs frequently in the data.
2. It links various data.
3. Because it is central, it explains much of the variation in all the data.
4. It has implications for a more general or formal theory.
5. As it becomes more detailed, the theory moves forward.
6. It permits maximum variation and analyses. (Strauss, 1987, p. 36)

BSPs are core variables that illustrate social processes as they continue over time, regardless of varying conditions (Glaser, 1978). For example, in Rew's (2003) article, "A Theory of Taking Care of Oneself Grounded in Experiences of Homeless Youth," the basic social process of taking care of oneself in a high-risk environment is identified and supported by three additional categories: becoming aware of oneself, staying alive with limited resources, and handling one's own health (p. 234).

CONCEPT FORMATION

Grounded theory requires that researchers collect, code, and analyze data from the beginning of the study. "The method is circular, allowing the researchers to change focus and pursue leads revealed by the ongoing data analysis" (Hutchinson, 2001, p. 223). Figure 7.1 illustrates the ongoing nature of data analysis in grounded theory.

Coding

During the conduct of a grounded theory investigation, the processes of data collection, coding, and analysis occur simultaneously. As they collect data through interviews, participant observation, field notes, and so forth, researchers begin to code data. They then examine data line by line, identify processes, and conceptualize underlying patterns. Coding occurs at three levels.

LEVEL I CODING. *Level I coding* requires that grounded theorists look for process. As they receive data, investigators apply a system of open coding; that is, they examine the data line by line and identify the processes in the data. It is critical to code each sentence and incident using as many codes as possible to ensure a thorough examination of the data. Researchers write code words in the wide margins of the field notes for easy identification.

In Level I coding, the codes are called substantive codes because they codify the substance of the data and often use the words participants themselves have used (Stern, 1980, p. 21). The two types of substantive codes

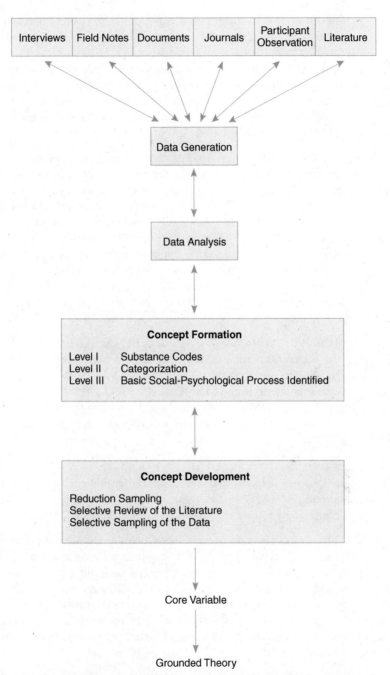

Figure 7-1. **Grounded theory and connections among data generation, treatment, and analysis.**

are (1) those from the language of the people who were observed or interviewed and (2) implicit codes constructed by researchers based on concepts obtained from the data (Mullen & Reynolds, 1978).

From the beginning of the study, grounded theorists attempt to discover as many categories as possible and to compare them with new indicators to uncover characteristics and relationships. They discard early codes if those codes lack foundation in the data and may add more codes as data gathering progresses (Mullen & Reynolds, 1978).

LEVEL II CODING. *Level II coding,* or *categorizing,* requires use of the constant comparative method in the treatment of data. Researchers code the data, compare them with other data, and assign the data to clusters or categories according to obvious fit. Categories are simply coded data that seem to cluster and may result from the condensing of Level I codes (Hutchinson, 2001; Stern, 1980). Deciding on specific categories is facilitated by questioning what each Level I code might indicate and then comparing each Level I code with all other Level I codes. This process enables researchers to determine what particular category would be appropriate for the grouping of similar Level I codes. Researchers then compare each category with every other category to ensure the categories are mutually exclusive.

LEVEL III CODING. *Level III coding* describes BSPs, which essentially is the title given to the central themes that emerge from the data. Questions suggested by Glaser and Strauss (1967) to describe BSPs include the following: What is going on in the data? What is the focus of the study and the relationship of the data to the study? What is the problem that is being dealt with by the participants? What processes are helping the participants cope with the problem?

Concept Development

Three major steps expand and define the emerging theory: reduction, selective sampling of the literature, and selective sampling of the data. Through these processes, the core variable emerges (Stern et al., 1982).

REDUCTION. During data analysis, an overwhelming number of categories emerge that researchers need to reduce in number. Comparing categories allows researchers to see how they cluster or connect and can be fit under another broader category (Stern et al., 1982). Category reduction is an essential component determining the primary social processes or core variables that trace the action in the social scene being investigated. The result of this reduction is a clustering of categories that, when combined, form a category of broader scope.

SELECTIVE SAMPLING OF THE LITERATURE. Stern (1980) has suggested that attempting a literature search before the study begins is unnecessary and perhaps may even be detrimental to the study. Reviewing the literature may lead to prejudgments and affect premature closure of ideas; the direction may be wrong; and available data or materials may be inaccurate (Stern, 1980).

Selective sampling of the literature is suggested and generally follows or occurs simultaneously with data analysis. The literature review helps researchers become familiar with works published on the concepts under study and fills in the missing pieces in the emerging theory. Referring to the example—How do nursing faculty address unsafe skill performance by nursing students?—that illustrated the development of the research question, investigators may review the published literature on the teaching of clinical skills, evaluation of those skills, or perhaps what constitutes unsafe performance. Depending on what additional data emerge, researchers will also need to review literature pertinent to those new concepts.

As theory begins to develop, researchers conduct a literature review to learn what has been published about the emerging concepts. They use the existing literature as data and weave the literature into a matrix consisting of data, category, and conceptualization. Literature, carefully scrutinized, helps expand the theory and relate it to other theories (Stern et al., 1982). The literature can fill in gaps in the emerging theory and add completeness to the theoretical description.

SELECTIVE SAMPLING OF THE DATA. As the main concepts or variables become apparent, comparison with the data determines under which conditions they occur and if the concepts or variables seem central to the emerging theory. Researchers may collect additional data in a selective manner to develop the hypotheses and identify the properties of the main categories. Through selective sampling, saturation of the categories occurs (Stern et al., 1982).

EMERGENCE OF THE CORE VARIABLE. Through the process of reduction and comparison, the core variable for the investigation emerges. "The concept of core variable refers to a category which accounts for most of the variation in a pattern of behavior and which helps to integrate other categories that have been discovered in the data" (Mullen & Reynolds, 1978, p. 282). Keating-Lefler & Wilson (2004) studied "The Experience of Becoming a Mother for Single, Unpartnered, Medicaid-Eligible, First-Time Mothers." The core variable was identified as "reformulating life." Following the emergence of the core variable, researchers begin the steps of concept modification and integration. Through the use of theoretical codes, the conceptual framework moves from a descriptive to a theoretical level.

Concept Modification and Integration

Concept modification and integration are accomplished as researchers continue to analyze data. Theoretical coding provides direction, and memoing preserves the researcher's thoughts and abstractions related to the emerging theory.

THEORETICAL CODING. *Theoretical coding* gives direction to the process of examining data in theoretical rather than descriptive terms (Stern, 1980). According to Stern (1980), this means applying a variety of analytical schemes to data to enhance their abstraction. Moving from descriptive to theoretical explanations, researchers examine all the variables that may affect data analysis and findings (Stern, 1980). During concept modification and integration, researchers use memoing to create a record of their ideas pertinent to the emerging theory.

MEMOING. *Memoing* preserves emerging hypotheses, analytical schemes, hunches, and abstractions. Researchers must sort memos into cluster concepts to tie up or remove loose ends. They write memos on file cards or paper or store them in computer files. During the process, it becomes clear how concepts fully integrate with one another and which analytical journey extends beyond the focus of the research report. Investigators set aside memos that do not fit until they write another focus of the study. Sorted memos become the basis for the research report (Stern, 1980).

Production of the Research Report

The research report for a grounded theory investigation presents the theory, which is substantiated by supporting data from field notes. The report should give readers an idea of the sources of the data, how the data were rendered, and how the concepts were integrated. A good report reflects the theory in ways that allow an outsider to grasp its meaning and apply its concepts.

EVALUATION OF GROUNDED THEORIES

Strauss and Corbin (1990) identified four criteria for judging the applicability of theory to a phenomenon: (1) fit; (2) understanding; (3) generality; and (4) control. If theory is faithful to the everyday reality of the substantive area and is carefully induced from diverse data, then it should fit that substantive area. If a researcher collected insufficient data and attempted closure too soon, then it is impossible to meet this criterion. Because it represents a reality, the grounded theory derived should be comprehensible to both the study participants and to practitioners with experience in the specific area studied. If the data on which the theory is based are comprehensive and the interpretations conceptual and broad, then that theory should be abstract enough and include sufficient variation so that it may apply to a variety of contexts related to the phenomenon under study, thus meeting the criterion of generality. The theory also should provide control with regard to action toward the phenomenon (Strauss & Corbin, 1990).

Chiovitti & Piran (2003) expanded on methodological issues related to authenticity and trustworthiness of data in grounded theory investigation. They describe eight steps to incorporate into a grounded theory investigation to enhance rigor:

1. Let participants guide the inquiry process.
2. Check the theoretical construction generated against participants' meanings of the phenomenon.
3. Use participants' actual words in the theory.
4. Articulate the researcher's personal views and insights about the phenomenon explored.
5. Specify the criteria built into the researcher's thinking.
6. Specify how and why participants in the study were selected.
7. Delineate the scope of the research.
8. Describe how the literature relates to each category that emerged in the theory. (p. 427)

Added to pre-established criteria, the work of Chiovitti & Piran (2003) can enhance the methodological soundness of a grounded theory investigation and can provide a guide for the constructive critique of published grounded theory research reports.

SUMMARY

G rounded theory plays a significant role in the conduct of qualitative research. The fundamental characteristics and application of the approach include issues related to refinement of the research question; determination of the sample; and data generation, treatment, and analysis. Applied to the profession of nursing, grounded theory can increase middle-range substantive theories and help explain theoretical gaps among theory, research, and practice. Grounded theory has continued to evolve and has become an extensively applied research approach. The methodology makes important contributions to nursing's development of a substantive body of knowledge, primarily due to its ability to develop middle-range theory, which can be tested empirically. Chapter 8 addresses grounded theory method as it has been applied in nursing education, practice, and administration.

References

Baker, C., Wuest, J., & Stern, P. N. (1992). Method slurring: The grounded theory/phenomenology example. *Journal of Advanced Nursing, 17,* 1255-1360.

Beck, C. T. (1993). Teetering on the edge: A substantive theory of postpartum depression. *Nursing Research, 42*(1), 42-48.

Beck, C.T. (2002). Releasing the pause button: Mothering twins during the first years of life. *Qualitative Health Research, 12*(5), 593-608.

Benoliel, J. Q. (1967). *The nurse and the dying patient.* New York: Macmillan.

Benoliel, J. Q. (1996). Grounded theory and nursing knowledge. *Qualitative Health Research, 6*(3), 406-428.

Blumer, H. (1969). *Symbolic intervention, perspective and method.* Englewood Cliffs, NJ: Prentice Hall.

Chiovitti, R., & Piran, N. (2003). Rigour and grounded theory research. *Journal of Advanced Nursing, 44*(4), 427-435.

Cutliffe, J. R. (2000). Methodological issues in grounded theory. *Journal of Advanced Nursing, 31*(6), 1476-1484.

D'Abundo, M., & Chally, P. (2004). Struggling with recovery: Participant perspectives on battling an eating disorder. *Qualitative Health Research, 14*(8), 1094-1106.

Dougherty, C. M., Pyper, G. P., & Benoliel, J. Q. (2004). Domains of concern of intimate partners of sudden cardiac arrest survivors after ICD implantation. *Journal of Cardiovascular Nursing, 19*(1), 21-31.

Fawcett, J. (1995). *Analysis and evaluation of conceptual models of nursing* (3rd ed.). Philadelphia: F.A. Davis.

Glaser, B. (1978). *Theoretical sensitivity.* Mill Valley, CA: Sociology Press.

Glaser, B. G., & Strauss, A. (1967). *The discovery of grounded theory: Strategies for qualitative research.* New York: Aldine.

Glaser, B. G. (1992). Emergence vs. forcing: Basics of grounded theory analysis. Mill Valley, CA: Sociology Press.

Hutchinson, S.A. (1992). Nurses who violate the Nurse Practice Act: Transformation of professional identity. *Image, 24*(2), 133-139.

Hutchinson, S. (2001). Grounded theory: The method. In P. L. Munhall (Ed.), *Nursing research: A qualitative perspective* (pp. 209-243). Sudbury, MA: Jones and Bartlett.

Keating-Lefler R., & Wilson, M. (2004). The experience of becoming a mother for single, unpartnered, Medicaid-eligible, first-time mothers. *Journal of Nursing Scholarship, 26*(1), 23-29.

Keddy, B., Sims, S. L., & Stern, P. N. (1996). Grounded theory as feminist methodology. *Journal of Advanced Nursing, 23*, 448-453.

McCann, T. V., & Clark, E. (2003a). Grounded theory in nursing research: Part I—methodology. *Nurse Researcher, 11*(2), 7-18.

McCann, T. V., & Clark, E. (2003b). Grounded theory in nursing research: Part II—critique. *Nurse Researcher, 11*(2), 18-28.

McCann, T. V., & Clark, E. (2003c). Grounded theory in nursing research: Part III—application. *Nurse Researcher, 11*(2), 29-39.

McCormack, D., & MacIntosh, J. (2001). Research with homeless people uncovers a model of health. *Western Journal of Nursing Research, 23*(7), 679-697.

Mead, G. H. (1964). *George Herbert Mead on social psychology.* Chicago: University of Chicago Press.

Meeker, M.A. (2004). Family surrogate decisions making at the end of life. Seeing them through with care and respect. *Qualitative Health Research, 14*(2), 204-225.

Mullen, P. D., & Reynolds, R. (1978). The potential of grounded theory for health education research: Linking theory and practice. *Health Education Monographs, 6*(3), 280-294.

Olson, K. (2002). Evolving routines: Preventing fatigue associated with lung and colorectal cancer. *Qualitative Health Research, 12*(5), 655-670.

Rew, L. (2003). A theory of taking care of oneself grounded in experiences of homeless youth. *Nursing Research, 52*(4), 234-241.

Robrecht, L. C. (1995). Grounded theory: Evolving methods. *Qualitative Health Research, 5*(2), 169-177.

Schatzman, L. (1991). Dimensional analysis: Notes on an alternative approach to the grounding of theory in qualitative research. In D. R. Maines (Ed.), *Social organization and social process: Essays in honor of Anselm Strauss* (pp. 303-314). New York: Aldine.

Stern, P. N. (1980). Grounded theory methodology: Its uses and processes. *Image, 12*(7), 20-23.

Stern, P. N., Allen, L. M., & Moxley, P. A. (1982). The nurse as grounded theorist: History, processes, and uses. *Review Journal of Philosophy and Social Science, 7*(142), 200-215.

Strauss, A. (1987). *Qualitative analysis for social scientists.* New York: Cambridge University Press.

Strauss, A., & Corbin, J. (1990). *Basics of qualitative research: Grounded theory procedures and techniques.* Newbury Park, CA: Sage.

Strauss, A., & Corbin, J. (1998). *Basics of qualitative research: Grounded theory procedures and techniques.* Newbury Park, CA: Sage.

Wuest, J. (1995). Feminist grounded theory: An exploration of the congruency and tensions between two traditions in knowledge discovery. *Qualitative Health Research, 5*(1), 125-137.

Grounded Theory in Practice, Education, and Administration

*A*s a means of studying nursing and the social processes that occur, grounded theory research creates opportunity for nurses interested in the approach to develop substantive theories regarding phenomena important to the clinical aspects of nursing as well as the administrative and educative processes that are inherent to the discipline.

In Chapter 7, methodological issues related to grounded theory investigations were described. This chapter examines grounded theory investigations in the areas of nursing practice, education, and administration. Two important questions guided the direction of this chapter: When should grounded theory be used? and How has the method been used to study issues in nursing education, administration, and practice? In this chapter, three published studies are reviewed using the guidelines for evaluating grounded theory research presented in Box 8.1. The critiquing guidelines offer specific directives for determining the quality of the grounded theory studies presented in this chapter and in the literature. A reprint of Meeker's (2004) article found at the end of this chapter assists readers in understanding the critiquing process. The chapter also provides readers with an overview of selected studies that highlight how nurse researchers have used grounded theory research in the investigation of phenomena important to nursing (Table 8.1).

CRITIQUE GUIDELINES

*S*trauss and Corbin (1990) indicate that "a qualitative study can be evaluated accurately only if its procedures are sufficiently explicit so that readers of the resulting publication can assess their appropriateness" (p. 249).

Box 8.1

Guidelines for Critiquing Research Using Grounded Theory Method

Focus/Topic

1. What is the focus or the topic of the study? What is it that the researcher is studying? Is the topic researchable? Is it focused enough to be meaningful but not too limited so as to be trivial?

2. Has the researcher identified why the phenomenon requires a qualitative format? What is the rationale for selecting the grounded theory approach as the qualitative approach for the investigation?

Purpose

1. Has the researcher made explicit the purpose for conducting the research?

Significance

1. Does the researcher describe the projected significance of the work to nursing?

2. What is the relevance of the study to what is already known about the topic?

Method

1. Given the topic of the study and the researcher's stated purpose, how does grounded theory methodology help to achieve the stated purpose?

2. Is the method adequate to address the research topic?

3. What approach is used to guide the inquiry? Does the researcher complete the study according to the processes described?

Sampling

1. Does the researcher describe the selection of participants and protection of human subjects?

2. What major categories emerged?

3. What were some of the events, incidents, or actions that pointed to some of these major categories?

4. What were the categories that led to theoretical sampling?

5. Did the research specify how and why participants were selected for the study?

Data Generation

1. Does the researcher describe data collection strategies?

2. Have participants been allowed to guide the direction of the inquiry?

3. How did theoretical formulations guide data collection?

Data Analysis

1. Does the researcher describe the strategies used to analyze the data?

   a. Has the theoretical construction been checked against the participants' meanings of the phenomenon?

   b. Are the researcher's views and insights about the phenomenon articulated?

   c. Has the literature been related to each category that emerged in the theory?

2. Does the researcher address the credibility, auditability, and fittingness of the data?

3. Does the researcher clearly describe how and why the core category was selected?

Box 8.1   (Continued)

Empirical Grounding of the Study: Findings

1. Are concepts grounded in the data?
2. Are the concepts systematically related?
3. Are conceptual linkages described, and are the categories well developed? Do they have conceptual density?
4. Are the theoretical findings significant? If yes, to what extent?
5. Were data collection strategies comprehensive and analytical interpretations conceptual and broad?
6. Is there sufficient variation to allow for applicability in a variety of contexts related to the phenomenon investigated?

Conclusions, Implications, and Recommendations

1. How does the researcher provide a context for use of the findings?
2. Are the conclusions drawn from the study appropriate? Explain.
3. What are the recommendations for future research?
4. Are the recommendations, conclusions, and implications clearly related to the findings?

Adapted from Chiovitti, R., & Prian, N. (2003). Rigour and grounded theory research. *Journal of Advanced Nursing Practice, 44*(4), 427–435, and Strauss, A., & Corbin, J. (1990). *Basics of qualitative research: Grounded theory procedures and techniques.* Newbury Park, CA: Sage.

If a grounded theory researcher provides this information, readers can use these criteria to assess the adequacy of the researcher's complex coding procedure. Detail given in this way would be supplemented with cues that could, in longer publications, at least be read as pointing to extremely careful and thorough tracking of findings of conscientious and imaginative theoretical sampling. (pp. 253–254)

Furthermore, they suggested that, in reality, "there may be no way that readers can accurately judge how the researcher carried out the analysis" (Strauss & Corbin, 1990, p. 253). Therefore, guiding criteria for evaluating grounded theory investigations are provided. Criteria can assist reviewers of grounded theory studies to search for the critical elements of the method (see Box 8.1). When reviewers are critiquing any published investigation, it is important to recognize that journal restrictions, page limitations, or other external forces beyond the author's control may have necessitated deletion of certain material, resulting in a limited critique of the research. Readers interested in more detailed discussion of method in a published study should contact the author.

Text continued on page 165.

Table 8.1 • Selective Sampling of Grounded Theory Research Studies

Author(s)	Date	Domain	Phenomenon of Interest	Sample	Data Generation	Findings
D'Abundo & Chally	2004	Practice	The process of recovery from eating disorders in women and girls	20 women and girls with eating disorders	Interviews, focus groups, and participant observation	A cyclical model of eating disorders referred to as the *eating disorder curve* is described. Development of eating disorders, how they increase in severity, and the process of recovery are detailed. The author describes components of the eating disorder curve as including increasing severity, the circle of acceptance, and decreasing severity.
Dougherty, Pyper, & Benoliel	2004	Practice	Domains of concern of intimate partners of sudden cardiac arrest (SCA) survivors during the first year after internal cardioverter-defibrillator (ICD) implantation	15 families	Data were collected from the SCA survivor and one intimate partner at five different times: hospital discharge; and 1, 3, 6, and 12 months. The first interview	Eight "domains of concern" were identified for intimate partners and included (1) Care of the survivor; (2) My (partner) self care; (3) Relationship; (4) ICD; (5) Money; (6)

				took place in the hospital, all subsequent interviews took place in the home of the participants. A total of 150 interviews were completed, yielding 176 hours of interview data. Interviews were audiotape-recorded, transcribed, and analyzed using constant comparative analysis.	Uncertain future; (7) Health care providers; and (8) Family. Five categories of strategies to deal with the domains of concern were identified: (1) Care of the survivor; (2) My (partner) self-care; (3) Relationship; (4) Uncertain future; and (5) Controlling the environment.
Judson	2004	Practice	The process of mothering a child who is dependent on parenteral nutrition	19 mothers of children who were currently or had been recently dependent on parenteral nutrition	In-depth interviews guided by a set of open-ended questions. Interviews lasted 60 to 90 minutes and were audiotaped and transcribed verbatim.	A Theory of Protective Care is described and composed of three phases: gaining control, taking control, and maintaining control. The categories of committing to care, watching over, challenging the

Table 8.1 • (Continued)

Author	Date	Domain	Phenomenon of Interest	Sample	Data Generation	Findings
						system, promoting normalcy, putting life into perspective, and celebrating the positive characterize the antecedents, strategies, and consequence of protective care.
McNeill	2004	Practice	Experiences of fathers who have a child with juvenile rheumatoid arthritis	22 fathers	Semi-structured interviews, tape-recorded and transcribed verbatim	Substantive theory of fathers' experiences addressing the impact of their child's juvenile rheumatoid arthritis, their adaptational responses, and the meanings they associated with their experiences. Fathers were profoundly affected, perceived their child's condition as a catalyst for meaningful involvement, experienced many

						emotions, and sought to adopt a positive approach to making sense of their child's experience. Fathers' efforts to be strong for others resulted in an overreliance on self-supporting strategies, particularly during periods of high stress. Given the nature of fathers' experiences and the extent of their involvement, greater attention by health care practitioners to fathers' adaptations by health care professionals is indicated.
Meeker	2004	Practice	The process of decision making for surrogates of terminally ill family members.	20 surrogates assisting terminally ill family members	Sixteen participants were interviewed, and four participated in focus groups. Interviews and focus groups were audiotaped and transcribed verbatim.	The basic social process identified was seeing them through with care and respect, during which time surrogates continuously synthesized the core values of caring for

Table 8.1 • (Continued)

Author	Date	Domain	Phenomenon of Interest	Sample	Data Generation	Findings
						their family member and respecting their family members' autonomy. The major categories of surrogate decision making during the process were Standing with the ill family member and Acting for the ill family member. Events reported in related categories were Brokering information and Working with family. A final category, Outcomes, reports consequences for the surrogate of having been a decision maker for a terminally ill family member.
Brown & Draye	2003	Practice, education	Pioneers' experiences of establishing the nurse practitioner (NP) role and their experiences in	50 middle-aged women currently	Interviews and focus groups to gather data about the nurses' early experiences	The central organizing theme was Advancing autonomy to make a difference. This

maintaining and building the NP role in the contemporary practice environment

practicing in Washington State who began the NP role during 1965–1979

theme was manifested through six broad themes: Breaking free; Molding the clay; Encountering obstacles; Surviving the proving ground; Staying committed; and Building the eldership. Autonomy was found to be requisite to practice to one's full potential and maintain commitment over time. The findings show the evolution of advanced nursing practice in the United States and provide guidance for nurses who are working to establish advanced practice nursing in other countries.

Table 8.1 • (Continued)

Author	Date	Domain	Phenomenon of Interest	Sample	Data Generation	Findings
Parry	2003	Practice	Meaning and impact of uncertainty in the lives of long-term survivors of childhood cancer	23 survivors. Participants were selected from a larger sample that participated in a quantitative study.	In depth semi-structured interviews, tape recorded and transcribed verbatim	Uncertainty was found to be a source of distress as well as a catalyst for growth. Participants noted a deeper appreciation for life, a greater awareness of purpose, and development of confidence, resilience, and optimism.
Dewar	2003	Practice	Examination of how individuals were able to live with catastrophic illnesses and injuries.	28 participants, all of whom were or had experienced a catastrophic illness	In-depth, semi-structured interviews, 60 to 90 minutes in length, tape-recorded and transcribed verbatim	A strategy called "boosting" was identified and describes the person's effort to improve self-esteem and adjust to the emotional, social, and physical effects associated with his or her disease or

						disability. Boosting had three major subcategories: Comparing self to others; Focusing on the positive; and Building up courage.
Jones, Zhang, & Meleis	2003	Practice	Experiences of two groups of immigrant Asian American women caring for older patients	22 Chinese American and 19 Filipino American women	In-depth, semi-structured interviews, tape-recorded and transcribed verbatim	Participants were found to be loyal to their traditional culture while adapting to new cultural expectations. Through difficulties encountered in meeting role expectations and coping with paradox, the women mobilized personal and family resources to transform vulnerability into strength and well-being.

Table 8.1 • (Continued)

Author	Date	Domain	Phenomenon of Interest	Sample	Data Generation	Findings
Milliken & Northcott	2003	Practice	Changes in parent's identity and caregiving during the erratic course of a child's mental illness	29 parent caregivers	In-depth, semi-structured interviews, tape-recorded and transcribed verbatim	The basic social problem identified in this study is that parents believe they have the right and responsibility to care for, protect, and make decisions for their children when they do not see them as capable of caring for themselves. Parents whose adult children suffer from mental illness engage in the basic social process of redefining their identity and adapting caregiving activities.

Text continued from page 155.

APPLICATION TO PRACTICE

*G*rounded theory research methods offer an important opportunity for nurses interested in examining clinical practice issues and developing substantive theory. An example of grounded theory research related to the practice arena is the study, "Family Surrogate Decision Making at the End of Life: Seeing Them Through With Care and Respect," by Mary Ann Meeker (2004), and this is the reference for critique in this section. This study provides an example of grounded theory research in the investigation of phenomena important to nursing practice. The Meeker (2004) article conveys the intensity and rigor of grounded theory method as it related to the "decision-making experiences of 20 surrogates who assisted terminally ill family members" (p. 204). The title and introduction clearly identify the focus of this grounded theory investigation. The statement of purpose further emphasizes the rationale for a qualitative design and the focus of the study. According to the author,

> Family surrogates play a pivotal role in health care decision making, yet little is known about their experiences and needs. Surrogates' participation has often been neglected in the clinical setting, and much of the research attention has been directed to assessing their ability to predict accurately their family members' choices. The purpose of this study was to investigate decision-making experiences and the social psychological processes family member surrogates use for health care decisions as they related to decision making with and for a terminally ill family member. (p. 205)

The literature review also supports the case for a grounded theory study. Further, the significance of the work to nursing and end-of-life care is abundantly clear. Meeker (2004) provides the reader with a comprehensive review of the literature and clearly makes the case for the findings of her study and their ability to contribute to an important aspect of nursing practice that requires further description and explanation.

The method used to conduct the inquiry is appropriate. Because of the reported intent to develop substantive theory about the participant experiences, grounded theory is particularly valuable. The philosophical underpinnings of grounded theory methodology are addressed in detail. Meeker (2004) discusses her application of grounded theory and how the basic social process in the experiences and interactions studied emerged.

Meeker (2004) describes the selection of participants and protection of human subjects in her article. "The purposeful sample consisted of 20 persons who had functioned in the role of family surrogate decision maker during the terminal phase of a family member's cancer illness" (p. 207). Meeker provides detailed information about how participants were recruited and notes that "sampling continued until theoretical saturation was reached and further data collection and analysis failed to contribute new information" (p. 207). This is consistent with grounded theory methodology and adds to the rigor of this investigation.

The data collection techniques applied in this study are consistent with a grounded theory investigation. The article clearly reports how theoretical formulations guided data collection.

> I offered participants the choice of individual interview or focus group interview. Sixteen persons participated in semi-structured individual interviews, and 4 persons participated in a focus group interview. (Meeker, 2004, p. 207)

Data analysis is consistent with grounded theory methodology, and strategies are described in detail. As data collection and analysis progressed, Meeker (2004) conducted theoretical sampling to provide data needed to fully describe the categories. A grounded theorist was consulted throughout the process. She further notes,

> I coded data using the constant comparative method of grounded theory. I accomplished initial coding of data by reviewing each transcript several times to identify and label data with substantive codes that described participant's perceptions and experiences. As analysis progressed, I grouped conceptually related codes into categories and elaborated the properties and dimensions for each category." (p. 208)

Meeker (2004) clearly describes how and why the core category was selected. The core variable is the goal of grounded theory and serves as the foundational concept for theory generation. The core variable must also link additional emergent categories. As the author reports, "The family surrogate decision maker's emic view forms the basis for the basic social process of Seeing Them Through With Care and Respect" (p. 208).

The substantive theory and major theoretical constructs were described in detail by Meeker (2004):

> Findings describe a basic social process of Seeing Them Through With Care and Respect, during which surrogates continuously synthesized the core values of caring for their family member and respecting their family member's autonomy. Surrogate narratives began with Learning the Diagnosis. The major categories of surrogate decision makers' activities during the process were Standing With and Acting for the ill family member. Events reported in two gating categories, Brokering Information and Working With Family, facilitated or impeded decision making. A final category, Outcomes, reports consequences for the surrogate of having been a decision maker.

A detailed discussion of the major categories is addressed by the author. By reading the report of findings presented by the author, the reader is immersed in the experience described. Meeker (2004) addresses authenticity and trustworthiness of the final analysis by conducting "a group discussion with 2 participants to share the results of the analysis and seek validation, clarification, and refinement from participants" (p. 208).

The findings noted by Meeker (2004) are limited to this study and reflect the need to repeat the investigation with different groups of women. Meeker has made an important contribution to nursing research in general and specifically to research related to end-of-life care. Her use of grounded theory methodology makes an important contribution to nursing theory development and offers detailed suggestion for continued research in this area. A major strength of this report lies not only in the detailed report of the findings but also in the detailed attention to the review of literature and method application. It is an excellent read for the researcher new to grounded theory, offering not only the opportunity to learn about concerns related to end-of-life care but also to learn about grounded theory.

APPLICATION TO EDUCATION

*N*ursing education continues to be an important area for the conduct of research and presents another context in which nurse researchers can conduct grounded theory investigations. However, few grounded theory studies exist solely in the domain of nursing education. The limited number of grounded theory studies in nursing education since the publication of the third edition of this text visibly illustrates this. Clearly, grounded theory has its place in research studies that focus on teaching-learning and offers the grounded theory researcher a rich opportunity for study. An example of the contribution grounded theory can make to nursing education is a study by Campbell (2003), "Cultivating Empowerment in Nursing Today for a Strong Profession Tomorrow." This article serves as the reference for critique in this section and was selected because it demonstrates the use of grounded theory in studying a nursing education issue. This study illustrates a good presentation of findings from a grounded theory investigation. Although it is used as an example relevant to education, the findings cut across the domains of administration and practice as well.

The purpose of Campbell's (2003) study was to explore processes related to empowerment and disempowerment among 16 participants from a baccalaureate nursing program within the context of the current nursing shortage. Campbell makes abundantly clear her rationale and purpose for this investigation. "Use of empowerment, in the context of understanding the cultural and organizational aspects of the nursing education environment, is paramount because this setting has the potential to influence individuals' beginning perspectives of nursing as a career" (p. 423). Further, "behaviors reflective of empowerment or disempowerment that may be exhibited by nurse educators and administrators can provide insight into the possibility of observing continued oppressive behaviors in the next generation of nurses" (p. 423). Campbell applied the concept of theoretical sampling as describe by Glaser and Strauss (1967). The interpretation of grounded theory presented by Streubert and Carpenter (1995) was applied.

The methodology is described in the article; however, more detail related to this aspect of the research process would have added to the quality of the article. The fact that the research was presented as a "brief" probably explains the absence of significant detail related to the method.

The data collection techniques reflect the process of theoretical sampling that is consistent with grounded theory methodology. It is not clear, however, how the emergence of major categories led to theoretical sampling. Nor is it clear how theoretical formulations guided data collection. This can probably be explained by imposed publication limitations and the fact that the author considers this a pilot study.

The author has described her findings in detail. "Cultivating" was constructed as the basic core category in the research. A description of how and why the core category was selected is provided. Within the context of the core category, the concept of empowerment is incorporated. A theoretical explanation of the concept of empowerment as it emerges internally and externally is describe in detail by the author. How students, faculty, and administration cultivate empowerment is addressed. What emerges most significantly from her discussion of the findings is the fact that despite nursing education's best efforts or intentions to cultivate a sense of empowerment in students, "intent does not necessarily produce the desired results" (Campbell, 2003, p. 424). Within the fluid process of Cultivating, the themes of Seeding, Grafting, Grounding, and Transforming are described. The findings presented are empirically grounded and systematically related.

Campbell (2003) does not address issues of credibility, auditability, or fittingness of the data. This would have added to the authenticity and trustworthiness of her findings. She does, however, provide an excellent context for the use of the findings, and the conclusions drawn have important implications for nursing education and practice. The study would be strengthened if the author had made a clearer connection between grounded theory methodology and her study. However, her concluding statement captures the essence of the study. Campbell (2003) concludes that nurses continue to treat one another negatively and that "All nurses must consciously decide to facilitate empowering experiences for the nursing students with whom they interact" (p. 426).

APPLICATION TO ADMINISTRATION

For previous editions of this text, it was extremely difficult to find grounded theory studies that reflected the area of nursing service administration. Again this is the case. The article selected to serve as the reference for this area cuts across administrative and practice domains. MacIntosh (2003) applies grounded theory methodology to a study that explores experienced nurses' perceptions of how they became professional. Her study, "Reworking Professional Identity," is grounded in the notion that "[i]n spite of professional socialization through nursing education programs, new graduates experience stress as they become working professionals" (p. 725). MacIntosh's article conveys the intensity and rigor of grounded theory method as it related to how nurses perceive themselves becoming professional.

The title and introduction clearly identify the focus of the qualitative investigation by MacIntosh (2003). The statement of purpose further emphasizes the rationale for a qualitative design and the focus of the study. According to MacIntosh (2003), "The purpose of this study was to explore how experienced nurses interpreted their development as professionals, what they identified about this as problematic and how they addressed the problems they identified" (p. 727). The author shares that although nursing education programs begin the socialization process, new nurses continue this process in the workplace where the ideals learned in school are very often challenged or met with resistance.

A qualitative format is important for this study, and the rationale for selecting grounded theory as the method for the investigation is stated. The philosophical underpinnings of grounded theory methodology are addressed. MacIntosh (2003) notes that the constant comparative method of data analysis described by Glaser (1978) was applied to this investigation. A particular strength of this study lies in the fact that the author provides a detailed account of method application. This is extremely helpful to the reader because it highlights the line of thinking by the author and the rigorous procedural steps of grounded theory investigations. This article is an excellent read for someone new to the method and interested in understanding its application to a particular area of inquiry. The data collection techniques applied in this study are consistent with grounded theory investigation.

Data were mainly collected through open-ended interviews to engage participants in dialogical interview relationships. Only six letters of invitation were sent to potential participants at one time to permit theoretical sampling throughout the data collection process. The researcher transcribed each interview verbatim and analyzed it before conducting additional interviews. The initial interview guide was modified when collected and analyzed data influenced the choice of questions for subsequent data collection. Simultaneous data collection and analysis (Glaser, 1978), substantive and theoretical coding (Beck, 1999), and constant comparative analysis (Glaser, (1978) identified relevant concepts, processes, connections and contextual connotations. Periodic review of all analyzed interviews provided perspective on all the data. No additional participants were sought when analysis indicated that data saturation had been reached. The findings were returned to the sample of participants in second interview. (p. 729)

Data analysis was consistent with grounded theory methodology. MacIntosh (2003) used the constant comparative technique to simultaneously collect, code, and analyze data. This is also very helpful to the reader, making clear how grounded theory methodology was applied in this investigation and allowing the reader to understand how issues of reliability and validity were addressed. All research activities, starting with data collection and continuing through the process of analysis, were done simultaneously, with the ultimate goal being discovery of the basic social-psychological problem or core variable (MacIntosh, 2003).

MacIntosh (2003) describes her findings in detail. She clearly describes how the core category was selected and the conceptual linkages associated:

The process that emerged in these data describe how experienced RNs address the problematic issues of dissonance as they become and sustain being professional. The name assigned to this iterative three-stage process is reworking professional identity. The three stages— assuming adequacy, realizing practice, and developing a reputation— occur when nurses encounter discrepancies that stimulate feelings of dissonance and work to develop strategies to address those discrepancies and reduce the dissonance. (p. 730)

Trustworthiness of the data was clearly addressed by MacIntosh (2003). The findings are theoretically significant. This research contributes to nursing knowledge about professional socialization. As MacIntosh notes,

... becoming professional involves more than graduating and earning the legal title nurse. [It indicates] the need to work consciously over a career to develop and maintain [nurses'] professional identity. This understanding can be useful in nursing education to help prepare nurse for workplace realities and to help nurses adopt active roles in developing their profession identity (p.740).

Her use of grounded theory methodology makes an important contribution to nursing theory development. Application to nursing administration is implied in that socialization takes place in the setting in which students ultimately practice. Nursing administration holds a stake in this professional socialization and must take active responsibility to ensure that the ideals instilled in nurses' educational programs can be upheld in their practice settings.

SUMMARY

G rounded theory as a qualitative research approach provides an excellent method of investigation for phenomena important to nursing. This chapter reviewed application of the method to areas important to nursing practice, education, and administration and offered selected examples of published research that applies the methodologies described in Chapter 7. There is a substantive body of knowledge emerging from grounded theory research. Recognizing the need for middle-range theory development in nursing, investigators should continue to apply this rigorous qualitative method to the investigation of phenomena important to nursing practice, education, and administration.

References

Brown, M. A., & Draye, M. A. (2003). Experiences of pioneer nurse practitioners in establishing advanced practice roles. *Journal of Nursing Scholarship, 35*(4), 391–403.

Campbell, S. L. (2003). Cultivating empowerment in nursing today for a strong profession tomorrow. *Journal of Nursing Education, 42*(9), 423–430.

D'Abundo, M., & Chally, P. (2004). Struggling with recovery: Participant perspectives on battling an eating disorder. *Qualitative Health Research, 14*(8), 1094–1106.

Dewar, A. (2003). Boosting strategies: Enhancing the self-esteem of individuals with catastrophic illnesses and injuries. *Journal of Psychosocial Nursing and Mental Health Services, 41*(3), 24–33.

Dougherty, C. M., Pyper, G. P., & Benoliel, J. Q. (2004). Domains of concern of intimate partners of sudden cardiac arrest survivors after ICD implantation. *Journal of Cardiovascular Nursing, 19*(1), 11–22.

Glaser, B. (1978). *Theoretical sensitivity.* Mill Valley, CA: Sociology Press.

Glaser, B. G., & Strauss, A. (1967). *The discovery of grounded theory: Strategies for qualitative research.* New York: Aldine.

Jones, P. S., Zhang, X. E., Meleis, A. (2003). Transforming vulnerability. *Western Journal of Nursing Research, 25*(7), 835–853.

Judson, L. H. (2004). Protective care: Mothering a child dependent on parenteral nutrition. *Journal of Family Nursing, 10*(1), 93–120.

MacIntosh, J. (2003). Reworking professional nursing identity. *Western Journal of Nursing Research, 25*(6), 725–741.

McNeill, T. (2004). Fathers' experience of parenting a child with juvenile rheumatoid arthritis. *Qualitative Health Research, 14*(4), 526-545.

Meeker, M. A. (2004). Family surrogate decision making at the end of life: Seeing them through with care and respect. *Qualitative Health Research, 14*(2), 204-225.

Milliken, P. J., & Northcott, H. C. (2003). Redefining parental identity: Caregiving and schizophrenia. *Qualitative Health Research, 13*(1), 100-113.

Parry, C. (2003). Embracing uncertainty: An exploration of the experiences of childhood cancer survivors. *Qualitative Health Research, 13*(1), 227-246.

Strauss, A., & Corbin, J. (1990). *Basics of qualitative research: Grounded theory procedures and techniques.* Newbury Park, CA: Sage.

Streubert, H., & Carpenter, D. R. (1995). *Qualitative research in nursing: Advancing the humanistic imperative.* Philadelphia: J. B. Lippincott.

Research Article

Family Surrogate Decision Making at the End of Life: Seeing Them Through With Care and Respect

Mary Ann Meeker

Family surrogate decision makers are pivotal in end-of-life decision-making processes. The author investigated decision-making experiences of 20 surrogates who assisted terminally ill family members for this grounded theory study. Findings describe a basic social process of Seeing Them Through With Care and Respect, during which surrogates continuously synthesized the core values of caring for their family member and respecting their family member's autonomy. Surrogate narratives began with Learning the Diagnosis. The major categories of surrogate decision makers' activities during the process were Standing With and Acting For the ill family member. Events reported in two gating categories, Brokering Information and Working With Family, facilitated or impeded decision making. A final category, Outcomes, reports consequences for the surrogate of having been a decision maker.

Keywords: terminal care; end-of-life decision making; family decision making

*E*nd-of-life (EOL) care in America has become a significant societal concern. With the increasing ability of medical science to sustain bodily functions (often in very technological ways) comes the need to make determinations about whether it is beneficial to do so. Highly sophisticated medical interventions, when applied to irrevocably progressive illnesses, might increase suffering of the individual as well as consume disproportionate amounts of finite health care resources. Difficult decisions must be made in complex situations. In recent decades, American culture has experienced a shift from acceptance of a paternalistic model of medical practice to an emphasis on patient autonomy (Yellen, Burton, & Elpern, 1992). In the United States, legal and bureaucratic structures focus on individual autonomy. However, the changing demographics of dying often include patients' being unable to speak for themselves. Decision-making responsibility usually falls to family members in those situations in which patients are no longer able to make their own decisions (High, 1994). Family surrogates play a pivotal role in health care decision making, yet little is known about

AUTHOR'S NOTE: The author gratefully acknowledges the assistance of Mary Ann Jezewski, R.N., Ph.D., and financial support from the National Institute of Nursing Research, 1F31 NR07569-01, 02; Sigma Theta Tau Gamma Kappa Chapter; and the Mark Diamond Research Fund of the University at Buffalo. Thanks are also extended to the family surrogate decision makers who participated in this study.
QUALITATIVE HEALTH RESEARCH, Vol. 14 No. 2, February 2004 204–225
DOI: 10.1177/1049732303260501

their experiences and needs. Surrogates' participation has often been neglected in the clinical setting, and much of the research attention has been directed to assessing their ability to predict accurately their family members' choices. The purpose of this study was to investigate decision-making experiences and the social psychological processes family member surrogates use for health care decisions as they related to decision making with and for a terminally ill family member.

Review of the Literature

The context of treatment decision making has changed over the past several decades. Progress in medical science has resulted in fewer natural limits on medicine's powers and abilities to prolong life (Veatch, 1998). As technological interventions have become more numerous, sophisticated, and effective, the nature of dying has changed. More potentially life-sustaining interventions are available, and more persons encounter protracted states of ill health in which they are unable to make health care choices for themselves. The need for surrogate decision making in health care arises more frequently, and the decisions are increasingly complex.

A second significant societal change is that the historical acceptance of paternalism in medical treatment decision making has given way to increasing concern with self-determination and the preservation of individual autonomy. Although advance directives (ADs) are regarded as "the next best way" of honoring patient self-determination when the patient lacks the capacity to exercise that self-determination directly, there remain many barriers to the creation and implementation of legally valid and effective advance directives. Only about 20% of Americans have formulated advance directives (Dexter et al., 1998; Goldblatt, 2001; Gross, 1998). The majority of those who formulate an advance directive designating a surrogate decision maker choose a family member, and when no directives are present, clinicians usually turn to family members. Thus, decision-making responsibility usually falls to a family member surrogate when a patient lacks decision-making capacity (High, 1994).

Although decision making by family member surrogates is a prominent reality in today's health care environment, family surrogates' decision-making voice within the health care system is weakened or, at least, brought into question based on empirical evidence that family surrogates cannot accurately predict the preferences of the patients they represent. In several studies, hypothetical vignettes were presented separately to patients and surrogates, and treatment decisions were elicited. The scenarios explored have often focused on life support decisions, especially those related to resuscitation and mechanical ventilation, and have most commonly been conducted with elderly patient populations (Ditto et al., 2001; Ouslander, Tymchuk, & Rahbar, 1989; Seckler, Meier, Mulvihill, & Paris, 1991; Tomlinson, Howe, Notman, & Rossmiller, 1990; Uhlmann, Pearlman, & Cain, 1988; Zweibel & Cassel, 1989). These concordance studies consistently revealed low-to-moderate accuracy between the patient's choice and the surrogate's prediction of that choice (Hare, Pratt, & Nelson, 1992; Seckler et al., 1991; Suhl, Simons, Reedy, & Garrich, 1994; Uhlmann et al., 1988; Zweibel & Cassel, 1989). Adding further concern about surrogate decision making are data revealing that surrogates' confidence in the accuracy of their choices was often higher than their measured accuracy (Hare et al., 1992; Tomlinson et al., 1990; Uhlmann et al., 1988).

In several studies, surrogates were more likely to choose interventions that the patient refused than to withhold wanted care (Ditto et al., 2001; Suhl et al., 1994; Tomlinson et al., 1990; Uhlmann et al., 1988). Some authors regard this as a "safer" error. Other investigators found inaccuracies equally divided between choosing in favor of unwanted care and withholding care the patient would choose (Seckler et al., 1991; Sulmasy, Terry, et al., 1998). Concerned with the potential of harm arising from family surrogates' limited predictive accuracy, several investigators compared the accuracy of family members to that of physicians. Physicians' predictions of patient choices were nearly always more discrepant from the patients' than those of family surrogates (Ouslander et al., 1989; Seckler et al., 1991; Uhlmann et al., 1988).

Patients and surrogates have reported using different decision-making criteria when presented with hypothetical scenarios. Libbus and Russell (1995) found that patients considered the ability to care for themselves to be most important, whereas surrogates rated amount of pain as their first criterion in whether to choose or forego a particular treatment. Patients ranked burden on family as third most important, but surrogates did not choose this criterion at all. These data on discrepant criteria employed to make a decision are similar to those found by others (Hare et al., 1992; Tomlinson et al., 1990).

One of the most consistent and clinically useful findings from this body of concordance studies was that prior discussion of EOL issues between patients and surrogates improved surrogate accuracy (Suhl et al., 1994; Sulmasy, Haller, & Terry, 1994; Sulmasy, Terry, et al., 1998). However, findings from a randomized controlled trial by Ditto and colleagues (2001) failed to demonstrate that surrogate accuracy was measurably improved by the presence of advance directives and/or discussion of those advance directives between patient and surrogate.

The issue of accuracy of prediction is only one element within a complex decision-making process. Despite the imperfect ability of family surrogates to match patient preferences (at least in hypothetical vignettes), family surrogates are usually the best available spokespersons, and their participation in decision making has become widely accepted over the past 10 years. According to Miles, Koepp, and Weber (1996), the validity of family surrogacy is not dependent on predictive accuracy. "The moral authority of a family proxy need not be contingent on their ability to recount or predict a patient's choice; the trust that lies behind their selection may justify their authority" (p. 1067).

The reported concerns, preferences, and needs of patients are broader than the issue of a substitute decision maker's predictive accuracy. Singer, Martin, and Kelner (1999) explored patients' criteria for quality EOL care. Two of the five most significant domains identified by these patients were family related. These areas of concern were relieving burden placed on loved ones and strengthening family relationships. Patients completing ADs viewed the advance-planning process both as a way to stay in control of their care and as a way to protect their families from excessive physical and emotional burdens (Martin, Emanuel, & Singer, 2000; Martin, Thiel, & Singer, 1999). The majority of patients studied placed greater value on discussing EOL care preferences with family members than with physicians.

Family members involved in health care decision making have consistently reported wanting as much information as possible about what was going on with the patient and what to expect (Jacobson et al., 1997; Tilden, Tolle, Garland, & Nelson, 1995). Family members valued consensus in making these difficult decisions and emphasized to researchers the importance of group versus individual decision making (Hanson, 1997; Pierce, 1999; Swigart, Lidz, Butterworth, & Arnold, 1996; Tilden et al., 1995). Many felt that the burden of functioning as the sole decision maker was too great. Nevertheless, legal and bureaucratic structures in the American health care system are oriented toward an individual decision maker. Clinical practice involves selecting a designated surrogate in those situations where the patient cannot make self-determined choices. Family member surrogates are called on to confront and somehow resolve the dissonance between a health care system reliant on individual decision makers and families' documented preference for group decision making. Clearly, great pressures can accompany this pivotal position. This study increases knowledge in the area of EOL decision making by my exploring the decision-making processes of family member surrogates as they respond to the needs of patients, other family members, and health care providers.

Method

To investigate EOL decision making from the surrogates' perspectives and understand the meaning of the role to them, I used grounded theory (Glaser & Strauss, 1967; Strauss & Corbin, 1998) for sample selection, data collection, and data analysis. Using grounded theory yielded a theoretical model explicating the basic social process inherent in the experiences and interactions of family surrogate decision makers.

I obtained approval to conduct this study from the Health Sciences Institutional Review Board of the University at Buffalo, the State University of New York, and obtained written informed consent prior to the start of each interview or focus group. I conducted all interviews and focus groups.

The purposeful sample consisted of 20 persons who had functioned in the role of family surrogate decision maker during the terminal phase of a family member's cancer illness. This study was restricted to those whose family member had died from cancer rather than from any progressive illness to increase homogeneity of the illness trajectory. I conducted the study in urban and suburban settings in western New York State. In addition to the availability of traditional hospital and home care services in this area, hospice care is available to qualified patients in their homes, in all area hospitals, and in a dedicated hospice inpatient setting. I recruited participants from bereavement support groups that are conducted on an ongoing basis by a grief counseling agency. A representative for this agency facilitated my access to these groups, securing the group members' permission for me to visit the group, describe the study, and invite participation. I also recruited participants by posting a notice to two University of Buffalo electronic mailing lists, yielding several responses. One participant was recruited through referral by another participant.

I offered participants the choice of individual interview or focus group interview. Sixteen persons participated in semistructured individual interviews, and 4 persons participated in a focus group interview. For the semistructured individual interviews, the interview guide began with a broad request to the participant to "tell me what happened during the time you were the surrogate decision maker for your (family member)." Further questions elicited data about the involvement of other family members in decision making, the role of health care providers, and how any difficulties that arose were handled. Sampling continued until theoretical saturation was reached and further data collection and analysis failed to contribute new information.

All interviews were audiotaped and transcribed verbatim. Beginning after the first interview, I coded data using the constant comparative method of grounded theory. I accomplished initial coding of data by reviewing each transcript several times to identify and label data with substantive codes that described participants' perceptions and experiences. As analysis progressed, I grouped conceptually related codes into categories and elaborated the properties and dimensions for each category. I conducted all data analysis, with methodological consultation provided by an expert grounded theorist.

As data collection and analysis progressed, I conducted theoretical sampling to provide data needed to describe the categories thoroughly. For example, because early participants were all reporting that other family members had been very supportive, I sought participants who had experienced conflict. I conducted the focus group after I had analyzed data from the first 10 individual interviews. Thus, I used the focus group interview for generating data to develop further and refine emerging categories and their properties. Following analysis of all data and initial model development, I conducted a group discussion with 2 participants to share the results of the analysis and seek validation, clarification, and refinement from participants.

Findings

The family surrogate decision makers' emic view forms the basis for the basic social process of Seeing Them Through With Care and Respect. All participants (20) in this study had served as surrogate decision makers for a family member who died from cancer. In two instances, two surrogates made decisions jointly for a family member and were therefore interviewed together. Thus, the narratives that constitute the data for this study describe experiences related to 18 dying family members (sometimes referred to as patients in this analysis). Of these 18 persons, 14 used hospice care at some point in the course of their illness. Nine patients died at home, and 9 died in an inpatient care setting. Of the 9 persons who died in an inpatient care setting, 5 died in hospice inpatient care, whereas 4 died in an acute hospital setting.

All participants except one were White. They ranged in age from 34 to 78 years, and the mean age was 56 years. Role relationships of surrogates and family members varied. In relationship to the patient, surrogates were daughters, wives, sisters, granddaughters, husbands, and sons. Sixteen participants were women. Nearly all participants were Christian. At the time of the interview, the interval since the death of the family member varied from 3 months to 8 years. The mean time elapsed since the family member's death was 3.3 years.

The family surrogate decision makers from this study engaged in a basic social process titled Seeing Them Through With Care and Respect. Table 1 provides an

Table 1 • Major Analytic Categories of Seeing Them Through

Learning the diagnosis	Standing with		Gating Categories		Acting For		Taking Leaving	Outcomes
			Brokering information[a]	Working with family[a]	Advocating	Protecting	Knowing/ preparing	Persisting concerns
Continued seeking	Active presence	Respect for person						
Shock	Supporting	Knowing/learning the family member's wishes			Accessing care	Treading lightly	Honoring the life	Satisfaction
Living fully in the interim	Vigilance	Empathizing/ understanding the meanings			Continuum of care	Taking over		Learning
					Hitting the wall			
					Honoring choices			

Note: Categories in italics are at the same level.
a. These are gating categories.

outline of the major analytic categories. Decision making was reported as an ongoing process, interwoven with the other activities and characteristics of the surrogates' lives rather than an isolated episode or event. Surrogates typically shifted into their role long before the patient's loss of capacity to self-determine. With this role assumption, the ill family member's needs and well-being became a primary focus in the surrogate's life.

Although the phases of Learning the Diagnosis and Taking Leave create the temporal boundaries of the process of Seeing Them Through, the phases of the theoretical model and activities described within it are not discrete and mutually exclusive, nor is movement through the process linear. During the course of Seeing Them Through, surrogate decision makers moved fluidly back and forth across the major categories. Standing With embodies the values and attitudes that prepared the surrogate for the activities of Acting For and that guided their choices and interventions in that phase. Exemplifying the integrated nature of the basic social process, surrogates often manifested the properties of Standing With and Acting For during the phase of Learning the Diagnosis.

Balancing Care and Respect

In the narratives of the family surrogate decision makers in this study, two common threads (respect and caring) provide a dialectic tension between the imperatives of caring for the ill family member and simultaneously respecting his or her self-determination. Much as providers sometimes struggle between honoring a patient's self-determination and acting beneficently, so, too, did the surrogates weigh and assess the pull of these two primary values. Consideration of both care and respect characterized all of the surrogates' reported activities in relationship to the ill family member. For most of the participants, care giving and decision making were inextricably intertwined. The surrogates consciously sought the optimal balance between respecting their family member's self-determination and providing for needed care. They attempted to allow and encourage the sick person to make his or her own choices to the extent he or she was able and desired to do so. Simultaneously, they attempted to facilitate or provide the amount and type of care needed. One surrogate exemplified this struggle as he described searching for the optimum level of involvement for his ill mother:

> I didn't want to over-interfere; I didn't want to be too pushy and say this is the way it should be and this is what I think. I didn't want to take away any of their [the parents'] independence or to think that now they're the kids and I'm trying to take over and make decisions, but it came to the point where I had to.

Learning the Diagnosis

The narratives of the family surrogates began at the time of the family member's cancer diagnosis. Learning the Diagnosis marked the entry point of the process of Seeing Them Through. This initial phase of the process was characterized by Continued Seeking, Shock, and Living Fully in the Interim. Many times, getting a diagnosis was complex, involving multiple providers, various difficulties, and much uncertainty.

Continuing seeking. This, when needed, was the strategy employed to learn the diagnosis. For example, one surrogate reported that she and her husband saw five physicians before a biopsy of a suspicious lump could be obtained and a diagnosis made.

Shock. The usual response to the diagnosis was Shock. Participants described their responses with language such as, "It was a shock to begin with," "It threw us for a loop," and "We were absolutely floored." Immediately following the patient's diagnosis, and within this context of Shock, surrogates and patients together sought information and made decisions about treatment options. Based on the information obtained, treatment or nontreatment decisions emerged from a synthesis of health care provider recommendations, level of trust in the provider, patient and surrogate prior experiences, and the anticipated extent of disruption of the patient's level of function and quality of life.

Living fully. Subsequent to the Shock of diagnosis and when the disease process afforded them enough time, many surrogates and patients took advantage of that time to do the things they wanted to do, manifesting Living Fully. "And I mean we went on vacations, we did everything." And another, "And we traveled, we did everything possible. We lived life to the fullest."

Standing With

During the process of Seeing Them Through, surrogates endeavored to Stand With the ill family member. Standing With was an orientation and a way of relating to the family member that was operative throughout the time from diagnosis until after the patient's death. Standing With encompasses the categories of Active Presence and Respect for the Particular Person.

Active Presence

Active Presence was an essential component of Standing With the ill family member throughout the course of the final illness and formed a key part of how the surrogates worked to sustain the ill family member during this time. Active Presence typically included being physically present, attentive, and responsive to needs, whether or not the surrogate decision maker was the primary caregiver. The two principal strategies for providing Active Presence were Supporting and Vigilance.

Support. Family surrogate decision makers attempted to Support the ill family member both physically and emotionally throughout the course of the illness. Surrogates attended visits to the physician and listened with the patient to information about the diagnosis and options for care. When the patient was cared for and died at home, the surrogate decision maker was usually the primary caregiver. As much as possible, surrogates did what was needed to meet their family members' needs. A strategy often seen in surrogates' efforts to Support their family members was to prioritize both the physical and emotional needs of the ill family member over their own needs. For example, one surrogate deliberately modulated her emotional response in deference to the patient's needs. She was furious with a physician who insisted the patient was getting well and that hospice care was inappropriate when it was very obvious that the disease was progressing and that the family member was dying, "which I was livid about but I didn't get too much into that because my energy needed to be open to what she needed, not to the jerk." Similarly, many surrogates reported neglecting their own need for sleep to stay available to their family member.

Vigilance. Active Presence also involved Vigilance, an ongoing monitoring of the ill family member's status and needs. Stated simply, surrogates paid attention to the family member, observing changes in status, responding to those changes when indicated and simply witnessing them when no helpful response was possible. One surrogate spent as much time as possible at the ill family member's hospital bedside, in her words, "watching over her."

Respect for the Particular Person

Respect for the Particular Person constituted the second major category of Standing With. Surrogates attempted to foster patient autonomy even though the family member's capacity for self-determination inevitably diminished as his or her illness progressed. Surrogates' Respect for their family member as a unique and valued individual was expressed through the properties of Knowing/Learning Patient Wishes and Empathizing. Surrogates attempted to ensure their own ability to honor the family member's wishes by Knowing and/or Learning what those wishes were. Empathizing and understanding the meaning to the patient of events and situations also conveyed surrogates' Respect for their family member.

Knowing/learning patient's wishes. For many surrogates, especially spouses, Knowing the patient was the primary source of information about their wishes. Surrogates described Knowing what the patient would want as simply going with the territory of being in a close relationship over many years. "My husband and I knew each other since the time we were five years old. We were always friends. So, I really had no hesitation in making these decisions for him at this time." Surrogates who were adult children of the patient also relied on their knowledge of the patient as a person. As expressed by a surrogate about her mother, "I pretty much knew what kind of woman she was and what she would go for and what she wouldn't."

Some surrogates came to know and understand the patient's wishes through recurring discussions of end-of-life care over time. Sometimes observing experiences of others triggered these conversations. One surrogate, talking about her mother, said, "She saw this woman that was in a wheelchair that was obviously mentally incapacitated and she said oh, she didn't want to be that person getting treatment, hooked up to an IV and whatever." For some patients and surrogates, these discussions were triggered by the illness experience. One husband related, "We had a lot of conversations like that. We would be sitting here watching TV, she would get tired, we'd just lay in bed, cat would get up there in between us. We'd talk about what she wanted to do." Similarly, another spouse surrogate reported, "We had talked about this in great depth. We kept saying, you know, this is what we would do. We don't want any extenuating circumstances, any feeding tubes, anything like that."

The third strategy for Knowing/Learning About the Patients' Wishes was to ask about them directly. The surrogates in this study wanted to be sure they understood the patient's wishes. As one surrogate commented, "I think that person has to be clear with what they want and they have to specifically tell you what they want."

Understanding and empathy. Surrogates frequently expressed Understanding of and Empathy for the ill family member, discerning the meaning of an experience or situation as assigned by the patient.

Out of their Respect for the unique person for whom they were caring, they considered how their family member would be likely to experience the particular situation. This enabled them to Stand With the family member more effectively. One surrogate declined to have her mother (for whom she was caring in her home) access hospice respite care despite the many care demands and the surrogate's own fatigue. Knowing her mother and understanding her concerns with being a burden, the surrogate perceived that her mother would have experienced being sent to another care setting for respite care as rejection. The surrogate resolutely declined to consider this option.

> That would have been some message to her that would have been a really hard thing for her, a really negative thing for her. She was always really careful about "not being a burden," as she put it, and that would have been some kind of rejection for me to do that to her or for her to go.

This surrogate's choice reflected Understanding the patient's meaning and also prioritizing the patient's needs above her own.

Sometimes, a surrogate decision maker was not able to understand the meaning of a situation or experience for the family member. When something did not "fit" with the surrogate's perception of his or her family member, the resulting confusion became a Persisting Concern. One surrogate, who described the ill family member as very realistic and accepting, reported that she hesitated to sign the Do Not Resuscitate (DNR) consent.

> But it bothers me, I don't know why she didn't want to sign it. She signed everything else, then maybe if I don't sign it, I'll live a little longer. Maybe that was the rationale behind it, I don't know. The only thing I can figure out, I don't know what was behind it.

Brokering Information

Brokering Information emerged as one of two transitional, or gating, categories in the process of Seeing Them Through. Brokering Information describes surrogates' activities in seeking and receiving information and the activities of conveying or providing information to others, including other family members and health care providers. In contrast to the patient-focused categories of Standing With and Acting For, the gating categories are not directly patient focused. Rather, they have a facilitating or hindering influence on the surrogate decision-making process as a whole. For example, when surrogates were able to obtain the information they needed and wanted, this information, considered in the light of respect for the particular person, guided the choices during the phase of Acting For. When surrogates encountered barriers to obtaining information, this difficulty impeded movement through the process of Seeing Them Through.

Obtaining information, conveying information to others, and using information to guide their decisions were important components of the surrogate's role. Sometimes, surrogates were involved as partners with the patient in pursuing needed information, and at other times they were representatives for the patient in this process. Surrogates would become intermediaries, seeking and obtaining information from providers and then conveying, interpreting, and explaining that information to the patient and/or other family members. Especially toward the time of death, surrogates sought information about what was going on and what to expect. Surrogates used this information to guide them and strengthen their capacity to continue to Stand With the patient through the final days and hours.

When needed, surrogates actively pursued medical information of two types: general background knowledge to enable them to understand events and options, and specific data from providers regarding patient status and choices. When there were knowledge deficits or barriers in either of these components, surrogates employed strategies both to improve their understanding independently and to obtain desired information from providers. On their own, surrogates read medical texts or searched the Internet for information. Some surrogates sought health care expertise within their personal network of friends and associates. "One of the biggest helps that I had was I had a friend that just graduated from pharmacy school." This surrogate sought guidance and clarification about medications, side effects, and interactions from this friend.

Health care providers, especially physicians, were the most common source of medical information specific to the ill family member's situation. When health care providers gave information to patients and surrogates in sufficient amounts and in a form that was meaningful to them, decision making was able to proceed smoothly, and surrogates perceived that they and the patients were being well cared for. Surrogates varied regarding the kind of information that was meaningful and useful to them. One surrogate wanted information in the form of statistical probabilities of various possible outcomes. Decision making was thwarted when he was unable to obtain this form of information. Some surrogates found it generally difficult to obtain information from providers. They reported things like "It was really hard to get answers sometimes" and "It was like pulling teeth to get answers from him sometimes."

Working With Family

The category Working With Family describes participants' experiences and interactions with family members other than the ill person for whom they were functioning as surrogate decision maker. Family members other than the ill person usually supported the family surrogate decision maker in the process of Seeing Them Through. However, difficulties sometimes arose in this area and made the process more difficult for the surrogate. The two gating categories, Brokering Information and Working With Family, share this characteristic of either supporting and sustaining the family surrogate decision makers in their role or, alternatively, creating barriers and obstructions, diverting energy and attention from the central tasks of Standing With and Acting For.

Other family members typically shared the journey of Seeing Them Through but played a less central role than that of the surrogate. Surrogates' interactions with other family members varied in two primary ways. The level of involvement on the part of other family members varied, and the extent to which the other family members agreed with the decisions of the surrogate varied. When family members were involved and supportive, group or consensual decision making occurred. Some families worked together, responding to the situation and making decisions as a group.

In other situations, family members were less closely involved in decision making but were supportive of the surrogate's decisions. For these families, an important part of the surrogate's role was conveying information to other family members. The surrogate kept them informed of changes and decisions. Emotional as well as instrumental support from other family members eased the burdens of seeing a family member through a terminal illness.

Many surrogates in this study reported high levels of supportiveness and assent on the part of family members regarding surrogate choices. As one surrogate stated, "My family was all very supportive of the decisions I made. No one thought I was out of line with what I was doing." Surrogates generally reported that family members were comfortable with them in the decision-making role. Surrogates' perceptions of the feelings of other family members included these comments from various participants: "They felt comfortable and confident and glad that they didn't have to do it," "I think that they were all glad to have someone doing this and taking charge of the situation," "I think partly because I had been in nursing . . . that seemed to reassure them that I would make the best kind of health decision."

Although reports of conflict among family members were rare, conflicts created obstacles and disruptions to the overall process of Seeing Them Through when they did occur. There were instances where other family members disagreed with the surrogate decision maker and argued for different choices. Strategies used in responding to disagreement from other family members included providing information about the patient's status and previously expressed wishes, Advocating for the patient, and Protecting the patient.

Acting For

As the demands of advanced illness increased and their family members' strength decreased, surrogate decision makers increasingly Acted For their ill family members. Acting For describes surrogates' interactions, primarily with health care providers, on behalf of the patient. During this phase, surrogates substituted for their ill family members. The two major properties emerging to characterize Acting For were Advocating and Protecting.

Advocacy

Surrogate decision makers generally perceived Advocacy as central and appropriate to their role and regularly Advocated for the needs and interests of their family member. The major properties of Advocating are Accessing Care and Honoring Choices. Frequently, Advocacy manifested as facilitating access to health care services in response to the family members' needs.

Accessing care. Accessing Care included choices about physicians, location for care, and symptom-relief interventions. Decisions included in Accessing Care varied dimensionally from major choices, such as aggressive versus palliative care, to day-to-day or hour-to-hour choices, such as when to phone the hospice nurse about a troublesome symptom. Some surrogates reported receiving very little guidance or assistance from health care providers in decisions related to Accessing Care. They found it necessary to Advocate quite proactively for their ill family members: "You know, it was just us [husband and daughter of the patient] deciding what to do."

Honoring choices. As surrogates Advocated for the well-being and needs of the family member, Honoring Choices was an important way in which they expressed this advocacy. Honoring Choices was a key influence in Accessing Care. In most cases, when the ill family members were able to make their own choices, this independence was preferred and sought by the surrogates. Sometimes, surrogates would offer advice or recommendations. The family member might follow the surrogate's advice or might not. Because they placed such importance on respecting the family members' self-determination, either choice was generally acceptable to the surrogate. As voiced by one, "She trusted me with those kinds of things, but she wouldn't always move on them, which was fine with me because really it is her decision."

As necessary, surrogates followed through on earlier decisions made by or with the ill family member: "That's just about what we did. We all had agreed on this." Although this study does not include data from the perspective of the patient, this is certainly one of the concerns about choosing a surrogate decision maker. People consider whether the surrogate will be able to honor their wishes. They wonder if the chosen surrogate will be able to follow through, possibly setting aside their own needs and their own grief (Jezewski & Meeker, 2003). The interview data revealed that Honoring Choices was a fully dimensionalized category, varying from a direct implementation of the family member's prior decisions, to honoring the patient's known goals and values in contradiction to prior written statements regarding the desirability of various interventions, to honoring the patient's choice not to choose.

Not everyone wanted to make autonomous choices during his or her final illness. As reported by her surrogate, one woman was aware of the extent of her illness and poor prognosis but wanted limited involvement in decision making. "She didn't want to make all of the decisions herself." Another surrogate reports that her sick husband did not want to know about his illness or medical outlook: "He wanted no reality about this; he just wanted me to take care of him and whatever happened, happened. After the chemo[therapy], he never made any decisions about his care." In both of these situations, surrogates were able to honor the family members' preferences not to make their own choices.

As surrogates accessed care with and for their ill family member, they encountered health care providers and services that varied greatly in quality. Providers' behaviors, as reported by surrogates, varied along a Continuum from inadequate to exemplary caring. The level of caring from providers had a profound effect on the comfort and satisfaction reported by surrogates, as well as on surrogates' perceived needs to Advocate for and Protect their family member. A smooth relationship with providers was characterized, minimally, by adequate caring on the part of the provider. In addition, an effective working relationship with providers was characterized, on the part of the patient-surrogate dyad, by a threshold level of respect and trust for the provider.

Complaints about providers were often related to impaired caring and, especially, failure to honor the individuality of the person. The extreme of inadequate caring was manifested as a failure to regard basic human dignity. When caring was insufficient for the surrogate to achieve respect for and trust in the provider, then surrogates tended to increase their Vigilance and increase their Advocacy in an attempt to Protect the patient from an uncaring provider or, at times, from an uncaring system. One surrogate reported a home visit by a hospice social worker who failed to provide a basic level of regard and courtesy. "She didn't have any knowledge of us at all. She really didn't know our names when she walked in." The surrogate declined further visits from this provider to Protect the dying family member from further distress.

When the level of professional care was sufficient, surrogates felt comfortable in allowing the provider to influence them and assist them in decision making. When care, respect, and trust were at threshold levels, then occurrences of conflict or discrepant perceptions between providers and surrogates could be negotiated and resolved. When a context of adequate caring was maintained, surrogates perceived difficulties as workable. Exemplary caring by providers resulted in surrogates' feeling supported and sustained, as well as feeling safe to express disagreement. When one surrogate perceived that whatever constituted life for her husband was no longer present and that the ventilator should be discontinued, the physician disagreed:

> I liked this doctor. I didn't agree with her, but I really liked her. She was a very kind and loving person. . . . She was the kind that when I said what I was going to do, we stood there and cried together. She was very loving. I just disagreed with her at this particular time.

This surrogate Advocated effectively and insisted that her decisions be honored. In addition to creating a safer environment for surrogates to act for the patient, exemplary caring enabled them to look back on their experiences with feelings of gratitude and comfort.

For most of the participants in this study who chose hospice care, doing so was precipitated by a crisis of some sort. They experienced a critical juncture of Hitting the Wall. Hitting the Wall was usually characterized by worsening symptoms for the ill family member and a concomitant insufficiency of care and resources. It was not unusual for the surrogate and/or his or her family member (as reported by the surrogate) to feel highly stressed by their circumstances or even desperate and overwhelmed. One surrogate could no longer manage physically to care for her husband as his mobility diminished. Describing her experience of Hitting the Wall, she reported talking to the doctor and saying,

> I don't know how to handle this anymore, you know, he can't get out of bed. I had the man next door come over and help me, and he says, you know, I mean he just about had to pick him up to go to the bathroom.

Protecting

As the family member's illness progressed, surrogates increasingly Acted For the patient by choosing action or, sometimes, inaction designed to Protect the ill family member. Surrogates made decisions whose primary intention was to insulate the dying family member from risk of harm or further harm, most often from health care providers. Despite a diversity of manifestations, these behaviors shared a predominant goal of safeguarding the family member. Varying with the situation as well as with the personality of the surrogate, the activities categorized as Protecting fell along a continuum anchored by the dimensions of Treading Lightly and Taking Over.

Treading lightly. Surrogates sometimes reported a perceived need to tiptoe, figuratively speaking, in relationship to the health care system or particular providers, relinquishing some of what they might like to have in an effort to avoid jeopardizing something even more critical to the patient's well-being. One surrogate found the conditions and environment of his wife's chemotherapy treatment to be "medieval" and yet would not consider changing physicians. He feared complaining or asking for things to be different, because pain relief was the highest priority and his wife's physician was reputed to be skilled and generous in providing adequate pain management. "You know, the thing about it, I was afraid to step on any toes because of the pain medications." Another surrogate voiced this same sense of vulnerability and the perceived need to Tread Lightly, "Boy, you are at their mercy, and if you don't say the right thing, you are afraid that they are going to withhold medication."

Taking over. Some surrogates reported very strong Protective efforts that can be categorized as Taking Over. Taking Over was manifested in both active and passive modes. One surrogate demonstrated both active and passive Taking Over in Protecting the family member and allowing for a peaceful death. This elderly patient was hospitalized and actively dying. Her husband was having a great deal of difficulty facing this impending loss. The surrogate decision maker (not the husband) allowed him to go home one evening, intentionally refraining from making him aware that his wife was dying. The surrogate knew the husband would insist on futile attempts at resuscitation and prolonging the patient's life. This surrogate Protected the dying family member by not speaking of what she knew to the husband, exemplifying a passive form of Taking Over.

In this same situation, the surrogate manifested an active form of Taking Over when she informed the nurses that the patient was dying, that they were to stay away from the room, and that there were to be no resuscitative efforts. Although there was no physician order indicating DNR, the nurses did not question these instructions. Despite considerable potential barriers, this surrogate effectively created a cocoon of peace and safety for the family member and then remained at the bedside, providing an Active Presence of care and reassurance and saying goodbye. At the time of interview, this surrogate expressed deep Satisfaction with having made this "letting go" decision as she did and having acted powerfully to Protect her family member.

When surrogates, despite their best efforts, were unable to Protect the patient from some perceived harm, they experienced the distress of Persisting Concerns. One surrogate was unable to Protect her family member from a lung biopsy she strongly believed to be inappropriate and harmful. The physician illegally and unethically obtained consent from the next of kin and failed to discuss the procedure with the designated proxy decision maker. Subsequent to this biopsy, the patient required mechanical ventilation until the time of her death.

Taking Leave

The final phase of Seeing Them Through was Taking Leave. This subprocess consisted of the categories of Knowing (Perceiving Terminality), Preparing for the Death, and Honoring the Life.

Knowing. Part of the context for surrogate activities throughout the process of Seeing Them Through was the surrogate's awareness that the patient was dying. However, this critical Knowing happened at different points in time, and for some it did not precede the actual death. One surrogate speaks about both the phase when he did not yet realize his mother was dying and later when he did. He described his feelings earlier in his mother's illness, saying, "I didn't realize the severity. So the way I felt at that point was, no, you're not going to die. We can't let that happen." Somewhat later, when he made the decision to call the hospice, he said, "I knew at this point it wasn't getting any better and she was declining really fast."

One surrogate experienced a sudden onset of Knowing. "One night, I was just sitting there and, all of a sudden, I just had this great realization that he was gone. Whatever made him alive wasn't there anymore." This surrogate went home for the night and returned the next morning to inform providers that all life-sustaining treatments, including mechanical ventilation, were to be discontinued.

Preparing for the death. Preparing for the Death was the component of Taking Leave that followed Knowing, or perceiving terminality. One surrogate bought burial plots where he knew his wife wanted to be buried. Although they had previously chosen the location together, the surrogate did not tell his wife when he carried out that decision. This activity was part of Preparing for her death and was also characterized by Protecting. In his words, "And I never told her after she got sick I went out there and bought two plots. I never told her that, but I knew where she wanted, I never told her that." The repetition in his report conveys the deliberateness with which he sought to Protect her from painful knowledge while making necessary preparations.

Honoring the life. Although none of the questions in the interview guide for this study dealt with funeral arrangements or experiences, surrogates nearly always spoke, unsolicited, about events subsequent to the death. What they reported was a carrying through of the category Respect for the Particular Person and Honoring Choices following the death. These were important closure events as their role as surrogate decision makers came to an end.

Outcomes

Several Outcomes were consequent to the experience of being a family surrogate decision maker as reported by the participants in this study. The most frequent and prominent of these Outcomes were Persisting Concerns, Satisfaction, and Learning.

Persisting concerns. For many persons in this study, an outcome of having been a family surrogate decision maker was the experience of persisting concerns. Persisting concerns were thoughts and feelings, memories about events during the time of decision making that still bothered the decision maker. This category includes anything that the participants identified as still being troubled by or still wondering about. For example, unanswered questions, guilt, and unresolved anger were all Persisting Concerns. Temporally, Persisting Concerns were part of the surrogate's continuing experience at the time of interview.

One surrogate worried that her mother might have given up and died quickly. The surrogate had spoken to her mother of needing to get care organized so she (the surrogate) could get back to her family in another state. "And I do feel really guilty about that. `Cause she just died so quickly and, you know, it is definitely something about her giving up." This surrogate identified a sense of having failed to provide Active Presence without limitations. "I wish I could just have given her the feeling that I was there for her."

Another surrogate was restricted by hospital staff from being at her family member's bedside as much as she wanted to be. She wished she had been more forceful in asserting her right to presence. "And I wasn't strong enough, you know."

When provider caring was inadequate, family surrogates reported painful memories, characterized by anger, regret, or disbelief. One surrogate, whose family member was sent for a CAT scan 2 days before her death, believed that the physician must have realized how close death was at that point. The surrogate could not comprehend the value of a scan and continues to regret that it was done. "I just don't know why he put her through that. . . .Why put her through that much more? It was really tough."

Some surrogates spoke about the process by which they resolved or determined to live with their Persisting Concern(s). They were able to acknowledge a painful sense of short coming and yet simultaneously regard the situation with a more accepting attitude that took account of the difficulty of the role, the impossibility of perfection, and the need to forgive oneself. As voiced by one of the participants,

> But knowing what I knew at the time, I did the best I could. I still rehash a lot of that. I always do the same thing at the end of the rehashing but knowing what I knew that day, I did what I really thought I should do and I wasn't going into things emotionally and that I was really trying to think them through and I think I did a good job. I think I did as good a job as anybody could have done. So, I forgive myself for the mistakes that I made.

Although this study did not include information from the perspective of the dying family member, Persisting Concerns were less when the family member was aware he or she was dying and was able to reach some level of acceptance of his or her situation, as reported by the surrogate decision makers. Those ill persons who acknowledged their impending death had the opportunity to express what they wanted, thus making it easier for the surrogate to Honor Their Choices. Indeed, one surrogate perceived that his wife's realistic attitude and acceptance of events was deliberately chosen to make things easier for him. "She accepted it [that the availability of effective treatment for her cancer was limited] like that. I think she was making it easier for me."

Satisfaction. Satisfaction, as an outcome, exists as a mirror image of Persisting Concerns. When surrogates felt that they had effectively fulfilled the requirements and criteria for Seeing Them Through, they experienced Satisfaction with the role. Despite the difficulties and challenges, none of the surrogate decision makers interviewed indicated they would have wished to decline the job. However, many were surprised by the demands and great responsibility involved.

Expressions of Satisfaction reflected the primacy of care and respect in the process of Seeing Them Through. When they were able to fulfill patients' preferences and wishes, surrogates expressed feelings of Satisfaction and consolation. One surrogate clearly expressed her Satisfaction and comfort in being able to Honor the patient's wishes, "And I had the, I don't know what you'd call it, good fortune or what, to know that what we did he approved of."

Similarly, when surrogates in some way provided excellent care, they experienced very positive feelings about having been able to do so. Sometimes family surrogate decision makers were able to facilitate healing in situations previously characterized by distress and discord. In these situations, surrogates experienced a profoundly meaningful level of Satisfaction. Following a difficult time characterized by conflict with the physician and his resistance to providing needed care, one surrogate, through her Advocacy and Protective efforts, was able to provide for a peaceful death for her family member:

> And that gave us back the feeling that we did make something right. . . .If I ever had to write a story about what was the best decision or what was one of the best things you ever did in your life, it would be to give my [family member] a quiet peaceful death with her family next to her.

Learning. Learning was another outcome experienced by family surrogate decision makers. Based on what they learned and experienced during their family member's illness, some decision makers would now do things differently. For some, future choices for themselves have been influenced. Others reported that they would apply what they learned during the experiences reported in the interview for this study in any future situations where they were again surrogate decision makers. Some participants reported attempts, since the death of their family member, to share what they learned during Seeing Them Through. They used their experiences to inform and help others. Those who had experienced high satisfaction with hospice care frequently reported suggesting this form of care to others.

Participants' changed personal attitudes and decisions occurred in both negative and positive dimensions. One surrogate would refuse all treatment if she were diagnosed with cancer because of her experiences with her husband. "Like I said, if I ever had cancer, I'll never have the treatment. Never. They don't take care of you." This surrogate was awaiting biopsy results at the time of the interview. Another surrogate expressed similar feelings. Having seen the consequences of his wife's chemotherapy, he would refuse cancer treatment for himself. In contrast, another surrogate experienced Learning something positive for himself: "I have no fear of dying now that I see the way she went."

Discussion and Implications of Seeing Them Through

When asked about their experiences as surrogate decision makers, participants in this study described a complex process of accompanying their family members through their final illness. Overall, their narratives described an experience of being drawn by unwanted circumstances into an arduous experience inevitably characterized by struggle and uncertainty. Ultimately, these surrogates can never know if they made the "right" decisions or the decisions their family members would have wanted them to make. Some remain unsettled by this uncertainty. All participants described a deeply felt sense of responsibility toward the family member and often characterized their role as surrogate decision maker with terms indicating weight and burden. The central importance accorded to the synthesis of care and respect in the thought processes and activities of family surrogate decision makers is unique to the basic social process of Seeing Them Through. The importance of care and respect in the basic social process enhances our understanding of the demands on and priorities of family surrogate decision makers by explicating the dialectic tension created by their commitment to these values.

Surrogate decision makers in this study moved seamlessly from making choices with the ill person to making choices for the ill person as the family members' needs and circumstances dictated. They synthesized the core values of care and respect in ways unique to each situation, patient, and relationship. In contrast to other studies of surrogate decision making, this study provides an enlarged and more inclusive view of surrogate decision making from the time of diagnosis through the patient's death. The process of Seeing Them Through was arduous yet compelling. None of the participants reported that they would decline the job if they had it to do over. This finding is consistent with that of Jacob (1998), who, in her study describing family member involvement in treatment withdrawal decisions, reported, "Although the emotional burden of responsibility for the decision was a common theme, no informant expressed a wish that he or she had not been involved" (p. 34). Seeing Them Through is characterized by effort and struggle. The process is also characterized by lasting, life-altering Outcomes for the surrogate decision makers.

The experiences and meanings of decision making for the participants in this study contrast with the perspectives presented in prior research focusing on particular decisions, such as consenting to a DNR order or ventilator withdrawal. The family surrogates in this study described decision making as one facet of a complex and consuming process of traversing the EOL phase with a family member. The surrogates' narratives reveal that they made multiple decisions, large and small, integral to their relationship with the family member and their commitment to easing EOL burdens to whatever extent they could. One participant contrasted health care providers' perceptions of decision making, for example, signing or not signing a DNR consent, with the actual experience of having been a surrogate decision maker. He stated, "But actually there are all these other decisions as well." Examples of these other decisions from his experience included whether to make a phone call summoning other family members, whether to bring the ill person to the hospital, and whether to administer or allow medication that would increase comfort but might hasten death.

Data from this study highlight the frequent neglect of the surrogate decision maker by health care providers. With the exception of hospice providers, health care providers generally remained focused on the needs of and interactions with individual patients and failed to grasp the importance of their relational context. As we are reminded by Brown and Stetz (1999), "Even though an individual person has the disease, whole families experience illness" (p. 195). Thus, it is important for health care providers to acknowledge the role and contributions of the family surrogate decision makers. Unless countermanded by the ill person, involvement of the surrogate needs to be integral to care throughout the course of illness and not just when the ill person approaches or enters a condition of incapacity. A synergy between providers and surrogate decision makers is possible that can enhance outcomes for both the patient and the surrogate as well as increase professional satisfaction for providers. Health care providers and surrogates share a common goal of supporting and assisting the ill person as well as possible through the final phase of life. Recognizing this common goal can facilitate what Emanuel (2001) has referred to as "synergistic empowerment" between providers and family members (p. 33).

Protection of individual autonomy in EOL decision making is multifaceted and complex. Findings from this study reveal several significant barriers, including disempowerment of surrogate decision makers in the health care setting. Providers often failed to regard surrogates as appropriate participants in decision making or to appreciate their multiple roles and the diverse array and magnitude of decisions the surrogates were involved in making. Surrogates frequently experienced vulnerability in relationship to providers, sensing a need to be cautious in their requests and interactions lest their family member's care be adversely affected.

Seeing Them Through involves great physical, emotional, and cognitive demands on family surrogate decision makers. Given this situation of heightened stress and vulnerability, as well as the surrogate's central role in assisting the patient, surrogate decision makers are legitimate recipients of professional care, yet rarely did they regard themselves as such, nor did, according to the surrogates, most providers. Clinicians' attention to the needs and roles of family surrogate decision makers can facilitate the process of Seeing Them Through. For example, information provided in meaningful (to the surrogate) and usable form is critical to the surrogate's effectiveness. Furthermore, through awareness of surrogates' perspectives, health care providers can help correct the imbalance of power that generates behaviors and compromises such as those of Treading Lightly.

Further study of family surrogate decision making processes is needed. The purposeful sample obtained for this study was racially and demographically homogenous and was restricted to persons whose family member had experienced death from cancer. Surrogate decision makers participating in this study were self-selected, and all data collection was retrospective. Future study could usefully include a prospective investigation of family surrogate decision-making processes and also include the perspectives of patients, nurses, physicians, and other involved family members. Such study could yield increased understanding of decision-making processes and the interactions and relationships of the persons involved in decision making. A fuller understanding of surrogates' experiences and needs is a critical prerequisite to effective interaction with and assistance for family decision makers. Both the protection of patient autonomy and improved health outcomes for surrogates depend on more sensitive engagement with family surrogate decision makers.

References

Brown, M. A., & Stetz, K. (1999). The labor of caregiving: A theoretical model of caregiving during potentially fatal illness. *Qualitative Health Research, 9*, 182–197.

Dexter, P. R., Wolinsky, F. D., Gramelspacher, G. P., Zhou, X. H., Eckert, G. J., Waisburd, M., et al. (1998). Effectiveness of computer-generated reminders for increasing discussions about advance directives and completion of advance directive forms: A randomized, controlled trial. *Annals of Internal Medicine, 128*(2), 102–110.

Ditto, P. H., Danks, J. H., Smucker, W. D., Bookwala, J., Coppola, K. M., Dresser, R., et al. (2001). Advance directives as acts of communication. *Archives of Internal Medicine, 161*, 421–430.

Emanuel, L. L. (2001). Palliative care: A weak link in the chain of civilized life. In D. N. Weisstub, D. C. Thomasma, S. Gauthier, & G. F. Tomossy (Eds.), *Aging:Decisions at the end of life* (pp. 31–47). Norwell, MA: Kluwer Academic.

Glaser, B. G., & Strauss, A. L. (1967). *The discovery of grounded theory: Strategies for qualitative research.* New York: Aldine.

Goldblatt, D. (2001). A messy necessary end: Health care proxies need our support. *Neurology, 56*(2), 148–152.

Gross, M. D. (1998). What do patients express as their preferences in advance directives? *Archives of Internal Medicine, 158*(4), 363–365.

Hanson, L. C., Danis, M., & Garrett, J. (1997). What is wrong with end-of-life care? Opinions of bereaved family members. *Journal of the American Geriatrics Society, 45*(11), 1339–1344.

Hare, J., Pratt, C., & Nelson, C. (1992). Agreement between patients and their self-selected surrogates on difficult medical decisions. *Archives of Internal Medicine, 152,* 1049–1054.

High, D. M. (1994). Surrogate decision-making: Who will make decisions for me when I can't? *Clinics in Geriatric Medicine, 10,* 445–461.

Jacob, D. A. (1998). Family members' experiences with decision making for incompetent patients in the ICU: A qualitative study. *American Journal of Critical Care, 7*(1), 30–36.

Jacobson, J. A., Francis, L. P., Battin, M. P., Green, D. J., Grammes, C., VanRiper, J., et al. (1997). Dialogue to action: Lessons learned from some family members of deceased patients at an interactive program in seven Utah hospitals. *Journal of Clinical Ethics, 8,* 359–371.

Jezewski, M. A., & Meeker, M. A. (2003). *Completing advance directives from the perspective of people with chronic illnesses.* Unpublished manuscript.

Libbus, M. K., & Russell, C. (1995). Congruence of decisions between patients and their potential surrogates about life-sustaining therapies. *Image: Journal of Nursing Scholarship, 27,* 135–140.

Martin, D. K., Emanuel, L. L., & Singer, P. A. (2000). Planning for the end of life. *Lancet, 356*(9242), 1672–1676.

Martin, D. K., Thiel, E. C., & Singer, P. A. (1999). A new model of advance care planning: Observations from people with HIV. *Archives of Internal Medicine, 159*(1), 86–92.

Miles, S. H., Koepp, R., & Weber, E. P. (1996). Advance end-of-life treatment planning: A research review. *Archives of Internal Medicine, 156,* 1062–1068.

Ouslander, J. G., Tymchuk, A. J., & Rahbar, R. (1989). Health care decisions among elderly long-term care residents and their potential proxies. *Archives of Internal Medicine, 149,* 1367–1372.

Pierce, S. F. (1999). Improving end-of-life care: Gathering suggestions from family members. *Nursing Forum, 34*(2), 5–14.

Seckler, A. B., Meier, D. E., Mulvihill, M., & Paris, B. E. C. (1991). Substituted judgement: How accurate are proxy predictions? *American College of Physicians, 115*(2), 92–98.

Singer, P., Martin, D. K., & Kelner, M. (1999). Quality end-of-life care: Patients' perspectives. *Journal of the American Medical Association, 281,* 163–168.

Strauss, A., & Corbin, J. (1998). *Basics of qualitative research: Techniques and procedures for developing grounded theory.* Thousand Oaks, CA: Sage.

Suhl, J., Simons, P., Reedy, T., & Garrick, T. (1994). Myth of substituted judgment: Surrogate decision making regarding life support is unreliable. *Archives of Internal Medicine, 154,* 90–96.

Sulmasy, D. P., Haller, K., & Terry, P. B. (1994). More talk, less paper: Predicting the accuracy of substituted judgments. *American Journal of Medicine, 96*(5), 432–438.

Sulmasy, D. P., Terry, P. B., Weisman, C. S., Miller, D. J., Stallings, R. Y., Vettese, M. A., et al. (1998). The accuracy of substituted judgments in patients with terminal diagnoses. *Annals of Internal Medicine, 128*(8), 621–629.

Swigart, V., Lidz, C., Butterworth, V., & Arnold, R. (1996). Letting go: Family willingness to forgo life support. *Heart & Lung, 25*(6), 483–494.

Tilden, V., Tolle, S., Garland, M., & Nelson, C. (1995). Decisions about life sustaining treatment: Impact of physicians' behaviors on the family. *Archives of Internal Medicine, 155*(6), 633–638.

Tomlinson, T., Howe, K., Notman, M., & Rossmiller, D. (1990). An empirical study of proxy consent for elderly persons. *The Gerontologist, 30*(1), 54–64.

Uhlmann, R. F., Pearlman, R. A., & Cain, K. C. (1988). Physicians' and spouses' predictions of elderly patients' resuscitation preferences. *Journal of Gerontology, 43*(5), 115–121.

Veatch, R. M. (1998). Ethical dimensions of advance directives and surrogate decision making in the United States. In H. M. Sass, R. M. Veatch, & R. Kimura (Eds.), *Advance directives and surrogate decision making in health care* (pp. 66–91). Baltimore, MD: Johns Hopkins University Press.

Yellen, S. B., Burton, L. A., & Elpern, E. (1992). Communication about advance directives: Are patients sharing information with physicians? *Cambridge Quarterly of Healthcare Ethics, 4,* 377–387.

Zweibel, N. R., & Cassel, C. K. (1989). Treatment choices at the end of life: A comparison of decisions by older patients and their physician–selected proxies. *The Gerontologist, 29,* 615–621.

Mary Ann Meeker, D.N.S., is a research assistant professor of nursing at the University of Buffalo, New York.

Ethnography as Method

As nursing research develops, so do the methods that are available to discover the meanings of health and illness as lived by individuals, families, and groups. Ethnography is an example of one of the methods that has received considerable attention, particularly as it relates to the culture of individuals and specifically how they experience their culture in times of health and illness. Nurses have used ethnography to study a variety of topics important to nursing, including the patterns that promote breast-feeding in one Native American community (Dodgson, Duckett, Garwick, & Graham, 2002); symptom concerns of women with ovarian cancer (Ferrell, Smith, Cullinane, & Melancon, 2003); and the experience of health care for Bosnian and Soviet refugees (Lipson, Weinstein, Gladstone, & Sarnoff, 2003). These are just a few examples of how nurses are using ethnography to better care for the people who are entrusted to their care. To fully understand why there is a demonstrated commitment to ethnographic research, it is important to look at the foundations of ethnography as a research method.

Social scientists share an interest in and a commitment to discovery. Anthropologists, as a particular group of social scientists, are committed to the discovery of cultural knowledge. Early in the history of the social sciences, individuals interested in culture found that the ways of traditional science were inadequate to discover the nuances of people who live together and share similar experiences. This inadequacy led to the beginnings of *ethnography*, a means of studying groups of individuals' lifeways or patterns. Sanday (1983) reports that ethnographic methods are not new. The ancient Greek Herodotus was an ethnographer who recorded variations in the cultures to which he was exposed. According to Sanday, Franz Boas's (1948) ethnographic examination of the Eskimo culture signaled the contemporary beginning of ethnographic study.

Anthropology is synonymous with the term *ethnography*. The product of anthropologists' work is ethnography (Muecke, 1994). As early as the 1960s, references can be found regarding the value of an ethnographic approach as a means to study nursing culture (Boyle, 1994; Leininger, 1970; Ragucci, 1972). Early nurse ethnographers embraced the methods of anthropology to study phenomena they perceived were irreducible, unquantifiable, or unable to be made objective. Leininger (1985) went beyond the borrowing of ethnographic methods to develop what she called "ethnonursing research." This chapter explores ethnography and discusses common elements of ethnographic methodology and its uses, interpretations, and applications.

ETHNOGRAPHY DEFINED

According to Spradley (1980), "Ethnography is the work of describing culture" (p. 3). The description of culture or the cultural scene must be guided by an intense desire to understand other individuals' lives so much that the researcher becomes part of a specific cultural scene. To do this, Malinowski (1961) believed that researchers must learn the "native's point of view" (p. 25). Spradley (1980), however, warned that ethnography is more than the study of the people; rather, "ethnography means learning from people" (p. 3). Spradley also pointed out that "the essential core of ethnography is this concern with the meanings of actions and events to the people [ethnographers] seek to understand" (p. 5).

Beyond Spradley's (1980) discussion of ethnography, there is a long-standing debate about what constitutes ethnography. Muecke (1994) suggested, "there is not a single standard form of ethnography" (p. 188). Boyle (1994) proposed that "the style and method of ethnography are a function of the ethnographer, who brings her or his own scientific traditions, training, and socialization to the research project" (p. 182). This debate has led to a certain amount of confusion about ethnography as a method and has further fueled arguments about the relative value of ethnography as rigorous science (Savage, 2000). More recently, Brink and Edgecombe (2003) suggested that there has been a "bastardization of [qualitative] research designs" (p. 1028), in particular, ethnography. Despite the disagreements and controversies surrounding the method, ethnography has and will continue to provide important information about the meanings, organization, and interpretations of culture.

According to Muecke (1994), the four major ethnographic schools of thought are (1) classical; (2) systematic; (3) interpretive or hermeneutic; and (4) critical. Classical ethnography requires that the study "include both a description of behavior and demonstrate why and under what circumstances the behavior took place" (Morse & Field, 1995, p. 154). Regardless of the school of thought or type of ethnography, use of the method requires considerable time in the field, constantly observing and making sense of behaviors.

The objective of *systematic ethnography* is "to define the structure of culture, rather than to describe a people and their social interaction, emotions, and materials" (Muecke, 1994, p. 192). The difference between classical and systematic ethnography lies in scope. Classical ethnography aims to describe everything about the culture. Systematic ethnography takes a focused look at the structure of the culture—what organizes the study groups' lifeways. Systematic ethnography is the framework used by Spradley, whose method of ethnographic inquiry is explored fully in this chapter.

The aim of *interpretive* or *hermeneutic ethnography* is to "discover the meanings of observed social interactions" (Muecke, 1994, p. 193). According to Wolcott (cited in Muecke, 1994), "Ethnography is quintessentially analytic and interpretive, rather than methodological" (p. 193). Interpretive ethnographers are interested in studying the culture through analysis of inferences and implications found in behavior (Muecke, 1994).

Critical ethnography is another type of ethnography Muecke (1994) described. It relies on critical theory (Fontana & Frey, 1994). Critical ethnographers do not believe there is a culture out there to be known but, rather, that researchers and members of a culture together create a cultural schema. Ethnographers subscribing to this tradition account for "historical, social and economic situations" (Fontana & Frey, 1994, p. 369) when reporting. Germain (2001) adds that "critical ethnography . . . is distinguished from conventional approaches by its focus on issues of injustice and social oppression" (p. 279). "Inherent in a critical approach is the understanding that through communicative practices and reflection, researchers and participants discern an absolute truth of the culture" (Manias & Street, 2001, p. 235).

These four types of ethnographies represent four philosophic positions. "All research proceeds from philosophy, articulated or not" (Germain, 2001, p. 279). Therefore, it is essential that researchers define their position before embarking on an ethnographic study. A researcher's philosophic stance determines what he or she will study as well as the framework for data collection and analysis.

In addition to the four types of ethnographies described, it is important to add the work of Leininger. Leininger (1985) identifies a specific approach to ethnography she calls ethnonursing that allows nurses to "study explicit nursing phenomena from a cross-cultural perspective" (p. 38). The goal is "to discover nursing knowledge as known, perceived and experienced by nurses and consumers of nursing and health services" (p. 38). The most significant contribution of Leininger's work is its focus on nursing as the phenomenon of interest.

Grbich (1999) also offers autho-ethnography as a type of ethnography that is gaining in popularity. Grbich states that this is the ethnography of personal experience. Using this approach, the "self is overtly and centrally positioned; the subjective experience is located culturally and theoretically; thick ethnographic description and other techniques of presentation capture its immediacy, combining its emotional, physical and cognitive aspects" (p. 167).

ETHNOGRAPHY ROOTS

*T*here is much debate about the historical beginnings of ethnography. Sanday (1983) proposed that ethnography began with Herodotus. Rowe (1965) suggests that the Renaissance marked the initiation of ethnography as a research method. Still others have indicated that Malinowski's (1922) study of the Trobriand Islanders marked the beginning of ethnography. Atkinson and Hammersley (1994) offer that the contemporary beginning of ethnography occurred late in the 19th century as individuals began to acknowledge cultural differences or "deviations from norms" (p. 249) and became interested in studying these deviations. "The application of ethnographic method by Western anthropologists and sociologists to the investigation of their own societies has been a central feature of twentieth-century social science" (Cole, cited in Atkinson & Hammersley, 1994, p. 250). Atkinson and Hammersley (1994) identified two key phases in the development of ethnography in the 20th century: "the work of the founders of modern anthropology and that of the Chicago school of sociology" (p. 250).

Boas, Malinowski, and Radcliffe-Brown, the founders of modern anthropology (Atkinson & Hammersley, 1994), were committed to anthropology as a science. These ethnographers focused on chronicling their descriptions of primitive cultures. "The prime motivation on the part of all three founders was the rejection of speculation in favor of empirical investigation, a theme that has always been a central characteristic of empiricism, but not exclusive to it" (Atkinson & Hammersley, 1994, p. 250).

The Chicago school's most striking feature was its limited "questioning of the relevance of natural science as a methodological model for social research" (Atkinson & Hammersley, 1994, p. 250). One of the most important influences of the Chicago school was the attempt by many scientists in the school to connect scientific and hermeneutic philosophies with pragmatic philosophies such as the one espoused by Dewey (Atkinson & Hammersley, 1994). According to Woods (1992), the University of Chicago scientists laid the foundation for field research. They saw the city as a "social laboratory" (Woods, 1992, p. 338) that exemplified all forms of human behavior and activity. It was here that the idea of "native" was expanded to include social groups of local importance.

Beyond these early developments, ethnography has expanded and developed to meet the needs of scientists using its varied forms. As Atkinson (1999) points out,

> . . . ethnography has always contained within it a variety of perspectives. As a whole, it has never been totally subsumed within a framework of orthodoxy and objectivism. There have been varieties of aesthetic and interpretive standpoints throughout nearly a century of development and change. (p. 465)

Today, it is the quest to discover cultures and behaviors different from the researcher's that drives the use of this method. It is an exciting, interactive, decidedly qualitative approach that appeals to its followers. As Hughes (1992) pointed out, "What is quintessentially distinctive about anthropology [and thus ethnography] is just [its] *species-centeredness* and holistic character" (p. 442).

FUNDAMENTAL CHARACTERISTICS OF ETHNOGRAPHY

Six characteristics are central to ethnographic research. Three can be claimed by other qualitative methods: (1) researcher as instrument; (2) fieldwork; and (3) the cyclic nature of data collection and analysis. The other three arguably are unique to ethnography: (4) the focus on culture; (5) cultural immersion; and (6) the tension between researcher as researcher and researcher as cultural member, also called *reflexivity*. These characteristics should be considered foundational to ethnographic research.

Researcher as Instrument

The study of culture requires an intimacy with the participants who are part of a culture. Ethnography as a method of inquiry provides the opportunity for researchers to conduct studies that focus on personal and sometimes intimate experiences of members of the culture, which is why the ethnographer becomes the conduit for information shared by the group. When anthropologists speak of researcher as instrument, they are indicating the significant role ethnographers play in identifying, interpreting, and analyzing the culture under study. The primary ways that researchers become the instruments are through interviewing, observing, recording of cultural data, and examining cultural artifacts.

More than just observing, researchers often become participants in the cultural scene. Atkinson and Hammersley (1994) suggest that "participant observation is not a particular research technique but a mode of being-in-the-world characteristic of researchers" (p. 249). Participant observation demands complete commitment to the task of understanding. The ethnographer becomes part of the culture being studied to feel what it is like for the people in the situation (Atkinson & Hammersley, 1994; Boyle, 1994; Sanday, 1983).

Ethnographic researchers, despite becoming part of the cultural scene, will never fully have the insider's (emic) view. The emic view is the native's view, which reflects the cultural group's language, beliefs, and experiences. The only way ethnographers can begin to access the emic view is by interviewing group members, observing their behavior, and collecting cultural artifacts.

The strength of participant observation is the opportunity to access information from the outsider's (etic) view. The etic view is the view of the outsider with interpretation. The essence of ethnography is determining what an observed behavior is or what a ritual means in the context of the group studied. Ethnography is the description and interpretation of cultural patterns.

Fieldwork

All ethnographic research occurs in the field. Researchers go to the location of the culture of interest. For example, Lipson and colleagues (2003) were interested in studying Bosnian and Soviet refugees' experiences with health care. Specifically, the researchers were interested in learning about the health, illness, and health care patterns of refugees in Northern California. The authors perceived this topic to be important for nursing. They took part in the informants' lives by going to their homes and participating in important community activities. These activities helped researchers better understand the culture of the people studied. Physically situating oneself in the environs of the study culture is a fundamental characteristic in all ethnographic work.

Cyclic Nature of Data Collection and Analysis

In ethnographic research, a question about the differences in human experience found in a culture usually different from one's own leads researchers to investigate those differences. As Agar (1982, 1986) has pointed out, one of the problems for ethnographers is that no clear boundaries exist between the similarities and differences in human experience. Data collected by ethnographers in the field to describe the differences and similarities lead to still other questions about the culture. Answering those questions leads to more questions. Therefore, the researcher is engaged in a continuous process of interviewing, observing, reviewing materials, analyzing those data, and returning to the field to do more interviews, conduct more observations, and collect additional artifacts. As Spradley (1980) and Spradley and McCurdy (1972) indicate, the study ends not because a researcher has answered all of the questions or completely described the culture, but because time and resources are exhausted.

Focus on the Culture

Unique to ethnography is the focus on the culture. Ethnography is the only research method whose sole purpose is to understand the lifeways of individuals connected through group membership. As Boyle (1994) stated, "Ethnography focuses on a group of people who have something in common" (p. 161). It is essential that ethnographic researchers strive to discover and interpret the cultural meanings found within a connected group. Unfortunately, culture is hard to define (Roper & Shapira, 2000). From a behavioral/materialistic perspective, culture is the way a group behaves, what it produces, or the way it functions (Roper & Shapira, 2000). From a cognitive perspective, "it is the ideas, beliefs and knowledge that are used by a group of people as they live their lives" (p. 3). According to Roper and Shapira (2000), the application of the two perspectives will help to demonstrate "what people know and believe and what they do" (p. 3).

Goodenough, as cited in Wolcott (2003), provides the following statement about culture:

> The culture of any society is made up of the concepts, beliefs, and principles of action and organization that an ethnographer has found could be attributed successfully to the members of the society in context of his dealings with them. (p. 5)

Wolcott sees the appeal of this definition in the fact that Goodenough views ethnographers as the individuals who attribute culture to a society. There are three reasons that Wolcott takes this position: (1) the value of ethnography is found in the adequacy of the explanation rather than in the method; (2) culture is not seen, it is inferred; and (3) the attention that ethnographers give culture is a job they have given themselves (p. 156). In light of these interpretations by Goodenough, it is the search for the meaning of culture that gives researchers the context in which to study and to offer their interpretations of what is seen.

Cultural Immersion

Another characteristic of ethnography is the depth and length of participation ethnographers must have with the culture under study. The researcher's participation has been called *cultural immersion*, which requires that researchers live among the people being studied. For example, if a nurse researcher is interested in studying the culture of families coping with human immunodeficiency virus in a family member, the researcher would need to immerse himself or herself in the lives of the families studied. The researcher would observe how each family functions inside and outside of the home, studying as many facets of their lives as the participants will allow. Participant observation would take months, if not a year or more, to complete. Based on interviews, observations, participation in the culture, and review of cultural artifacts, the nurse researcher would interpret and draw conclusions about the culture based on his or her discoveries while collecting data.

Reflexivity

Reflexivity describes the struggle between being the researcher and becoming a member of the culture. It also has been described as the need to have an ongoing conversation about the experience while simultaneously living the moment (Coffey, as cited in Pellat, 2003, p. 28). Although it is important for the researcher to remain objective and stay focused on the research, on some level, the researcher becomes a member of the culture. Through this type of participation, researchers must realize that they alter the culture and have the potential to lose their objectivity more than is typical in the conduct of research. Because of the prolonged involvement as a researcher and participant in the group, it is extremely difficult to maintain a *completely* detached view. Allen (2004) points to the tremendous difficulty in trying to maintain an outsider relationship when one is both a researcher and a nurse. She further questions the value of such separation.

The tension between researcher as pure researcher and researcher as participant has been discussed in many forums. How does one discover the emic perspective—the insider's view—without becoming a part of the culture? The struggle for objectivity in collecting and analyzing data while being so intimately involved with the group is a characteristic unique to ethnography. More than just objectivity is of concern, however. Also critical is the necessity for the researcher to be fully aware of the fact that just by being present in the culture, it is changed.

SELECTION OF ETHNOGRAPHY AS METHOD

One of the goals of ethnography is to make explicit what is implicit within a culture (Germain, 1986). "Ethnography aims to get at the implicit or latent (backstage) culture in addition to the explicit, public, or manifested (front-stage) aspects of culture" (Germain, 2001, p. 284). Cultural knowledge requires an understanding of the people, what they do, what they say, how they relate to one another, what their customs and beliefs are, and how they derive meaning from their experiences (Goetz & LeCompte, 1984; Spradley, 1980; Spradley & McCurdy, 1972; van Maanen, 1983). With these goals in mind, nurses interested in exploring cultures or subcultures in nursing or nurse-related cultures have the world available to them for study. Within the profession of nursing, there are many undiscovered cultures. An example of cultural practices within nursing that is implicit and has been made explicit through research (Wolf, 1988) is nursing rituals. Wolf (1988) discovered the rituals that nurses use to enable and protect them in their work with clients. Similarly, in Wright's (2002) study of hospice nurses, the author examines the qualities of the participants to better understand how those qualities enhance patient care. In her research, she provides a look at how what is implicit is made explicit within a culture. The use of the ethnographic approach provides nurses with the opportunity to explore the holistic nature of society and to ask questions relevant to nursing practice. The naturalistic setting in which ethnographic research is carried out supplies nurses with the view of the world as it is, not as they wish it to be. Fundamentally, entrance into the naturalistic setting in which the research participants live with as little interference as possible from outside sources provides a rich data source for exploring many nursing practice issues.

Nurses conducting ethnographic research must accept reflexivity as part of the research design. Reflexivity allows nurses to explore cultures within the paradigm of nursing, which values the affective and subjective nature of humans. The duality of being both researcher and participant provides opportunities to capitalize on insights derived from datum sources. "'Meaning' is not merely investigated, but is constructed by [the researcher] and informant through active and reciprocal relationships and the dialectical processes of interaction" (Anderson, 1991, p. 116). Anderson (1991) added that "field work is inherently dialectical; the researcher affects and is affected by the phenomena (s)he seeks to understand" (p. 117). Reflexivity therefore leads to a greater understanding of the dynamics of particular phenomena and relationships found within cultures.

When choosing ethnography as the approach to study a particular culture or subculture, the nurse should ask several important questions. Do I have the knowledge and skill necessary or the research support available to conduct a credible study? Do I have the time to conduct this study? Do I have the resources to carry it out? Will the data collected bring new insights to the profession? If the nurse researcher answers *yes* to these questions, then his or her study has the potential to contribute significantly to the nursing profession.

In addition to answering the preceding questions, nurses interested in ethnography should know why the approach may be useful. Spradley (1980) identified four primary reasons for using ethnography to study a particular culture. The first is to document "the existence of alternative realities and to describe these realities in [the terms of the people studied]" (p. 14). Much of what individuals know about other cultures they interpret based on their own culture. This way of thinking is limiting in that it promotes the idea that one truth—and thus, one reality—exists. For ethnographers, a description of alternative realities provides a rich and varied landscape of human interaction. Coming "to understand personality, society, individuals, and environments from the perspective of other than professional scientific cultures ... will lead to a sense of epistemological humility" (Spradley, 1980, p. 15).

A second reason, according to Spradley (1980), for using the ethnographic approach is to discover grounded theories. Through description of culture, researchers are able to discover theories that are indigenous to the culture (Grant & Fine, 1992). Foundational to grounded theorists' research is a belief that the only useful theory is one that is grounded in the beliefs and practices of individuals studied. The principle that research should be based on the beliefs and practices of individuals (cultural groups) studied is also foundational to the work of ethnographers. The major difference between the conduct of ethnographic and grounded theory research is that ethnographers wishing to develop grounded theory will advance the description and interpretation of cultural observations to a level that yields a description of basic social-psychological process. For a full discussion of grounded theory, see Chapter 7.

Germain (2001) supports the development of theory as a natural outcome of ethnographic study. She offers that "ethnography contributes descriptive and explanatory theories of culture and cultural behaviors and meaning. Within the ethnography may be identified other middle-range theories such as typologies and hypotheses for further study" (p. 281).

A third reason for choosing ethnography is to better understand complex societies. Early anthropologists believed that the ethnographic method was ideally suited to the study of non-Western cultures. Today, anthropologists see the value of using ethnography to study subgroups of larger cultures—both Western and non-Western. Examples can be found in nursing in the works of Haglund (2000) and Lipson and colleagues (2003).

The fourth reason Spradley (1980) offers for using the ethnographic approach is to understand human behavior. Human behavior has meaning, and ethnography is one way to discover that meaning. Such discovery becomes particularly important when nurses look at the clients' health and illness behaviors. Understanding how and why cultural groups such as Hispanics, elderly people, abused women, or the Amish behave in health and illness situations can assist nurses who care for these groups to better provide interventions so that they may enhance the health-related strategies already in use by the groups.

When nurses decide they will use ethnography to study a culture of interest, a parallel consideration will be whether they will conduct a micro- or macro-ethnographic study. Leininger (1985) called these study types "mini" or "maxi," respectively. Regardless of the terminology, the intent has to do with the scale of the study. A *micro-* or *mini-ethnography* is generally of a smaller scale and is narrow or specific in its focus. Schulte's (2000) ethnographic study of the culture of public health nurses in a large, Midwestern, urban health department is an example of a micro-ethnography. The study focused on one organization, a particular group of employees, and occurred during a 6-month period. Therefore, the study was considered a micro-ethnography because of its description of only one group, public health nurses, within one health department, and with a limited time in the setting.

Increasingly, nurse researchers are using the term *focused ethnography* to identify their small-scale ethnographies. Focused ethnographies have as their focal point a distinct problem that is studied within a single context with a limited number of individuals.

Focused ethnographies share with classical ethnographies a commitment to conducting intensive participant observation activities within a naturalistic setting, asking questions to learn what is happening, and using other available sources of information to gain as complete an understanding as possible of people, places and events of interest. (Roper & Shapira, 2000, p. 7)

Dodgson and co-researchers' (2002) study of sociocultural patterns that promote breast-feeding and weaning in an indigenous community is an example of a focused ethnography. In this study, the researchers focused on breast-feeding practices of the Ojibwe, a native American group living in the Minneapolis–St. Paul area of the United States. The individuals interviewed and the subject matter were very focused.

A *macro-* or *maxi-ethnography* is a study that examines the culture in a broader context, extends over a longer period, and is most often reported in book form. Magilvy and Congdon's (2000) and Lipson's (2001) ethnographies are examples of this type of study. These researchers observed a significant number of individuals over a period of several years with a larger scope.

Spradley (1980) further delineated the scope of ethnographic studies by placing them on a continuum. On one end are micro-ethnographic studies that examine a single social situation (nurses receiving report on one unit); multiple social situations (critical care nurses participating in a report on three intensive care units); or a single social institution (the American Cancer Society of Philadelphia). Moving on the continuum closer to macro-ethnographic studies, Spradley included multiple social institutions (American Cancer Societies of Florida); a single community study (Chinatown in San Francisco); multiple communities (Hispanic communities in East Los Angeles); and a complex society (tribal life in Africa).

ELEMENTS AND INTERPRETATIONS OF THE METHOD

A number of individuals have described ethnographic research methods. Early ethnographic reports were written by individuals who documented their observations of the cultures they encountered. Although many of these individuals were not trained anthropologists, they gave rich and vivid accounts of the lives of the people they met. Sanday (1983) pointed out that these recorders were not participants in paradigmatic ethnography. *Paradigmatic ethnography* consists of the range of activities completed by a trained ethnographer, including observing, recording, participating, analyzing, reporting, and publishing experiences with a particular cultural group. Sanday offered three traditions within paradigmatic ethnography: (1) holistic; (2) semiotic; and (3) behavioristic.

The *holistic ethnographic interpretation* is the oldest tradition. The commitment of researchers in this tradition is to "the study of culture as an integrated whole" (Sanday, 1983, p. 23). According to Sanday, the ethnographers who ascribed to this approach included Benedict (1934), Mead (1949), Malinowski (1922), and Radcliffe-Brown (1952). Although all four ethnographers varied in their focus, their underlying commitment was to describe as fully as possible the particular culture of interest within the context of the whole. For instance, "Mead and Benedict were interested in describing and interpreting the whole, not in explaining its origin beyond the effect of the individual on it" (Sanday, 1983, p. 25). Radcliffe-Brown and Malinowski were not committed to the "characterization of the cultural whole but to how each trait functions in the total cultural complex of which it is part" (Sanday, 1983, p. 25). Although the focus of both sets of ethnographers was different, the underlying commitment to viewing the culture as a whole was preserved.

The *semiotic interpretation* focuses on gaining access to the native's viewpoint. Like the researchers committed to holistic interpretation, the major anthropologists in this tradition did not share epistemologies. The two major followers of this tradition are Geertz (1973) and Goodenough (1970, 1971). According to Sanday (1983), Geertz views the study of culture not as a means to defining laws but as an interpretative enterprise focused on searching for meaning. Furthermore, Geertz believes that the only way to achieve cultural understanding is through *thick descriptions*, large amounts of data (descriptions of the culture) collected over extended periods. According to Geertz, the analysis and conclusions offered by ethnographers represent fictions developed to explain rather than to understand a culture.

Goodenough (1970, 1971) is an ethnographer who embraces the semiotic tradition. He does so through what has been described as *ethnoscience*, "a rigorous and systematic way of studying and classifying emic (local or inside) data of a cultural group's own perceptions, knowledge, and language in terms of how people perceive and interpret their universe" (Leininger, 1970, pp. 168–169). "Ethnoscience [is] viewed as a method of developing precise and operationalized descriptions of cultural concept" (Morse & Field, 1995, p. 29). Ethnoscience also is called ethnosemantics or ethnolinguistics to emphasize the focus on language.

According to Sanday (1983), Geertz's commitment is to the "notion that culture is located in the minds and hearts of men" (p. 30). Culture is described by writing out systematic rules and formulating ethnographic algorithms, which make it possible to produce acceptable actions such as the "writing out of linguistic rules that makes it possible to produce acceptable utterances" (Sanday, 1983, p. 30).

"The differences between Geertz and Goodenough are not in aim but in the method, focus, and mode of reporting" (Sanday, 1983, p. 30). Both ethnographers are committed to the careful description of culture. Geertz's method and reporting are viewed as more of an art form compared with Goodenough's method, in which the focus is on rigorous, systematic methods of collecting data and reporting findings.

The third interpretation is the *behaviorist approach*. Ethnographers using this approach are most interested in the behavior of members of a culture. The main goal "is to uncover covarying patterns in observed behavior" (Sanday, 1983, pp. 33-34). This approach is deductive. Ethnographers subscribing to this interpretation look specifically for cultural situations that substantiate preselected categories of data. Use of this interpretation deviates radically from the intent of the other two interpretations, which rely solely on induction.

Leininger (1978, 1985), a nurse anthropologist, developed her own interpretation of ethnography: ethnonursing. *Ethnonursing*, according to Leininger, is "the study and analysis of the local or indigenous people's viewpoints, beliefs, and practices about nursing care behavior and processes of designated cultures" (Leininger, 1978, p. 15). The goal of ethnonursing is to "discover nursing knowledge as known, perceived and experienced by nurses and consumers of nursing and health services" (Leininger, 1985, p. 38). The primary function of Leininger's approach to ethnography is to focus on nursing and related health phenomena. This approach has been an important contribution to the nursing field. Many nurse ethnographers subscribe to Leininger's philosophy and apply her method of inquiry.

SELECTING ETHNOGRAPHY

When individuals choose to conduct ethnographic research studies, usually they have decided there is some shared cultural knowledge to which they would like access. The way individuals access cultural knowledge is by making *cultural inferences*, which are the observer's (researcher's) conclusions based on what the researcher has seen or heard while studying another culture. Making inferences is the way individuals learn many of their own group's cultural norms or values. For instance, if a child observes another child being scolded for talking in class, the observer—without being told—concludes that talking in class can lead to an unpleasant outcome. Therefore, the child learns through cultural inference that talking in class is unacceptable. Ethnographers follow this same process in their observations of cultural groups. According to Spradley (1980), ethnographers generally use three types of information to generate cultural inferences: cultural behavior (what people do); cultural artifacts (the things people make and use); and speech messages (what people say).

A significant part of culture is not readily available. This information, called *tacit knowledge*, consists of the information members of a culture know but do not talk about or express directly (Hammersley & Atkinson, 1983; Spradley,

1980). In addition to accessing explicit or easily observed cultural knowledge, ethnographers have the responsibility of describing tacit knowledge.

Understanding the Researcher's Role

To access explicit and tacit knowledge, researchers must understand the role they will play in the discovery of cultural knowledge. Because the researcher becomes the instrument, he or she must be cognizant of what the role of instrument entails. The role requires ethnographers to participate in the culture, observe the participants, document observations, collect artifacts, interview members of the cultural group, analyze, and report the findings. This role requires a significant commitment to the research that should not be taken lightly. In addition, it requires that researchers regularly reflect on the impact their participation in the culture has on the data and analysis.

The step-by-step method of collecting, analyzing, and presenting ethnographic research, according to Spradley (1980), is presented to educate readers. Although Spradley's is not the only ethnographic approach available, it is presented because of its explicitness, clarity, and utility for novice ethnographic researchers.

Spradley (1980) identifies 11 steps in the conduct of ethnographic research. Box 9.1 summarizes these steps. The processes for data generation, treatment, analysis, and interpretation are discussed within the context of the steps identified.

Gaining Access

One of the first considerations when initiating an ethnographic study is to decide on the *aim*. Based on the *aim* of the inquiry, researchers can decide

---

Box 9.1

Steps for Conducting Ethnographic Research

1. Do participant observation.
2. Make an ethnographic record.
3. Make descriptive observations.
4. Make a domain analysis.
5. Make a focused observation.
6. Make a taxonomic analysis.
7. Make selected observations.
8. Make a componential analysis.
9. Discover cultural themes.
10. Take a cultural inventory.
11. Write an ethnography.

the scope of the project. Will the aim be to focus on a particular group or a particular problem of a group? Will you use a focused, micro- or mini-ethnography approach? Will you examine a single social situation? Multiple social situations? A single social institution? Multiple social institutions? A single community study? Multiple communities? Complex societies?

Once researchers have decided on the scope of the project, their next step is to gain access to the culture. Because ethnography requires the study of people, the activities in which they are involved, and the places in which they live, to conduct the study, researchers will need to gain access to the culture. This may be the most difficult part of the study. Because researchers are not usually members of the group studied, individuals in the culture of interest may be unwilling or unable to provide the access required. In other instances, researchers may be studying social situations that do not require a group's permission. For instance, if researchers are interested in the culture of individuals who come to the local pharmacy to obtain their medications, permission may not be required. However, if they are interested in studying the culture of health professionals in an outpatient clinic, permission is necessary.

Access is easiest when researchers have clearly stated the study purpose and have shared how they will protect the participants' confidentiality. In addition, offering to participate in the setting may enhance researchers' abilities to gain entry to social situations. If, for example, a researcher wishes to study the culture of health professionals working in an outpatient clinic, his or her willingness to participate by offering "volunteer" services while in the setting may improve the chances of obtaining admission. As a "volunteer," the researcher not only has the opportunity to make observations but also will become part of the culture after remaining on the scene for an extended period. Each organization or institution will have its policies and procedures, some more clearly delineated than others. It is strategically important that you ascertain early what those involved require both formally and informally to gain access. Gaining access using the appropriate procedures will begin to build the trust needed to be successful in the field.

Making Participant Observations

Actual fieldwork begins when researchers start asking questions about the culture chosen. Initially, the ethnographer will ask broad questions of the setting. Using the outpatient clinic as an example, the researcher might ask: Who works in the clinic? Who comes to the clinic for care? What is the physical set-up of the clinic? Who provides the care to clients who come to the clinic?

In addition to asking questions, the researcher will begin to make observations. There are three types of observations: descriptive, focused, and selective (Spradley, 1980). *Descriptive observations* start when the researcher enters the social situation. The ethnographer will begin by describing the social situation, getting an overview of the situation, and determining what is going on. After completing this type of observation, the researcher will conduct more focused descriptive observations. These observations are generated from questions the researcher asked during the initial descriptive phase. For example, while in the clinic the researcher discovers that nurses are responsible for health teaching. A *focused observation* is required to look specifically at the types of health teaching done by the nurses in the setting. Based on this focused observation, the researcher conducts a more *selective observation*. For example, the researcher observes that only two out of the seven nurses in the clinic conduct any health teaching with clients with acquired immunodeficiency syndrome (AIDS). A selective interview or observation involving the two nurses will address additional questions about why clinic staff members behave as they do.

Neophyte ethnographers should not be led to believe that they conduct observations and interviews in the linear manner just described. Rather, broad, focused, or selective questions may arise out of any observation. Furthermore, the intent of an observation is not to merely "look at" something. More accurately, through observation while in the setting, researchers look, listen, ask questions, collect artifacts, and analyze data collected in a cyclic manner.

At any given time, ethnographers may be more or less involved in the social situation. For example, when the outpatient clinic is busy, the researcher as volunteer may be quite involved as a participant in the culture. At times of lesser traffic, the researcher may spend more time observing or interviewing. Explicit rules for when to participate and when to observe are not available. Researchers, the *actors* (members of the culture studied), and the activity determine the degree of participation in the social situation.

Roper and Shapira (2000) offer that "relying on personal observations alone can be misleading" (p. 70). It will be essential that all interpretations of observations be validated through other collected information. The researcher must be always aware of the fact that all individuals view social situations through their own cultural lenses. Therefore, cross-comparison of data is fundamental. Brink and Edgecombe (2003) recently observed the number of published ethnographic studies that use only one data collection strategy. It is critical for the neophyte ethnographer to understand the necessity of using varying data collection strategies to provide a rich cross-comparison of information collected.

Making the Ethnographic Record

On completion of each observation, ethnographers are responsible for documenting the experience. Documents generated from the observations are called *field notes*. Researchers may manage field notes by handwriting and storing them manually or by using computer programs to store and categorize data. A number of data storage, retrieval, and analysis software programs are available (see Chapter 3). Researchers who do not have a computer or are more comfortable documenting their observations in writing may use handwritten notes they organize in file boxes. These notes will chronicle what the researchers have seen and heard, answers to questions they asked, and created or collected artifacts. In addition, the field notes can be used to describe the researchers' reflections on what is seen and heard and how their presence may be affecting the data collection.

In the clinic, for example, the researcher may observe the physical layout. Based on the observation, the researcher may ask questions related to what happens in each room. A floor plan (artifact) may become part of the record. The researcher may also take photographs to document the colors of the clinic or the decorations used. These artifacts may offer important insights as the study continues.

It is important throughout the study—but especially in the beginning— not to focus too soon and also not to assume that any comment, artifact, or interaction is incidental. Researchers should document experiences to create a thick or rich description of the culture. In the outpatient example, the researcher should document the colors of the clinic. This observation may seem incidental; however, if a staff member later reports that it is important to maintain a calm atmosphere in the clinic because of the types of clients seen, then the choice of the color may be an artifact that supports this belief system.

In addition to recording explicit details of a situation, ethnographers also will record personal insights. A wide-angle view of the situation will provide the opportunity to detail what participants have said and to share what may be implicit in the situation. Using a wide-angle lens to view a situation provides ethnographers with a larger view of what is actually occurring in a social situation. For example, if an ethnographer is interested in observing a change-of-shift report and attends the report with the purpose of investigating the nurses' interactions, the researcher may miss valuable information regarding the report. With a wide-angle approach, the ethnographer would observe all individuals, activities, and artifacts that are part of the social situation, rather than merely focus on the interactions between the nurses in the report. Attention to all parts of the social situation will contribute to a richer description of the cultural scene. Once the researcher has a good grasp of the *wide-angle view*, then more focused and selective observations can take place.

Spradley (1980) offers three principles researchers should consider as they document their observations: "the language identification principle, the verbatim principle, and the concrete principle" (p. 65). The *language identification principle* requires that ethnographers identify in whose language the text is written. Spradley (1980) has pointed out that the most frequently recorded language is the *amalgamated language* (see Example 9.2), that is, the use of the ethnographer's language as well as the informants' language. For example, a nurse ethnographer recording his or her observations of a clinic day might choose to mix the answers to questions with personal observations. Such mixing may create problems when data analysis begins because the researcher can lose sight of the cultural meaning of the observation. To minimize the potential of this happening, entries should identify the person making the remarks. Example 9.1 illustrates the correct way to record field notes. In Example 9.2, the record does not describe how the researcher obtained specific information. It is difficult to decipher whether the notes are the researcher's interpretations or whether the researcher obtained the information directly from the informants.

Example 9.1

Field Note Entry No. 1	July 2, 2005

| Ethnographer | Today when I visited the clinic, I noticed that the walls were painted blue. I asked the receptionist who had done the decorating. |
| Receptionist | "We had several meetings with the decorator." |

Example 9.2

Field Note Entry No. 1	July 2, 2005

Today I observed the clinic waiting area. The area is painted in a pale blue. The chairs are wood and fabric. The fabric is a white-and-blue print, which contrasts with the wallpaper. The waiting area is very busy. The colors have an effect on the clients. They come in looking very harassed, then they fall asleep. A decorator helped with the colors.

Although Example 9.1 is a limited notation, readers can get a sense of how researchers should report field notes to facilitate analysis. In this example, the receptionist's response gives the ethnographer clear information about the decorating. The use of the word *we* in Example 9.1 gives the researcher insight into the interactions occurring among staff members. Although Example 9.2 offers significant information, the researcher will find it difficult, after long months of data collection, to return to this note and distinguish his or her insights from factual information obtained from the informants.

The reporting of the receptionist's comments in Example 9.1 reflects the *verbatim principle*, which requires ethnographers to use the speaker's exact words. To adhere to this principle, researchers may use audiotaping, which not only offers ethnographers verbatim accounts of conversation but also affords them an extensive accounting of an interaction that will provide the material for intensive analysis. Documenting verbatim statements also provides researchers with a view of native expressions. In Example 9.1, the use of verbatim documentation allows the researcher to gain insight into the language. The receptionist's use of the word *we* to describe the activities with the decorator may provide valuable insights into the culture of the clinic. The *concrete principle* requires that ethnographers document without interpretation what they have seen and heard. Generalizations and interpretations may limit access to valuable cultural insights. To reduce interpretation, researchers should document observations with as much detail as possible. Example 9.3 offers an example of concrete documentation without interpretation or generalization. In this example, documentation is clear. The researcher has recorded facts and conversation verbatim.

Example 9.3

Field Note Entry No. 1	July 2, 2005

The clinic waiting area is painted ocean blue. The ladder-back chairs are light brown wood with upholstered seats. The fabric on the seats is an ocean blue-and-white checkered pattern. There are two small 2-ft by 3-ft by 2½-ft brown wooden tables between the six chairs in the waiting room. There are two chairs along one wall with a table in the corner. Then, two chairs along the second wall with another table in the corner. The third wall has the two remaining chairs. The room is an 8-ft by 9-ft rectangle. Each table has a ginger jar lamp. The lamp base and shade are white. The fourth wall has a door and window in it. The draperies on the window are floor length and match the pattern on the chairs.

Individuals enter the clinic, approach the receptionist, state their names, sit in the chairs, and close their eyes. Some patients snore.

Ethnographer   "The colors in this room are great. Everything seems to go together so well. Who did the decorating?"

Receptionist   "We had several meetings with the decorator."

Making Descriptive Observations

Every time ethnographers are in a social situation, they generally will make descriptive observations without having specific questions in mind. General questions, which guide this type of observation, are *grand tour questions*. For example, a grand tour question that might initiate a study of a particular clinic is the following: How do people who live in this neighborhood receive health care? Remembering that the primary foci of all observations include the actors, activities, and artifacts will assist in the development of grand tour questions.

Spradley (1980) has identified nine major dimensions to any social situation:

1. *Space* refers to the physical place or places where the culture of interest carries out social interactions. In the outpatient clinic example, space would include the physical layout of the care delivery site.

2. *Actors* are people who are part of the culture under investigation. In the clinic example, the nurses, physicians, clients, maintenance workers, secretarial and receptionist staff, and family members of clients in the clinic would be the actors.

3. The *activities* are the actions by members of the culture. In the clinic example, activities would include the treatments provided to clients and conversations between cultural group members.

4. *Objects* in the clinic example would include artifacts such as implements used for care, pamphlets read by clients, staff records, and meeting minutes. Any inanimate object included in the space under study may give insight into the culture.

5. Any single action carried out by group members is an *act*. An example of an act observed in the clinic would be the locking of the medicine cabinet.

6. An *event* is a set of related activities carried out by members of the culture. In the clinic example, the ethnographer one day may observe the staff giving a birthday party for a long-time client.

7. It is important that the researcher document the *time* he or she made observations and when activities occurred during those times. In addition to recording time, the researcher must relate the effect time has on all nine dimensions of social situations.

8. *Goal* relates specifically to what group members hope to achieve. The clinic example illustrates how painting the clinic blue may be a way for the staff to relate their intention to create a calming effect on clients, who often must wait long periods.

9. The researcher should also record *feelings* for each social situation, including the emotions expressed or observed. For example, during the staff-given birthday party for a long-time client, the ethnographer might observe tears from the client, cheers by the staff, and anger by a family member. Recording feelings provides a rich framework from which to make cultural inferences.

The nine dimensions can be useful in guiding observations and questions related to social situations. It is beneficial to plot the nine dimensions in a matrix (Spradley, 1980) to contrast each dimension. For example, in addition to describing the space where the culture carries out its interactions, researchers should relate space to object, act, activity, event, time, actor, goal, and feelings. What does the space look like?

> What are all the ways space is organized by objects? What are all the ways space is organized by acts? What are all the ways space is organized by activities? What are all the ways space is organized by events? What spatial changes occur over time? What are all the ways space is used by actors? What are all the ways space is related to goals? What places are associated with feelings? (Spradley, 1980, pp. 82–83)

Critical ethnographers would add the dimensions of social and political climate to Spradley's (1980) list. It is extremely important that researchers consider issues of power, social class, and politics to get a full view of the culture. In the clinic example, the researcher might ask the following questions: Why are women the providers of intimate care? Does the male doctor ultimately make all the decisions? If so, why? Once researchers have collected data on all dimensions and have related each piece of data to other information, they can begin to focus further observations.

Making a Domain Analysis

Throughout data collection, ethnographers are required to analyze data. Analyzing data while in the field helps to structure later encounters with the social group of interest. Ethnographic data "analysis is a search for patterns" (Spradley, 1980, p. 85). These patterns make up the culture.

To begin to understand cultural meaning, ethnographers must analyze social situations they observe. A social situation is not the same as the concept of culture but, rather, "refers to the stream of behavior (activities) carried out by people (actors) in a particular location (place)" (Spradley, 1980, p. 86). Analysis of the social situation will lead to discovery of the cultural scene. *Cultural scene*, an ethnographic term, refers to the culture under study (Spradley, 1980). The first step in analysis is to do a domain analysis. Ethnographers doing a domain analysis focus on a particular situation.

In the outpatient clinic example, the category—people in the clinic—is the first domain the researcher must analyze. The researcher should ask, Who are the people in the clinic? Reviewing the field notes, the people in the clinic should be easy to identify (Figure 9.1). Spradley (1980) has suggested it is important to identify the semantic relationships in the observations made. For example, x is a kind of y: Nurses are kinds of people in the clinic. Furthermore, the researcher can do another analysis to explore the types of nurses who work in the clinic. Hammersley and Atkinson (1983) have approached analysis somewhat differently. They recommend researchers generate concept categories, refining them further into subcategories. Regardless of the method used, it is essential that researchers work to discover the cultural meaning for people, places, artifacts, and activities. Creating as extensive a list as possible of categories will assist in discovery. To maintain inclusiveness, return to the dimensions described earlier in this chapter. Generating domain analyses leads ethnographers to ask additional questions and make further observations to explore the roles and relationships of the cultural group members.

Making Focused Observations

Based on the completed domain analysis, ethnographers will need to make new observations and collect additional material. The domain analysis should

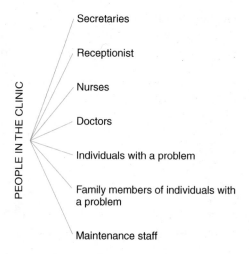

Figure 9.1.

be the impetus for the next round of observations. Researchers identify the domain categories that need development and then return to the research site. In the clinic example, based on the identification of different types of nurses in the clinic, the ethnographer would want to focus on the different types of nurses and discover their specific roles and activities. This information can provide important insight into the culture.

Making a Taxonomic Analysis

The taxonomic analysis is a more in-depth analysis of the domains researchers have previously selected. Researchers are searching for larger categories to which the domain may belong. In the clinic example, "nurses in the clinic" is a category identified in the domain analysis. Nurses are a type of people in the clinic. In addition, there are other types of nurses. Nurses can be categorized based on their educational backgrounds: licensed practical nurses (LPNs), registered nurses (RNs), nurse practitioners (NPs), and clinical nurse specialists (CNSs). These categories may be broken down further based on the focus of clients for whom the nurses care in the particular culture under study (Figure 9.2).

On completion of this analysis, ethnographers will look for relationships among the parts or relationships to the whole. Based on these new categories, researchers will make additional observations and ask more questions. In the clinic example, the researcher might ask, Why do the RNs have the primary responsibility for care of the clients with AIDS and sexually transmitted

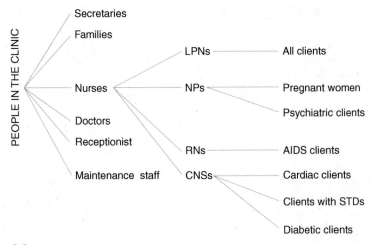

Figure 9.2.

diseases (STDs)? Are there different types of AIDS clients, and are they cared for by specific RNs? Are AIDS clients treated differently from the clients with STDs? Are other nurses consulted regarding the care of these two groups of clients? Are the nurses able to select the types of clients for whom they care?

Clearly, the researcher will generate a number of questions from this taxonomic analysis of the concept *nurse*. In addition to using a reductive exercise, ethnographers should try to discover whether there are larger categories for which they have not accounted. In the clinic example, are the people in the clinic part of a larger system? If the clinic is affiliated with a hospital or a community-based organization, then the answer is *yes*. The nurse ethnographer will then need to ask further questions based on this association and conduct focused interviews to validate whether the previously derived larger or smaller categorizations are accurate.

Making Selective Observations

Through selective observations, researchers will further refine the data they have collected. Selective observations will help to identify the "dimensions of contrast" (Spradley, 1980, p. 128). Spradley offers several types of questions that will help researchers discern the differences in the dimensions of contrast. The *dyadic question* seeks to identify the differences between two domains. The question is, In what way are these two things different? In the clinic example, one of the questions the researcher should ask is, In what ways are NPs and CNSs different? *Triadic contrast questions* seek to identify how three categories are related. The researcher in the clinic example might ask, Of the three—NPs, CNSs, and RNs—which two are more alike than the third? *Card-sorting contrast questions* allow ethnographers to place the domains on cards and sort them into piles based on their similarities. This also can be managed by specific computer software applications (see Chapter 3). By identifying the similarities, the contrasts become easily recognizable. Asking these questions of the available data will lead ethnographers to the setting to ask still other questions.

Making a Componential Analysis

"Componential analysis is the systematic search for attributes associated with cultural categories" (Spradley, 1980, p. 131). Boyle (1994) indicates that componential analysis has two objectives: to specify the conditions under which participants name something and to understand under what conditions the participants give something a specific name. Componential analysis is language driven.

During this stage of analysis, researchers are looking for units of meaning. Each unit of meaning is considered an attribute of the culture. Again, researchers are searching for missing data. During componential analysis, they examine each domain for its component parts and ask questions to identify the dimensions of contrast. Based on the identification of missing data, the researchers will make selected observations. Table 9.1 is an example of simple componential analysis that illustrates dimensions of contrast based on the sorting of people who work in the outpatient clinic. In the clinic example, the ethnographer is able to determine that unlicensed personnel do not provide health care. This analysis helps the researcher to begin to identify a hierarchical structure. He or she must validate conclusions through selective interviews and observations. The purpose of using this process is to search for contrasts, sort them out, and then group them based on similarities and

	Dimensions of Contrast		
Domain	*Licensed*	*Supervised Personnel*	*Health Care Provider*
Doctors	Yes	No	Yes
Nurses	Yes	Yes	Yes
Receptionist	No	Yes	No
Maintenance staff	No	Yes	No
Secretaries	No	Yes	No

Table 9.1 • Dimensions of Contrast

differences. This activity provides ethnographers with important information regarding the culture under study.

To fully carry out a componential analysis, ethnographers should move through the process in a sequential manner. The eight steps of the procedure are as follows: (1) select a domain for analysis (people who work in the clinic); (2) inventory previously discovered contrasts (some members are licensed, have supervisors to whom they report, and provide health care); (3) prepare the worksheet (this is called a *paradigm*); (4) classify dimensions of contrast that have binary values (licensed, yes or no); (5) combine related dimensions of contrast into ones that have multiple values (doctors and nurses are licensed personnel who provide health care); (6) prepare contrast questions for missing attributes (Are doctors the owners of the clinic because they appear not to have a reporting relationship?); (7) conduct selective observations and interviews to discover missing data and confirm or discard hypotheses; (8) prepare a complete paradigm (Spradley, 1980). "The final paradigm can be used as a chart in [the] ethnography" (p. 139). Although every attribute will not be discussed on the chart, important ones can be, allowing ethnographers to present a large amount of information in a concise and clear manner (Spradley, 1980).

PERFORMING DATA ANALYSIS

*A*lthough data analysis occurs throughout data collection, the next two stages—discovering cultural themes and taking a cultural inventory—focus solely on data analysis.

Discovering Cultural Themes

The discovery of cultural themes requires ethnographers to carefully examine the data collected and identify recurrent patterns. Whether tacit or explicit, the patterns constitute the culture.

To complete the theme analysis, researchers must become immersed in the data, which requires focused concentration over an extended period. The purpose of immersion is to identify patterns that have not become apparent at the particular point in the study or to explore patterns that may have been generated previously to ensure their soundness. Spradley (1980) identified six universal themes that may be helpful during this stage of data analysis. These themes are not meant to explain all patterns, but they do provide a place to begin. The universal themes are (1) social conflict; (2) cultural contradiction (What types of conflicts are occurring between people in social situations?); (3) informal techniques of social control (Is there information derived from the cultural group that appears contradictory?); (4) management of interpersonal relationships (Are there informal patterns of behavior that result in social control?); (5) acquisition and maintenance of status (How do group members conduct their interpersonal relationships?); and (6) problem solving. Researchers then write an overview summary of the cultural scene to help identify themes they have not yet discovered.

Taking a Cultural Inventory

Completing a cultural inventory is the first stage in writing an ethnography. The inventory provides the opportunity to organize collected data. A cultural inventory involves listing cultural domains; listing analyzed domains; collecting sketch maps, which are drawings of places or activities; listing themes; completing an inventory of examples; identifying organizing domains; completing an index or table of contents; completing an inventory of miscellaneous data; and suggesting areas for future study (Spradley, 1980).

Interpreting the Findings

The purpose of an ethnographic study is to describe the culture. It is important to remember that no two researchers would likely describe a culture in the same way, because of the unique attributes and values of researchers' cultures, the period in which the study was conducted, and the information gathered by the researchers. Perhaps, some researchers would argue, these are reasons why qualitative methods and, in particular, ethnography can never be viewed as science. On the contrary, these are precisely the reasons why ethnography and other qualitative methods are science. What most qualitative methods of research seek to do is share a context-bound view of phenomena; in this case, the phenomenon is the culture of a group. Because culture is ever-changing and dynamic, the discoveries of today are applicable within context. These discoveries bring important insights; they do not pretend to bring forward *the* truth but, rather, *a* truth. So, as ethnographers begin to write the study findings, they must remember that, if they used appropriate rigorous methods to collect and analyze data, then the product is one view of a truth.

"In the course of the final analysis, comparisons with existing ethnographies and other midrange theories are made. Existing theories may be supported or refuted and new midrange theories, in addition to the descriptive and explanatory theory of culture (the ethnography) may be induced" (Germain, 2001, p. 297). Once researchers have completed the inventory, interpreted the findings, and compared their work to the literature, they are ready to write the ethnography.

Writing the Ethnography

The purpose of writing an ethnography is to share with people what the researcher has learned and to attempt to make sense out of the cultural patterns that present themselves. To do so, an ethnographer must ask, For whom am I writing? Based on the answer to this question, the document will look different. If writing for a scholarly community, details will be important. If writing for the popular press, insights with exemplars will be most useful. If writing for an organization in the form of a formal report, the researcher must pay attention to those details that reflect the concerns that directed the inquiry.

One of the best ways to know what to write is to look for examples of what has been written. Ethnographers may choose to report natural history organized chronologically or spatially, or they may choose to organize information based on significant themes (Omery, 1988). A review of published texts that chronicles macro-ethnographies or scholarly journals that have published focused or micro-ethnographies will provide good examples of how to organize the final ethnographic report. Every detail or idea may not be collapsible into one journal article or one book. Focusing on aspects of the research for several books or articles may be the only feasible way to report the findings of an ethnographic study.

Researchers may write several drafts until the document accurately reflects the culture. They may recruit researcher colleagues to critique their work. Colleagues can help neophyte researchers discover whether they have appropriately covered the topic.

ETHICAL CONSIDERATIONS

*T*he protection of study participants is important regardless of the research paradigm, whether it is a qualitative or quantitative approach, phenomenology, grounded theory, ethnography, action, or historic. Because ethics is covered broadly in Chapter 4, this section shares unique ethical issues specific to ethnography.

When conducting ethnographic research, researchers by virtue of their roles as participant-observers are in a unique position to fit in. Researchers live among the people and therefore have the ability to be invisible at times in the researcher capacity. The invisible nature of researchers has significant value in data collection but can present potential dilemmas from an ethical standpoint. The important elements in conducting any type of research study are to inform participants fully about the matter to which they are consenting, inform participants that they can withdraw from the study at any time for any reason, reduce all unnecessary risks, ensure that the benefits of the study outweigh the risks, and ensure that the researchers who will be conducting the study have appropriate qualifications (Lipson, 1994).

Informed consent is an ethical principle that requires researchers to obtain voluntary consent, including description of the potential risks and benefits of participation. Munhall (1988) recommends using "process consent" (p. 156) rather than the traditional consent signed in the beginning of most studies and not revisited unless participants question their obligations related to the study. *Process consent* or "consensual decision-making" (Ramos, 1989, p. 61) means that researchers renegotiate the consent as unforeseen events or consequences arise (Munhall, 1988; Ramos, 1989). By providing the opportunity to renegotiate the consent and be part of the decision making as the study develops, ethnographers afford participants the chance to withdraw or modify that to which they initially agreed.

Lipson (1994) suggests that consent in the field becomes somewhat more difficult. For instance, the researcher secures consent before formal fieldwork begins. Some time passes, and the researcher is in the field at the time an unexpected event occurs, such as the birth of a child. Although it is important that the researcher inform the group that he or she is chronicling this event for research purposes, it would be intrusive to address consent at that point. One way to handle this situation would be for the researcher to inform participants at a later time that the birth experience gave him or her insight into cultural values. If objections are raised, the researcher would be unable to erase the memory of the event; however, to protect the informants, he or she would not include those data in the study. Covert participation in all research is regarded as a violation of individuals' rights. Therefore, ethnographers should always be forthright with their intentions.

Risk is another major concern. Researchers should never put a participant group in danger for data collection purposes. For example, the researcher in the field may discover that some young men are staging a gang fight in which they plan to use weapons. Believing that it would be important to learn more about conflict and how the group handles it, the researcher plans to go as an observer. In this situation, the risk to the people involved far outweighs the goal to observe how the group handles conflict. Intervention is necessary. How the researcher intervenes should be determined by a number of factors. A research mentor is invaluable in helping the novice researcher sort out when and how to intervene. Too many variables are involved to offer a simple answer. The important principle is that the researcher should not engage in data collection to achieve his or her own goals when significant risk to research participants is involved.

Another principle described by Lipson (1994) is the researcher's qualifications. Usually, Institutional Review Boards will assess the researcher's qualifications based on review of the submitted research proposal. An unqualified researcher can do substantial damage to a culture. It is essential that, even as a neophyte ethnographer, one clearly understands what it is he or she is doing and the potential risks in conducting a study without adequate sensitivity and knowledge.

Roper and Shapira (2000) also suggest that researchers adopt specific strategies to address ethical dilemmas. The ones recommended are to

deliberately evaluate their own effects on the research process by consciously identifying biases brought to the field and also emotional responses resulting from their experiences.

Next, . . . come up with an explicit description of their role during data collection. Finally, . . . establish mechanisms that guarantee honest and trustworthy research relationships. (p. 114)

Goodwin, Pope, Mort, and Smith (2003) also address the inherent problems for researchers who conduct research in a setting in which they have worked or have familiarity. In this case, the authors suggest that the role of researcher is frequently overlooked. When this occurs, sensitive information may be shared in the presence of the researcher when viewed as a practitioner rather than in the role of researcher. As a practitioner, other professionals may consider sensitive information confidential. As a researcher, however, the level of confidentiality may be compromised. There is no "right" way to handle this situation. However, Goodwin and colleagues suggest that the researcher has the responsibility to be as overt as possible in the research role.

It is important that all qualitative researchers—but, in particular, ethnographers—be aware of and knowledgeable about their responsibilities to research participants. Specifically, because of the intimate nature of the relationships that develop when ethnographers live among study participants, these researchers have a duty to inform and protect informants.

SUMMARY

*T*his chapter discussed the ethnographic approach to research and presented issues related to selection of the method, interpretations of the approach, application of the approach, and interpretation of the findings. A thorough explanation of how to conduct ethnographic research has been shared to provide a framework from which to conduct the first ethnographic inquiry.

Ethnography offers a significant research approach to individuals interested in learning about culture, willing and able to report data in narrative format, comfortable with ambiguity, able to build trusting relationships, and comfortable working alone (Germain, 1986). The study of culture, whether in a well-known nursing unit or in a country whose health practices are unknown, offers exciting discovery opportunities. Nurse researchers who choose to use this approach will find that the focus of the study will become an intimate part of their daily existence until they have fully explored, described, and interpreted that focus. The nature of the study, the proximity to participants, and the opportunity to bring forth a view of an undescribed or underdescribed culture provide a wonderful opportunity for nurse researchers who have the tenacity to listen and observe. It is a great privilege to be allowed an opportunity to view another's culture, one that nurses interested in ethnography should value.

Chapter 10 provides a review of research that uses the ethnographic approach. It is hoped that the review will further assist those individuals interested in the approach to understand the method and will provide concrete criteria from which to judge the merits of published reports.

References

Agar, M. H. (1982). Toward an ethnographic language. *American Anthropologist, 8*(4), 779-795.

Agar, M. H. (1986). *Speaking of ethnography*. Newbury Park, CA: Sage.

Allen, D. (2004). Ethnomethodological insights into insider-outsider relationships in nursing ethnographies of healthcare settings. *Nursing Inquiry, 11*(1), 14-24.

Anderson, J. M. (1991). Reflexivity in fieldwork: Toward a feminist epistemology. *Image, 23*(2), 115-118.

Atkinson, P. (1999). Ethnography: Post, past, and present. *Journal of Contemporary Ethnography, 28*(5), 460-470.

Atkinson, P., & Hammersley, M. (1994). Ethnography and participant observation. In N. K. Denzin & Y. S. Lincoln (Eds.), *Handbook of qualitative research* (pp. 248-261). Thousand Oaks, CA: Sage.

Benedict, R. (1934). *Patterns of culture*. New York: Houghton Mifflin.

Boas, F. (1948). *Race, language and culture*. New York: Macmillan.

Boyle, J. S. (1994). Styles of ethnography. In J. M. Morse (Ed.), *Critical issues in qualitative research methods* (pp. 159-185). Thousand Oaks, CA: Sage.

Brink, P. J., & Edgecombe, N. (2003). What is becoming of ethnography? *Qualitative Health Research, 13*(7), 1028-1030.

Dodgson, J. E., Duckett, L., Garwick, A., & Graham, B. L. (2002). An ecological perspective of breastfeeding in an indigenous community. *Journal of Nursing Scholarship, 34*(3), 235-341.

Ferrell, B., Smith, S., Cullinane, C. & Melancon, C. (2003). Symptom concerns of women with ovarian cancer. *Journal of Pain and Symptom Management, 25*(6), 528-538.

Fontana, A., & Frey, J. H. (1994). Interviewing: The art of science. In N. K. Denzin & Y. S. Lincoln (Eds.), *Handbook of qualitative research* (pp. 361-376). Thousand Oaks, CA: Sage.

Geertz, C. (1973). *The interpretations of culture*. New York: Basic Books.

Germain, C. P. (1986). Ethnography: The method. In P. L. Munhall & C. J. Oiler (Eds.), *Nursing research: A qualitative perspective* (pp. 147-162). Norwalk, CT: Appleton-Century-Crofts.

Germain, C. P. (2001). Ethnography: The method. In P. L. Munhall (Ed.), *Nursing research: A qualitative perspective* (3rd ed.). Sudbury, MA: National League for Nursing.

Goetz, J. P., & LeCompte, M. D. (1984). *Ethnography and qualitative design in educational research*. Orlando, FL: Academic Press.

Goodenough, W. (1970). *Description and comparison in cultural anthropology*. Chicago: Aldine.

Goodenough, W. (1971). *Culture, language and society*. Reading, MA: Addison-Wesley.

Goodwin, D., Pope, C., Mort, M., & Smith, A. (2003). Ethics and ethnography: An experiential account. *Qualitative Health Research, 13*, 567-577.

Grant, L., & Fine, G. A. (1992). Sociology unleashed: Creative directions in classical ethnography. In M. D. LeCompte, W. L. Millroy, & J. Preissle (Eds.), *The handbook of qualitative research in education* (pp. 405-446). San Diego, CA: Academic Press.

Grbich, C. (1999). *Qualitative research in health: An introduction*. London: Thousand Oaks.

Haglund, K. (2000). Parenting a second time around: An ethnography of African American grandmothers parenting grandchildren due to parental cocaine abuse. *Journal of Family Nursing, 6*(2), 120-136.

Hammersley, M., & Atkinson, P. (1983). *Ethnography: Principles in practice*. London: Tavistock.

Hughes, C. C. (1992). "Ethnography": What's in a word—Process? Product? Promise? *Qualitative Health Research, 2*(4), 439-450.

Leininger, M. (1970). *Nursing and anthropology: Two worlds to blend*. New York: Wiley.

Leininger, M. (1978). *Transcultural nursing: Concepts, theories and practices*. New York: Wiley.

Leininger, M. (1985). Ethnography and ethnonursing: Models and modes of qualitative data analysis. In M. Leininger (Ed.), *Qualitative research methods in nursing* (pp. 33-71). Orlando, FL: Grune & Stratton.

Lipson, J. G. (1994). Ethical issues in ethnography. In J. M. Morse (Ed.), *Critical issues in qualitative research methods* (pp. 333-355). Thousand Oaks, CA: Sage.

Lipson, J. G. (2001). We are the canaries: Self-care in multiple chemical sensitivity sufferers. *Qualitative Health Research, 11*(1), 103-116.

Lipson, J. G., Weinstein, H. M., Gladstone, E. A., & Sarnoff, R. H. (2003). Bosnian and Soviet refugees' experiences with health care. *Western Journal of Nursing Research, 25*(7), 854-871.

Magilvy, J. K., & Congdon, J. G. (2000). The crisis nature of health care transitions of rural older adults. *Public Health Nursing, 17*(5), 336-345.

Malinowski, B. (1922). *Argonauts of the Western Pacific*. London: Routledge & Kegan Paul.

Malinowski, B. (1961). *Argonauts of the Western Pacific*. New York: Dutton.

Manias, E., & Street, A. (2001). Rethinking ethnography: Reconstructing nursing relationships. *Journal of Advanced Nursing, 33*(2), 234-242.

Mead, M. (1949). *Coming of age in Samoa*. New York: New American Library, Mentor Books.

Morse, J. M., & Field, P.A. (1995). *Qualitative research methods for health professionals*. Thousand Oaks, CA: Sage.

Muecke, M.A. (1994). On the evaluation of ethnographies. In J. M. Morse (Ed.), *Critical issues in qualitative research methods* (pp. 187-209). Thousand Oaks, CA: Sage.

Munhall, P. L. (1988). Ethical considerations in qualitative research. *Western Journal of Nursing Research, 10*(2), 150-162.

Omery, A. (1988). Ethnography. In B. Sarter (Ed.), *Paths to knowledge: Innovative research methods for nursing* (pp. 17-31). New York: National League for Nursing.

Pellatt, G. (2003). Ethnography and reflexivity: Emotions and feelings in fieldwork. *Nurse Researcher, 10*(3), 28-37.

Radcliffe-Brown, A. R. (1952). *Structure and function in primitive society*. London: Oxford University Press.

Ragucci, A. T. (1972). The ethnographic approach and nursing research. *Nursing Research, 21*(6), 485-490.

Ramos, M. C. (1989). Some ethical implications in qualitative research. *Research in Nursing and Health, 12*, 57-63.

Roper, J. M., & Shapira, J. (2000). *Ethnography in nursing research*. Thousand Oaks, CA: Sage.

Rowe, J. H. (1965). The Renaissance foundation in anthropology. *American Anthropologist, 67*, 1-20.

Sanday, P. R. (1983). The ethnographic paradigm(s). In J. Van Maanen (Ed.), *Qualitative methodology* (pp. 19-36). Beverly Hills, CA: Sage.

Savage, H. (2000). Ethnography and health care. *British Medical Journal, 321*(7273), 1400-1403.

Schulte, J. (2000). Finding ways to create connections among communities: Partial results of an ethnography of urban public health nurses. *Public Health Nursing, 17*(1), 3-10.

Spradley, J. P. (1980). *Participant observation*. New York: Holt, Rinehart & Winston.

Spradley, J. P., & McCurdy, D. W. (1972). *The cultural experience: Ethnography in complex society*. Prospect Heights, IL: Waveland Press.

van Maanen, J. (1983). The fact of fiction in organizational ethnography. In J. van Maanen (Ed.), *Qualitative methodology* (pp. 36-55). Beverly Hills, CA: Sage.

Wolf, Z. R. (1988). *Nurses' work, the sacred and the profane*. Philadelphia: University of Pennsylvania Press.

Woods, P. (1992). Symbolic interactionism: Theory and method. In M. D. LeCompte, W. L. Millroy, & J. Preissle (Eds.), *The handbook of qualitative research in education*. San Diego, CA: Academic Press.

Wollcott, W. F. (2003). Ethnographic research in education. In C. F. Conrad, J. G. Haworth, & L. R. Lattuca (Eds.), *Qualitative research in higher education: Expanding perspectives* (2nd ed). Saddle River, NJ: Pearson Education.

Wright, D. J. (2002). Researching the qualities of hospice nurses. *Journal of Hospice and Palliative Nursing, 4*(4), 210-216.

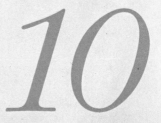

CHAPTER 10

Ethnography in Practice, Education, and Administration

*A*s a means of studying nursing and the cultural practices imbedded within it, ethnography creates unlimited prospects for nurses interested in using this approach. The study of patterns within a culture provides an excellent opportunity to describe the practices of the people for whom nurses care, to understand the health-related phenomena of people within various cultures, and to examine nursing's own unique culture. Ethnography provides a chance to explore both the clinical aspects of nursing and its administrative and educative patterns and lifeways.

This chapter provides an overview of ethnographic studies that have explored cultures of interest to nursing. In addition, it critiques ethnographic studies that reflect clinical nursing practice, nursing education, and nursing administration to provide readers with examples of published works and the contributions these works have made to the field. The ethnographic studies examined in this chapter have been critiqued using the guidelines in Box 10.1. The critiquing guidelines offer specific directives for determining the quality of the ethnographic works presented in this chapter and in the literature. The questions in Box 10.1 are specific to ethnographic research and reflect the most important aspects researchers must evaluate in an ethnographic report. A reprint of Sterling and Peterson's (2003) article found at the end of this chapter assists readers in understanding the critiquing process. Table 10.1 summarizes a recent series of ethnographic studies representing the areas of nursing education, administration, and practice.

APPLICATION TO PRACTICE

*E*thnographic research methodology offers an exceptional opportunity for nurses interested in examining clinical practice issues. Whether the

Text continued on page 232.

Box 10.1

Criteria for Critiquing Ethnographic Research

Focus

1. What is the culture being studied?
2. What is the focus or scope of the study?
3. What is the purpose of the study?

Method

1. How does ethnography fulfill the purpose of the study?
2. Is the study conducted in the field?
3. What guidelines have been established for participant consent?
4. How has the researcher protected study participants' rights?

Sampling

1. Why is the group selected to inform the study appropriate?
2. Does the researcher discuss how key informants are selected and why?

Data Collection

1. What strategies were used to collect data?
2. How do the strategies selected fully inform the study?
3. What was the researcher's role in the study?
4. How has triangulation of data sources (observation, interview, collection of artifacts) enhanced credibility of findings?
5. Is time in the field adequate to meet the purpose of the study?

Data Analysis

1. What strategies were used to analyze data? Were they consistent with the method?
2. How is the cyclic nature of data collection or data analysis reported?
3. Based on the report, can another researcher follow the logic of the researcher's conclusions?

Rigor

1. How has the researcher maintained his or her "objectivity"?
2. How has the researcher documented the authenticity of the data?
3. What role do the informants play in validating the researcher's findings?

Findings

1. Do the findings make clear a description of the culture studied?
2. In what context are the findings presented?
3. Are findings presented in a rich narrative format providing readers with a "feel" for the culture?
4. Do the findings go beyond the description to explain why particular aspects of the culture are as they are?
5. Are the findings reported in a systematic way, such as by themes?

Conclusions

1. How do the conclusions relate to the findings of the study?
2. What is the relevance of the findings to nursing, and how can they be used in practice?
3. What future directions for research are offered?

Table 10.1 • Selective Sampling of Ethnographic Studies

Author(s)	Domain	Culture	Focus	Data Collection Strategies	Data Analysis
Bent (2003)	Practice	One San José Spanish-speaking community	Relationships among health, environment, and culture	Interviews Participant observation Artifacts Field notes	Narrative analysis Relational analysis Examination of metaphor Content analysis
Cleary (2003)	Administration	Mental health nurses in New South Wales on a mental health unit	Mental health nurses' reconstruction of practice after policy changes	Participant observation Interview Discussion groups	Morse (1994) cognitive processes
Ferrell, Smith, Cullinane, & Melancon (2003)	Practice	Women with ovarian cancer	Symptoms concerns	Correspondence from women with ovarian cancer	Content analysis
Hem & Heggen (2003)	Practice	Psychiatric nurses in Norwegian psychiatric hospital	Contradictory demands on psychiatric nurses	Participant observation Narrative interviews Fieldnotes	Exemplary case
Kirkham (2003)	Administration	Two large acute care hospitals	Uncover social practices and processes that structure intergroup relations in health care provision	Interviews Participant observation Review of relevant texts	Not defined
Lesser, Oakes, & Koniak-Griffin (2003)	Practice	Adolescent mothers in an HIV education program	Response to HIV education program	Participant observation	Content analysis

Table 10.1 • *(Continued)*

Author(s)	Domain	Culture	Focus	Data Collection Strategies	Data Analysis
Lipson, Weinstein, Gladstone, & Sarnoff (2003)	Practice	Bosnian and Soviet refugees who use Santa Clara County Health Services	Experience with health care	Participant observation Interviews Focus group	Theme and category analysis
Mohr (2004)	Administration	A developing family support program	Understanding group development	Participant observation Interviews	Content analysis Thematic analysis
Pasco, Morse, & Olson (2004)	Practice Administration	Filipino Canadians receiving care in Canadian hospitals	Describe cultural values that guide Filipino Canadians in their interactions with Canadian nurses	Interviews Field notes Diary	Not defined
Nichols (2004)	Administration	Native American nurse leaders	Understand leadership development of Native American nurses	Focus group	ETHNOGRAPH 5.0
Shelton (2004)	Practice	Minority youth receiving mental health services through juvenile justice system	Explanatory model of minority youth receiving mental health services through the juvenile justice system	Focus group Observation	Grounded theory techniques described by Strauss & Corbin (1990)

Sterling & Peterson (2003)	Practice	African American women caregivers for children with asthma	Attributes and characteristics of African American women caregivers of children with asthma	Interviews Participant observation Fieldwork	QRS NUD*IST4
Tuohy (2003)	Education	Students caring for the elderly	Communication patterns between the elderly and student nurses	Participant observation Semi-structured interviews	Latent theme analysis
Ward-Griffin, Bol, Hay & Dashnay (2003)	Practice Administration	Families and nurses in long-term care facilities	Examine relationships between nurses and family members in long-term care facilities	Focused interviews	NUD*IST

Text continued from page 227.

interest is in studying Bosnian and Soviet refugees' experience of health care (Lipson, Weinstein, Gladstone, & Sarnoff, 2003), detained young offenders in need of mental health care (Shelton, 2004), or African-American women caregivers of children with asthma (Sterling & Peterson, 2003), ethnographic research provides the framework for exploring the richness of nursing and nursing-related phenomena. Sterling and Peterson's study of African-American women caregivers of asthmatic children is the reference for critique in this section.

It is important to point out that it is not unusual for ethnographic researchers who publish ethnography in a research journal to focus on only one facet of a larger study. Because of the significant amount of information generated in a long-term cultural study, many ethnographies are published as books. When researchers choose to publish their ethnographic work in a journal, the scope of the report must meet the page guidelines of the selected journal. Sterling and Peterson's (2003) study is an example of a portion of a larger study that is published as an article.

Sterling and Peterson (2003) clearly identify the culture studied. The authors state that the culture is African-American women who are primary caregivers for children with asthma. The scope of the study is not stated but could be described as a focused ethnography in light of its specific concentration on the characteristics of caretaking by African-American women. The researchers state that the purpose of the study is "to describe the attributes and characteristics of African American women who were the primary caregivers of children with asthma" (p. 32).

Sterling and Peterson (2003) do not explicitly state why they believe ethnography is the preferred method to study this culture. The report would be stronger if this information had been included. The informants are appropriate. They are all either mothers or grandmothers who are responsible for caring for their asthmatic child relatives. Sterling and Peterson identify the women primary caregivers as key informants but do not explain why. It can be surmised that they were chosen because of the focus of the study.

The research was conducted over a 1-year period in two geographic locations (Pacific Northwest and Gulf South) and included the use of formal and informal interviews, participant observation, and field notes for data collection. These are all appropriate methods of data collection in an ethnographic study. The addition of artifacts as part of data collection would add important information to the data set and enhance data triangulation. The authors also report participation in family activities, including church services, basketball games, family meals, graduation, and shopping. Participation in the types of activities described is a good way for researchers to obtain rich data at times when participants are more likely to be spontaneous and candid. However, these informal sessions also have the potential to create ethical dilemmas. Sterling and Peterson (2003) state that participants signed informed consent forms before the study began; however, there is no description of process consent. Process consent allows researchers and participants to renegotiate consent if unforeseen events or consequences arise (Munhall, 1988; Ramos, 1989). Process consent becomes especially important when participating in and observing close family interactions.

The investigators report data were analyzed using QRS NUD*IST4, which is code-based, theory-building software (Morison & Moir, 1998). Sterling and Peterson (2003) add that "coded data were clustered into broad categories, and data were further organized into meaningful and related themes" (p. 34). In addition, a number of references are made to the cyclic nature of data collection in this study. For example, "data were collected, transcribed, and analyzed, they were presented to families for validation and more input . . . input provided guidance for additional data collection" (p. 34). These are appropriate data collection and analysis strategies for ethnographic research studies.

Rigor was demonstrated by time in the field, collecting data in a cyclic manner to verify findings, sharing findings with participants throughout the study and choice of informants. There is no mention of the researchers using journals as a strategy for maintaining an objective eye on data collection or analysis. This would be a beneficial addition to the report.

The researchers do a good job of describing the culture studied. Six themes are used to organize the presentation of the findings. The researchers present rich narrative to illustrate each theme.

Sterling and Peterson (2003) do not overstate their findings. They tell the reader that their findings are not generalizable. They offer a set of clinical implications to demonstrate the usefulness of the findings to nursing. They also share future research directions, including the importance of investigating the women's emic view of themselves. The recommended direction for future research leads to a question about what was the intent of the current study if not to understand the emic view of the women who informed it. This study is well presented and offers its readers a good perspective on what the characteristics are of these African-American women who care for a child with asthma.

APPLICATION TO EDUCATION

*N*ursing education presents another context in which nurse researchers can conduct ethnographic studies. The teaching and learning environment, including the way students, faculty, health care providers, and clients relate to one another in clinical settings, creates its own culture. Few published studies have specifically illustrated the lifeways of students and faculty. The limited number of studies in nursing education since the publication of the last edition of this text clearly illustrates this. Only one ethnographic study of nursing education was found since the publication of the last edition of this text, despite an extensive electronic literature search. Clearly, ethnographic research has a role in the teaching and learning process and offers the qualitative education researcher rich opportunities. The article "Student Nurse–Older Person Communication" (Tuohy, 2003) serves as the reference for critique in this section. It was selected because it demonstrates the use of ethnography in studying a type of student learning experience.

In the article, Tuohy (2003) clearly identifies that the purpose of the study is to "ascertain how student nurses communicate with older people" (p. 19). The focus is also clear. The author is interested in communication between nursing students and the elderly. Tuohy states that the focus of the study is limited and she therefore reports it as a mini-ethnography. A mini-ethnography as described in the preceding chapter is of a smaller scale and is narrow or specific in its focus. In this case, the author tells us that she is interested in communication between nursing students and older persons. However, the findings section reports only data representative of the students' interactions with the elderly. The reader is left with an incomplete understanding of the culture studied. Because the study is an ethnography, it is vitally important to clearly state the culture being studied. This is as important in a mini-ethnography as it is in a traditional or classical ethnography. In a mini-ethnography, the focus may be on a distinct problem, and the researcher may collect data from a smaller group of people; however, the purpose of all ethnography is the description of behavioral patterns of individuals and groups within a specific culture (Agar, 1986; Bernard, 1994; Roper, & Shapira, 2000).

Tuohy (2003) reports that the reason she chose ethnography is because it is "useful for studying the culture and social organization of groups" (p. 20). She further adds that "ethnography enables culturally specific care to be identified" (p. 20). This study was appropriately conducted in the wards where the students practiced.

The reference to comments made by the "ethics committee" (p. 21) and references to the participants' rights being ensured through informed consent illustrate attention to human subjects protection. Tuohy states that there were concerns by the ethics committee that the participants were students of the researcher. She reports that she dealt with this by regularly reminding the students that their participation was voluntary and that they could withdraw from the study at anytime without affecting their grades. It is difficult to convey fully to students the "voluntary" nature of their participation when the power relationship of student and teacher exists. It would have been better to use data collection strategies that eliminate the power dynamic created in this situation between students and tutor.

Tuohy (2003) reports that the study participants included eight second-year diploma preregistration students who had completed modules on communication. There is no mention of the elderly individuals who were part of the communication process. Despite the author's reference to ethnography being the selected research method because of its usefulness in studying culture and social organization, there is no description of the elderly who were involved in the communication with the students. It is difficult to understand why Tuohy did not select phenomenology as the preferred method given that her data collection strategies and analysis of findings report only on the students' perceptions rather than the culture that exists as a result of the dynamic relationship created by the communication between the students and the elderly people they cared for. Tuohy also makes reference to the importance of identifying key informants but does not describe whom the key informants of the study are. An assumption that can be drawn is that she sees the nursing students as the key informants, which may be the reason that only their comments about communication are exclusively reported.

The methods of data collecting included participant observation and semi-structured interviews. Tuohy (2003) uses her observations to place the communication examples she reports in context. For instance, when she shares the theme "types of communication," she describes for the reader that "task related communication" occurs when the students are engaged in task-related activities such as morning bathing. Tuohy states that her time in the field may be a limitation of the study. There is a notation in the study—(38h). The reader is lead to conjecture that this reference means the researcher spent 38 hours in the field. Without clear statement of the time in the field, the reader would be unable to determine whether the time in the field was adequate and would have to agree with the study author that the time may have limited the findings. There are no references in the report of how data sources were triangulated to add to the credibility of the study.

Data were analyzed using latent thematic analysis. Tuohy (2003) shares Morse and Field's definition of latent thematic analysis to help the reader unfamiliar with this term. There is no specific description of the cyclic nature of data collection and analysis. It is also reported that "opinions of two nursing colleagues were sought with regard to data analysis, and a clear audit trail of the data collection and analysis was presented" (p. 21). From this the reader can infer that the two nursing colleagues were able to follow the line of reasoning presented to them.

Tuohy (2003) discusses the rigor of the study using the term *trustworthiness*. The ways trustworthiness is addressed in this study are through

> keeping records of data collection and analysis, and obtaining verification of interview transcripts from the participants. Furthermore, the opinions of two nursing colleagues were sought with regard to data collection and analysis, and a clear audit trail of the data collection and analysis was presented. (p. 21)

The researcher clearly identifies that her presence during the interactions and her note taking may have influenced the nature of the communication between the student and the older adult, and there is no reference to how she limited the effect.

The researcher clearly states that the findings of the study are not generalizable in light of the scope of the study. From this the reader can infer the author understands that the findings are context bound. Tuohy (2003) does provide some illustrative examples of student communication with the elderly. It is difficult from the themes presented to grasp fully the culture of the study. Part of this is related to earlier comments about the focus being exclusively on the students rather than the culture. The definition of culture requires a full understanding of the lifeways of a group—focusing exclusively on the students' perceptions of the communication experience is limited given that communication requires a sender and a receiver. The presentation of the findings does provide the reader with a set of organizers that helps to explain the students' perceptions.

The findings are presented in context. Tuohy (2003) tells the reader what the relationships of the findings are to the existing literature on student communication. She also offers a number of recommendations for enhancing communication between students and the elderly. She does not offer directions for future research.

APPLICATION TO ADMINISTRATION

*I*n previous editions of this text, it was extremely difficult to find ethnographic studies that reflected the area of nursing administration. This is not the case for this edition. A broad definition of nursing service administration was used to include any type of ethnographic study that was clearly not patient or student focused. This provided a rich source of ethnographic studies, including studies on patient satisfaction as a framework for hospital reform (Rankin, 2003), relationships between families and nurses in long-term care facilities (Ward-Griffin, Bol, Hay, & Dashnay, 2003), and the development of mental health support groups (Mohr, 2004). Cleary's (2003) research on the challenges of mental health care reform in New South Wales is critiqued to demonstrate the application of ethnography in nursing administration. Table 10.1 offers examples of other ethnographic research studies, including those published in the area of nursing administration.

Cleary (2003) states that her investigation was "concerned with the way mental health nurses' construct their practice in an acute inpatient psychiatric unit in light of the current challenges, demands and influences brought about by service reforms of the 1990s" (p. 139). The scope of the study is not reported; therefore, the reader is left to speculate on its scale. The culture under study is nurses practicing in a 22-bed admission unit of a public psychiatric facility in New South Wales.

The researcher reports that she used the method of interpretive ethnography described by Geertz. This particular approach was selected "because of its orientation to understanding shared meanings of mental health nurses and how meaning is constructed through culturally shared beliefs and practices in the context of an acute inpatient setting" (Cleary, 2003, p. 140). The study was conducted in the field: in this case, on the inpatient psychiatric unit over a 5-month period. The research was approved by the Area Health Service and the University Ethics Review Committee. There is no mention of any special protection for participants in the study. As stated earlier, establishing the option for process consent is an important strategy to ensure that human subjects are always aware of their right to control the information included as data.

The participants in the study are nurses working on the unit. Given that these are the individuals who have the responsibility for caring for psychiatric patients under the new mental health reforms, they are appropriate to inform the study. There is no reference to key informants in the report. The reader can conclude that the key informants are the nurses who shared their stories; however, in most ethnographic studies, there are particular individuals who serve as information gatekeepers and are key to gaining access to the appropriate individuals on the scene.

Data were collected using participant observation, interviews, and discussion groups over a 5-month period. Cleary (2003) worked part-time as a "buddy" to nurses on the unit to gain access and collect data in a way that minimized disruption. This strategy proved effective given that it led to many informal, spontaneous conversations during patient care. "The range of data sources and data methods enabled comparisons of data and highlighted areas for further consideration, exploration and clarification" (p. 141). From this statement, it is clear that data were collected in a cyclic way that moved from collection to analysis to collection and back to analysis.

Data analysis was described as consisting of four cognitive processes outlined by Morse: comprehending, synthesizing, theorizing, and recontextualizing the data collected. As presented, it is difficult to ascertain how the researcher arrived at her conclusions. Offering an example of how the process was used would be very helpful to the reader.

There is no explicit description of how rigor was addressed. It can be implied that based on the amount of time in the field and the cyclic nature of data collection, some attention to rigor occurred. The report would be stronger if Cleary (2003) addressed how the researcher maintained her objectivity and how she assured the authenticity of the data collected, and described the role of informants in validating the findings.

Cleary (2003) presents the majority of the findings as her commentary on data analysis. The presentation is organized around four major areas: relationships with patients, power and relationships, restrictions, and getting better and nursing rewards. There are less informant quotes presented in the article than are usual in ethnographic reports. The presentation of the findings is conclusive. Based on the report, the reader has a clear understanding of the "perceptions, motives and viewpoints of mental health nurses" (p. 141).

The findings are offered in context. Cleary (2003) specifically states that the findings are "context bound" (p. 145). She adds, however, that they are noteworthy and that they "resonate with the literature and research relating to acute in-patient facilities" (p. 145). As stated earlier, the findings are offered in four distinct areas. The researcher does not label them as themes.

The conclusions of the study are appropriate given the findings. Cleary (2003) discusses the relevance of the findings to what is already known on the topic and offers, based on the comparability of the findings to the literature and other research, that they could be viewed as useful in practice. She concludes the report by suggesting that her research "provides a platform for educators, leaders, managers and clinicians to develop further research to test emerging models of care delivery and to explore clinical and educational strategies to address the issues identified" (p. 145). Cleary's (2003) research adds to the ethnographic database in mental health nursing and provides solid evidence about the way nurses are adjusting to changes in mental health policy and practice.

SUMMARY

*T*his chapter reviewed samples of published ethnographic research in the areas of nursing practice, education, and administration. Each critique presents the strengths and limitations of the ethnographic research included. The reviewed authors have contributed to the literature and provided readers with an opportunity to become part of the culture or subculture they studied.

Ethnographic research and the studies that use ethnography as a method add to the richness and diversity of the human experience by allowing readers to share in the lives of the people studied. As nurse researchers become more comfortable with multiple ways of knowing and multiple realities, they will benefit by participating in the creation and dissemination of the knowledge imbedded in the cultural realities that are a person's life.

References

Agar, M. H. (1986). *Speaking of ethnography*. Newbury Park, CA: Sage.

Bent, K. N. (2003). "The people know what they want": An empowerment process of sustainable, ecological community health. *Advances in Nursing Science, 26*(3), 215–226.

Bernard, H. R. (1994). *Research methods in anthropology: Qualitative and quantitative approaches* (2nd ed.). Thousand Oaks, CA: Sage.

Cleary, M. (2003). The challenge of mental health care reform for contemporary mental health nursing practice: Relationships power and control. *International Journal of Mental Health Nursing, 12*, 139-147.

Ferrell, B., Smith, S., Cullinane, C., & Melancon, C. (2003). Symptom concerns of women with ovarian cancer. *Journal of Pain and Symptom Management, 25*(6), 528-538.

Hem, M. H., & Heggen, K. (2003). Being professional and being human: One nurse's relationship with a psychiatric patient. *Journal of Advanced Nursing, 43*(1), 101-108.

Kirkham, S. R. (2003). The politics of belonging and intercultural health care. *Western Journal of Nursing Research, 25*(7), 762-780.

Lesser, J., Oakes, R., & Koniak-Griffin, D. (2003). Vulnerable adolescent mothers' perceptions of maternal role and HIV risk. *Health Care for Women International, 24*(6), 513-528.

Lipson, J. G., Weinstein, H. M., Gladstone, E. A., & Sarnoff, R. H. (2003). Bosnian and Soviet refugees' experiences with health care. *Western Journal of Nursing Research, 25*(7), 854-871.

Mohr, W. K. (2004). Surfacing the life phases of a mental health support group. *Qualitative Health Research, 14*(1), 61-77.

Morison, M., & Moir, J. (1998). The role of computer software in the analysis of qualitative data: Efficient clerk, research assistant or Trojan horse. *Journal of Advanced Nursing, 28*(1), 106-116.

Munhall, P. L. (1988). Ethical considerations in qualitative research. *Western Journal of Nursing Research, 10*(2), 150-162.

Nichols, L. A. (2004). Native American nurse leadership. *Journal of Transcultural Nursing, 15*(3), 177-183.

Pasco, A. C. Y., Morse, J. M., & Olson, J. K. (2004). Cross-cultural relationships between nurses and Filipino Canadian patients. *Journal of Nursing Scholarship, 36*(3), 239-246.

Ramos, M. C. (1989). Some ethical implications in qualitative research. *Research in Nursing and Health, 12*, 57-63.

Rankin, J. M. (2003). 'Patient satisfaction': Knowledge for ruling hospital reform: An institutional ethnography. *Nursing Inquiry, 10*(1), 57-65.

Roper, J. M., & Shapira, J. (2000). *Ethnography in nursing research*. Thousand Oaks, CA: Sage.

Shelton, D. (2004). Experiences of detained young offenders in need of mental health care. *Journal of Nursing Scholarship, 36*(2), 129-133.

Sterling, Y. M., & Peterson, J. W. (2003). Characteristics of African American women caregivers of children with asthma. *MCN: The American Journal of Maternal Child Nursing, 28*(1), 32-38.

Tuohy, D. (2003). Student nurse-older person communication. *Nurse Education Today, 23*(1), 19-26.

Ward-Griffin, C., Bol, N., Hay, K., & Dashnay, I. (2003). Relationships between families and registered nurses in long-term-care facilities: A critical analysis. *Canadian Journal of Nursing Research, 35*(4), 150-174.

Research Article

Characteristics of African American Women Caregivers of Children With Asthma

Yvonne M. Sterling, DNSc, RN, C, and Jane W. Peterson, PhD, RN

ABSTRACT

Purpose: *To describe the attributes and characteristics of African American women who were the primary caregivers of children with asthma. Methods: Descriptive qualitative ethnography. Data collection consisted of formal interviews, participant observation, and fieldnotes. Each study participant was formally and informally interviewed (audiotaped) during a 1-year period. The researchers also observed and participated in family activities in various naturalistic settings.*

Results: *Six themes emerged that depict the characteristics of these women: (1) Knowledge about the child's asthma; (2) Gatekeepers to the child's care; (3) Being religious; (4) Support; (5) Roles as teacher, counselor, and advisor to the child; and (6) Self-sufficiency and industriousness.*

Clinical Implications: *Nurses should use the information in this study to examine the ways in which they interact with caregivers of asthmatic children. The caregivers personal beliefs, need for information, and previous experiences with asthma and family illness should be assessed. These mothers and grandmothers should be respected as the gatekeeper to the family's healthcare. Nurses should be nonjudgmental and supportive of caregivers when they express their religious beliefs and practices. Nurses who understand how mothers cope can reinforce these coping skills and provide better nursing care.*

Key Words: *African American caregivers; Asthma, Childhood chronic illness; Ethnography.*

*A*sthma is the most common chronic illness in childhood in the United States. Approximately 5 million children have asthma; it is a leading cause of disability and is the most frequently cited reason for school absences (Centers for Disease Control and Prevention [CDC], 1999; 2000). Death rates for children with asthma nearly doubled between 1980 and 1993 (National Institute of Allergy and Infectious Diseases [NIAID], 2000). Asthma is more prevalent in African American children than in Caucasian children, causing more severe disability, more frequent hospitalizations, and 4 to 6 times more death (NIAID, 2000). Thus, the burden of this disease is borne disproportionately by African American families, particularly those living in the inner city (Wade et al., 1997).

Data presented in this article are part of a larger study, "Explanatory Models of Asthma by African American Families and Their Children (Peterson, Sterling, & Stout, in press). Here we discuss the attributes of the African American women who were the primary caregivers of children with asthma. The emergent themes presented reflect the women's attributes, roles, and beliefs that frame and guide their lives as they manage their children with asthma. Their lives as they described them inevitably influenced the development of their explanatory models of asthma, and affected the lives of their children with asthma as well as the rest of the family system. The resulting data thereby revealed a richer portrait of these women as primary caregivers of children with asthma and as family members.

How Caregivers Cope With Asthma

Although descriptions of parental coping with chronically ill children abound, the literature about the experiences of African American family caregivers of chronically ill children is extremely limited, except for parents of children with sickle-cell disease. Investigators commonly include African American parents in their studies of children with chronic conditions, but the unique responses of those parents are often embedded in the reported research findings, and therefore, are difficult to separate and thus understand more fully (Sterling, Peterson, & Weekes, 1997).

The literature contains many descriptions of the coping strategies of parents with chronically ill children in general, and asthmatic children in particular. Kurnat and Moore (1999) stated that the chronic and episodic nature of asthma places excessive demands on the parent's time and energy. Horner (1998) found that "family caring" influences the quality of life of the child with asthma. *Family caring* is defined as the strategies enacted by parents to deal with a child's emerging health needs and asthma episodes while promoting his or her healthy development (p. 358). In a 1994 study of African American and Hispanic caretakers of asthmatic children, Mailick, Holden, and Walther found that the caregivers most frequently used active coping strategies including practicing religion and seeking emotional support.

In their 1997 multisite study of inner city children with asthma and their caretakers, Wade et al. found that 75% of the children's multiple caretakers were women. Using a battery of structured instruments, the researchers found that the caretakers demonstrated high levels of asthma knowledge, were motivated to manage the child's asthma but experienced multiple stressful events (p. 272).

Parental ability to cope with a child's illness has also been studied by Grus et al. (2001) of primarily Hispanic and black parents of children with asthma. They found that parents who reported less ability to manage their child's asthma effectively were also more likely to experience asthma-related morbidity.

Method

The study's design was descriptive and qualitative involving an ethnographic approach. Study participants were recruited from several clinical and from professional referrals in two cities located in the Pacific Northwest and the Gulf

South. Participants signed a consent form and then data collection began, which consisted of interviews, participant observation, and fieldnotes. Both formal interviews (those with a purpose, structure and appointed time) and informal interviews (casual, nonscheduled conversations) occurred over a 1-year period. Examples of questions asked of all participants were: "*Tell me about your experience with your child's asthma. Why did it start when it did? How does it work? What are your chief problems?*" The primary caregivers were initially contacted and interviewed by the researchers, and then other family members were identified as key informants. Multiple interviews were conducted with key informants during the course of the study. The researchers also observed and participated in family activities (e.g., church services, basketball games, family meals, graduations, shopping) in various naturalistic settings such as the participants' homes, clinics, sports events, churches, and schools. The researchers' observations were recorded as fieldnotes. Pseudonyms were assigned to all study participants to protect their identities.

Formal interviews were audiotaped and transcribed verbatim by a professional transcriptionist. The transcribed interviews and fieldnotes were imported into a computer software program, QSR NUD*IST4 for data management and analysis. Transcriptions were coded separately by each researcher in her respective city and were compared for agreement. Coded data were clustered into broad categories, and data were further organized into meaningful and related themes. As data were collected, transcribed, and analyzed, they were presented to families for validation and more input, maintaining their emic perspective. That input provided guidance for additional data collection. This process continued until the participants provided no new information; thus, redundancy provided the criterion for ending data collection. The credibility and truth value of data was achieved by the researchers' direct involvement in the family's lives over a long period of time and the selection of participants who were involved in the asthmatic child's life. Additionally, obtaining data from each participant in different circumstances, repeatedly seeking and confirming their explanations and actions, and the constant comparison of observations with interviews enhanced this study's rigor (Germain, 2001).

Sample

The study group was comprised of 19 women living in two cities, one located in the Pacific Northwest ($n = 9$) and the other in the Gulf South ($n = 10$). The women (age range 31–74 years) were primary caregivers of children, aged 9 to 12 years (mean age 10.73, SD 1.32) who had been diagnosed with asthma at least 1 year previously. The asthmatic condition was rated "severe" in 26% of the children, and "moderately severe" or "not severe" in 74% of the children.

Findings

Six themes were discovered that described the characteristics of the primary caretakers of children with asthma:

1. They have knowledge about the child's asthma and possess skills in asthma management.

Having knowledge refers to being informed and skilled. Such knowledge includes administration of medications and treatment regimens for the control of acute episodes, and also preventive care and symptom management, as well as evaluation of treatment effectiveness. The magnitude of the mothers' knowledge about the child's asthma varied and seemed related to their experience with asthma and length of time since the child's diagnosis. One mother stated: *"I know what to do to help her. If I first catch it when she first starts coughing, I'm in control of it. But if I let her...like she'll come to me and say, 'I can't breathe,' then I know I've taken too long to care for her."*

Other comments included, *"You have to do prevention. And wheezing—-you know you need to give her treatments. So I've learned that I don't always wait for the cough,"* and *"I think bein' able—knowing more about it, how it works, what can trigger it and all that."* Pamela, a registered nurse, discussed her sister, the mother of a child with asthma: *"I think she is more comfortable and she understands a lot more, she knows what she needs to do and she does it and she doesn't waste time."*

2. The women are gatekeepers to the child's care in that they monitor, facilitate, and provide direct care for the child with asthma.

For example, Kate explained her role as gatekeeper: *"If the doctor say this and I say: 'Well, did you tell her she did so and so?' You know, I was giving her this medicine and this was working, you know. When a man brings [children to the doctor, at least my husband], I have to write details, I have to write it down. I've been to the doctor with them all these years, so I know the doctor."*

Another mother, Phyliss, noted, *"I believe in preventive medicine. I don't believe in treating people after they're sick. Let's try to prevent 'em from getting sick. I have these kids on vitamins. I put...[my son with asthma] on vitamins. I had him on vitamins since he was, I think, 5 years old. I had a [talk] with the pediatrician, you know. 'Shouldn't he be on vitamins?' 'No,' [he responded]. The hell with that. I put Alex on vitamins and he rarely catches a cold...Chrissie is my child. Alex's my child. I will decide what is best for 'em."*

3. They are religious, meaning they have faith in God.

The mothers expressed faith in God as the source of strength for dealing with a child who has asthma and with other perceived stressors. To promote their beliefs, the study participants engaged in religious activities such as reading spiritual materials, praying, attending church, and participating in church-related activities. Their comments included the following: *"Prayers, prayers. Talkin' to Jesus. I ask Him to give me the strength, the wisdom, and the knowledge to do what I can for Him...and He helps me."*

One mother stated, *"I put my faith in God. The best teacher is Jesus. I put myself in His hands."*

Another mother said, *"I would go with the Pastor and we would take the elderly that couldn't come, communion on the first Monday. We call and we check on different members when we don't see them in church."*

4. Family and friends are supportive, assisting the caregivers in managing the child's asthma as well as providing transportation, information, comfort, communication, and facilitating venting of feelings.

Support of family and friends was commonly noted. Lisa said, "*I talk with my older sisters and, you know, we just talk. And sometimes certain things people say to you...really boosts you up and help you move on.*"

Darylyn noted, "*My dad was very, very supportive when it came down to Nicole. My dad brought me there...was sick hisself. He'd say, 'You gonna be all right baby.' He'd look at me and he'd say, 'Baby, you are gonna be all right and this baby is going to be all right.'*"

Marisa reported, "*Lots of times I call my sister...and my mom's a retired nurse and my sister's a nurse. My sister, she'll come and help because I think she went through it with her son when he was young.*"

One grandmother relied on her daughter, the aunt of the child with asthma. "*She [aunt] always tells [her niece, Pearl], 'I gonna teach Pearl how to do it herself,' so that's what she does. Pearl lives between her grandmother and her godmother. Her grandmother feels strongly that 'she [Pearl] needs to know what to do.' I think that's why she's doing so well, because we have Jasmine in our life and she knows about it.*"

Fathers also support the women caregivers in many ways. When asked to name a person he admires, one father immediately named his wife: "*She has so much courage. Faced with her own illnesses, asthma and diverticulitis, she carries on cheerfully and watches over our son with asthma.*"

5. The women operate in the roles of teacher, counselor, and advisor to the child regarding asthma management, peer relationships, and school activities.

An important role for the caregivers was as teacher and advisor to the child. The role was extended by giving guidance to friends and relatives about appropriate childcare. Regarding this role one mother stated, "*Right now, I am trying to use subliminal, you know, messages with her to tell her that you are breathing fine, that you can do this. And I say, 'Your mind got to start controlling your body.'*
Like my psych classes I've taken. You know, just trying to use mind over matter."

Another mother reported, "*I always tell her to calm down, tell her to calm down. And I have to tell her, 'Well, just don't worry about it. Try to make things better. You know, just do it, which you're supposed to do anyway. Keep tryin' at it.'*" For one mother, even the healthcare at the community clinic sees her as an advisor to them. "*We are going to be running out of Maxair soon. I will call up [the community clinic] and tell them to get me another prescription. But if I have questions, I would actually call up the research center, because the clinic told me not too long ago I actually know more about asthma now than they do.*"

6. They are self-sufficient and industrious as evidenced by their independence and autonomy.

These women reported being (and were observed to be) self-sufficient and industrious (i.e., independent and autonomous) in managing personal and family life. Twelve (63%) of the women held full- or part-time jobs. One mother reported that she was continuing her education while managing her family. Another mother, unable to work a traditional job because of her child's severe asthma, sold "cold cups" (frozen Kool-Aid) to assist her husband in generating money. Regarding that activity she stated, "*You really can't work because you have Dez (the child with asthma) to look after so I sell cold cups.*"

Another mother cogently remarked, "*I'm not used to laying around the house doin' nothin'. I'm used to movin' around. I'm a workaholic. I used to work for the school board. I was there whether they need it or not, I was there.*"

One mother described herself as follows: "*Sometimes it is better to do something myself than to ask for help...It is hard for me to ask for help. I [do] not like to be dependent on others.*"

Despite their industriousness, the women all had tenuous health histories. One mother had both asthma and diverticulitis. Another mother with asthma was hospitalized several times during the data collection phase of our study. One mother, who is also diagnosed with glaucoma, reported: "*My blood pressure is the creepy kind. It can go up and I don't know it, although I am taking the medicine like I should.*"

Another mother discussed her health status: "*But then I will stop runnin' with him [her son with asthma], then I run for me cause I suffer with asthma. I didn't suffer with it when I was small, but I got it once I got grown, I start suffering with asthma.*"

Discussion

Taylor (1998) suggests that there is a black feminist perspective that is most appropriate for the study of the complexities of African American women's lives. The novelist Alice Walker (1983) has called this perspective "womanist," stating that the experiences of African American women are unique and significantly divergent from those of white women, and incorporate the complexity of life as an African American woman, mirroring both the language and tenets of the African American community (p. 56).

Hudson-Weem's (1993) definition of womanism goes beyond Walker's (1983) original definition in that it includes all women of African American descent, reflects Afrocentric beliefs, and is paramount to understanding the "Africana" woman. Hudson-Weems' definition incorporates several characteristics, including being family-centered, spiritual, respectful of elders, adaptable, ambitious, mothering, and nurturing. Her definition is congruent with the descriptions of the women in our study. They are family-centered as the gatekeepers of family health matters, and are religious and nurturing mothers, especially to the child with asthma.

The women caregivers in our study had varying degrees of knowledge about asthma and skills in asthma management. They could articulate knowledge about the child's asthma triggers, symptom management, medication effects, and protocols for episodic care. Nonetheless, they did express the need for more information about their child's treatment regimen and expressed fears and anxieties about the child's future. These findings resemble those from the studies of Kurnat and Moore (1999) and Kieckhefer and Ratcliffe (2000). Horner (1998) found that parents, including those of African descent, learned about their children's asthma patterns, symptoms, and medications as a means of gaining control over the child's condition. Similar to the participants in MacDonald's (1996) study, the women caregivers in our study acquired knowledge about the child's asthma and were proactive in improving the child's health.

As gatekeepers of healthcare, the women in our study were the major caregivers of family members in times of illness. Friedman (1998) wrote that "It has become increasingly clear that in most families an important role subsumed under the mother position is that of health leader and caregiver" (p. 309). Many researchers have described the role of religion and faith in God in the lives of African American women. Edwards (1993) and Davis (1998) both found that African American women find great strength in faith and belief in a higher power related to health and illness. Additionally those women talked about God's ultimate control over illness and death and of God's healing power (p. 35). Rogers-Dulan and Blacher (1995) noted that although religion has become less important than it was, the African American church and family remain strongly linked. The finding of having support highlights the importance of familial social support across the life course within African American families. Historically, African Americans have been more likely than Caucasians to rely on extended family support (Taylor, Jackson, & Chatters, 1997). Within the social networks of African Americans, family members have been the primary source of support. During a crisis, most African Americans turn to family, friends, religion, or religious groups before seeking help from professional or social service agencies (Rogers-Dulan & Blacher, 1995). Grandmothers in African American families have been instrumental in providing for the needs of various family members, especially young unmarried mothers and their children (Taylor et al., 1997). In our sample of women, two grandmothers were primary caregivers of the child with asthma.

Krulik et al. (1999) has reported on the health problems for mothers of chronically ill children, including maternal depression and physical illness. In her introduction to *The Black Women's Health Book: Speaking for Ourselves*, White (1990) commented that for generations, black women have taken care of everything and everyone but themselves, and that establishing their own well-being as a priority is essential. In support of White's comments Friedman (1998) noted that the mother has been observed to assume the sick role only when absolutely mandatory, and then only reluctantly. Ahijevych and Bernhard (1994) found health-promoting behaviors of African American women were less intensive than those of other groups of women. Research findings in that area are conflicting and warrant more research, particularly to determine the effects of the child's chronic condition on the mother's health promotion and maintenance behaviors.

In examining all the themes found in this study, we conclude that "system of asthma" is an overriding theme. The women caregivers live in a system of asthma where various family members, including the affected child's siblings, parents, grandparents, and cousins have been diagnosed as having asthma. One pertinent comment regarding that system was, "*and it seems to me, just looking at this—most of this asthma stuff seems to be on our family.*" Most families in both cities included here reported other children and close relatives who experienced episodes of asthma. This phenomenon is not unusual. Sander (1998) described her family of four children, three of whom had asthma. Sander also noted that she, too, had asthma. Asher and Price (1998) found all of the mothers in their study reported some member of the extended family as having had asthma.

Implications for Nursing

Although the findings of our study are not generalizable to the general population of African American caregivers of children who have asthma, the implications for nursing

Table 1 • Suggested Clinical Implications	
Theme	*Implications*
Caregiver Knowledge	Assess caregivers' level of knowledge and sources of information about asthma. Design interventions to increase knowledge and necessary skills based on caregivers' learning needs. Provide educational opportunities for primary caregivers when possible.
Support	Identify sources and quality of support within family and community including child's school.
Faith/Religion	Recognize and respect caregiver's faith and religion as major coping strategy. Determine how their system of faith, including religious community, plays a role in family healthcare (e.g., beliefs about healing, use of medications).
Industrious/Gatekeepers	Determine the extent of caregiver roles and responsibilities and employment status; impact on ability/time to manage child with asthma. Provide assistance as necessary including referrals to appropriate resources.
Health Status	Recognize health status of primary caregivers and significant family members. Determine impact on child's asthma management. Develop appropriate interventions including necessary referrals for caregiver health management.

are worth noting (see Table 1). Nurses should assess the caregivers knowledge, not only when the child is initially diagnosed, but also during each healthcare visit. Nurses should also determine other sources of information and provide asthma educational opportunities for all caregivers when possible. The ability to cope with the child's asthma and other perceived stressors is strongly influenced by the mother's religious faith. In light of this well-documented fact, nurses should be sensitive, nonjudgmental, and supportive of parents when they express their religious beliefs and practices. Additionally, being a caregiver of a child with asthma is only one aspect of these women's lives. They may have other children with asthma, meaning that they may have multiple medications to administer and frequent trips to undertake to schools and to healthcare facilities for primary and acute episodic care as they attend to the "family affair" of asthma. Nurses should assess the family's health status including that of all primary caregivers and the impact of their health status on their ability to manage the child with asthma.

Conclusion

The women caregivers in this study live in a family system consisting of multiple members, and often have asthma and other health conditions themselves. Their lives are influenced by their cultural world view, and they should be described from this perspective. More research is needed that provides an emic view (the view they have of themselves) as they manage a child with asthma. Understanding them and their world is key to establishing credible interventions, that promote successful asthma management and optimal outcomes for their children. †

Yvonne M. Sterling is a Professor, Department of Family Nursing, Louisiana State University Health Sciences Center School of Nursing, New Orleans, LA. She can be reached c/o Louisiana State University Health Sciences Center, School of Nursing, 1900 Gravier Street, New Orleans, LA 70118 (e-mail: ysterl@lsuhsc.edu).

Jane W. Peterson is a Professor of Nursing and Anthropologist, Seattle University School of Nursing, Seattle, WA. This study was supported by NIAID, NIH as a Research Supplement for Underrepresented Minority Investigators to Grant No. U01 A13961.

References

Ahijevych, K., & Bernhard, L. (1994). Health-promoting behaviors of African American women. *Nursing Research*, 43(2), 86–89.

Asher, M., & Price, J. (1998). Childhood asthma: Parents' views of professional advice. *Community Practitioner*, 71(5), 177–178.

Centers for Disease Control and Prevention (CDC). (2000). Measuring childhood asthma prevalence before and after the 1997 redesign of the National Health Interview Survey-United States. *Morbidity and Mortailty Weekly Report*, 49(40), 908–911, October 13, 2002.

Centers for Disease Control and Prevention (CDC). (1999). *National Center for environmental health*. Retrieved March 2002 from http://www.cdc.gov.nceh/

Davis, R. (1998). Coming to a place of understanding: The meaning of health and illness for African American women. *The Journal of Multicultural Nursing & Health*, 4(1), 32–41.

Edwards, K. (1993). Low-income African American women expressions of their health management. *The Association of Black Nursing Faculty Journal (ABNF)*, 4(1), 17–19.

Friedman, M. (1998). *Family nursing: Research, theory & practice*. Stamford, CT: Appleton & Lange.

Germain, C. (2001). *Ethnography*. In Munhall, P. Nursing research. A qualitative perspective (3rd ed.) Boston: Jones and Bartlett Publishers.

Grus, C., Lopez-Hernandez, C., Delamater, A., Appelgate, B., Brito, A., Wurm, G., et al. (2001). Parental self-efficacy and morbidity in pediatric asthma. *Journal of Asthma*, 38(1), 99–106.

Horner, S. (1998). Catching the asthma: Family care for school-aged children with asthma. *Journal of Pediatric Nursing*, 13(6), 356–366.

Hudson-Weems, C. (1993). *Africana womanism: Reclaiming ourselves*. Troy, MI: Bedford.

Kieckhefer, G., & Ratcliffe, M. (2000). What parents of children with asthma tell us. *Journal of Pediatric Health Care*, 14, 122–126.

Krulik, T., Turner-Henson, A., Kanematsu, Y., Al-Ma'aitah, R., Swan, J., & Holiday, B. (1999). Parenting stress and mothers of young children with chronic illness: A cross-cultural study. *Journal of Pediatric Nursing*, 14(2), 130–140.

Kurnat, E., & Moore, C. (1999). The impact of a chronic condition on the families of children with asthma. *Pediatric Nursing*, 25(3), 288–292.

Mailick, M., Holden, G., & Walther, V., (1994). Coping with childhood asthma: Caretaker views. *Health & Social Work, 19*(2), 102–111.

MacDonald, H. (1996). "Mastering uncertainty:" Mothering the child with asthma. *Pediatric Nursing, 22*(1), 55–59.

National Institute of Allergy and Infectious Diseases (NIAID). (2000). *NIAID fact sheet.* Retrieved January 2000 from http://www.niaid.nih.gov/factsheets/allergystat.htm

Peterson, J., Sterling, Y., & Stout, J. W. (in press). Explanatory models of asthma from African American caregivers of children with asthma. *Journal of Asthma.*

Rogers-Dulan, J., & Blacher, J. (1995). African American families, religion and disability: A conceptual framework, *Mental Retardation, 33*(4), 226–238.

Sander, N. (1998). Belief systems that affect the management of childhood asthma. *Immunology and Allergy Clinics of North America, 18*(1), 99–112.

Sterling, Y., Peterson, J., & Weekes, D. (1997). African American families with chronically ill children: Oversights and insights. *Journal of Pediatric Nursing, 12*(5), 292–299.

Taylor, J. (1998). Womanism: A methodologic framework for African American women. *Advances in Nursing Science, 21*(1), 53–64.

Taylor, R., Jackson, J. & Chatters, L. (1997). *Family life in black America.* Thousand Oaks, CA: Sage Publications.

Walker, A. (1983). *In search of our mother's gardens: Womanist prose.* New York: Harcourt Brace Jovanovich.

Wade, S., Weil, C., Holden, G., Mitchell, H., Evans, E., Kruszon-Moran, D., et al. (1997). Psychosocial characteristics of inner-city children with asthma: a description of the NCICAS psychosocial protocol. *Pediatric Pulmonology, 24*, 263–276.

White, E. (1990). *The black women's health book: Speaking for ourselves.* Seattle, WA: Seal Press.

ONLINE

Allergy & Asthma Network/Mothers of Asthmatics, Inc.:

www.aanma.org

American Academy of Asthma

Allergy and Immunology:

http://www.aaaai.org

American Lung Association:

http://www.lungusa.org/

Asthma & Allergy Foundation of America:

www.aafa.org

School Asthma Allergy.com:

http://schoolasthma.com

11

Historical Research Method

*N*ursing care for patients always includes acquiring a nursing history. If nurses did not collect background data, they would—through ignorance—greatly jeopardize decisions regarding a client's current health care needs and future chance of achieving a higher level of wellness. A historical understanding also is crucial to providing nursing care because of nursing's essential holistic nature. Looking at the whole person requires recognition of multiple factors that influence the individual. Similarly, decisions related to the nursing profession, such as the current shortage, risk failure and inadequacy of response if the profession ignores its history.

In a recent editorial in *Nursing History Review* (*NHR*), D'Antonio (2004) questions whether nurse historians are "in the process of proclaiming history as an overarching intellectual paradigm for a practice discipline that draws its strengths from its contextual specificity and ideological flexibility" (p. 1). History may serve as a "new paradigm for nursing knowledge" (p. 1). D'Antonio's editorial sets the stage for this chapter on historical research method. Nurses need knowledge to practice. Their social contract with society and commitment to provide culturally competent care requires in-depth knowing and understanding. History allows us to look at events in the past from a variety of lenses, thus allowing us to interpret data in a number of different ways. The ability to examine past events gives meaning and texture to the care nurses provide, influences the way we educate new nurses, and provides the background to influence public and political support.

All knowledge has a historical dimension; conversely, history provides individuals with a way of knowing. Tholfsen (1977) explained that "the past is present in every person and in the cultural and institutional world that surrounds [them]" (p. 248). This means, Tholfsen continued, that historians must know the historical conditions of the period they are studying.

Knowledge of the past helps to inform research designs that include explanatory background necessary to establish an understanding of the phenomenon under study. Selecting historical research design as the research method of choice requires that researchers understand what history is; possess an understanding of various social, political, and economic factors that affect events, ideas, and people; have interest in the subject; and be creative in their approaches (Christy, 1978; Rines & Kershner, 1979).

Historical research provides a critical way of knowing. There are, however, many ways to study the past, and, depending on the framework used, the understanding will differ. For example, the way we have studied nursing over time has changed, alternating from the presentation of nursing heroines to the more recent use of a social feminist framework. Connolly (2004) asks us to broaden the study of history and writes that political history along with social history can provide important data needed for arguing the case from a political perspective for more nurses and other important related health care issues. "Nurse historians have expertise linking the stories of individual patients and nurses to their larger institutional framework, a natural link to the broader political context" (Connolly, 2004, p. 18).

Yet, historians can more easily explain why they do historical research than the steps involved in doing it. Even with the various tools and approaches available, there remains a certain "inexactness with which historians define, delineate and defend their particular research methodology" (D'Antonio, 2005, p. 1). The inability to clearly explain the process leads to a "methodological vulnerability" (p. 1) that in turn makes it more difficult to explain and understand what a historian does, ultimately jeopardizing the ability to pass this knowledge on to future historians (D'Antonio, 2005).

Throughout this chapter and Chapter 12, the reader will learn about the steps involved in historical research methodology. However, learning to do historical research requires an understanding and acceptance of the often circuitous nature of the process. In an attempt to demonstrate the number of ways historical research has been defined, refined, and applied over time, the sections Historical Research Defined and Historical Research Traditions will help to illustrate the iterative and nonlinear aspects of the process.

HISTORICAL RESEARCH DEFINED

*M*any definitions and explanations exist related to the meaning and nature of history. Austin (1958) defined *history* as "an integrated, written record of past events, based on the results of a search for the truth" (p. 4). Kruman (1985) explained history as "facts (ideas, events, social, and cultural processes) filtered through human intelligence" (p. 111). Kruman referred to an *objective relativism* that permits the objective reality of one historian to coexist with different historical interpretations of others, thus promoting change in ideas and advances in historical inquiry. Matejski (1986) conceived of history "as a past event, a record, or account of something that has happened" (p. 175). Furthermore, Matejski described history as a field of study with its own set of criteria and methods that enable researchers to collect data and interpret findings. Having its own method that has often borrowed from other disciplines, historical inquiry examines the interactions of people, activities, and "multiple variables" (Matejski, 1986, p. 177) that affect human thought and activity. The narrative that results from a historian's findings must creatively weave many factors into a readable and interesting story.

Historical research opens windows into the past, creating new ideas and reshaping human thinking and understanding. Ashley (1978) explained the crucial role historical research plays in the foundation of nursing scholarship by defining history as "the study of creative activity in human behavior [that] gives one the courage to create and respond to what is new without fear of losing one's identity with the whole of humanity" (p. 28). As Lynaugh (1996) suggested, history becomes "our source of identity . . . it helps us gain identity and personal meaning in our work, improves our comprehension and our planning, and validates social criticism" (p. 1).

Like nursing, history is an art and science. Olson (2000) stresses the link between the art and science of history and calls for a dialogue among historians to include quantifiable data along with qualitative data. Olson further notes that "quantifiable information from public and private records is often crucial to uncovering the seemingly hidden history of women (p. 138). Demonstrating the use of numbers to explain past phenomena, Olson examined the school records of the St. Luke's Hospital Training School for Nurses between the years 1892 and 1937. These records provided the quantifiable data that told a "story" about those who attended this Midwest school. The discipline of history requires the use of scientific principles to study the interrelationship of social, economic, political, and psychological factors that influence ideas, events, institutions, and people. Yet, to explain the findings of historical inquiry while balancing the rigors of scientific inquiry and the understanding of human behavior, historical researchers must revert to the "art of contemplation, speculation, and of interpretation" (Newton, 1965, p. 24).

Researchers who choose historical methods must exhibit more than just a curiosity about the past. Researchers formulate a thesis about the relationship among ideas, events, institutions, or people in the past. Chronologically ordering events over time does not explain the established links and ties. Probing for explanations between historical antecedents requires questioning, reasoning, and interpreting. Christy (1978) explained that "healthy skepticism becomes a way of life for the serious historiographer" (p. 6). Historians seeking to discover meanings in the past must sift through data and examine each piece closely for clues.

D'Antonio (1999) speaks of the use of cross-disciplinary interpretation in the writing and rewriting of nursing history. This "'two-way street' between the historical traditions of nursing and those of the liberal arts" (p. 268) has led to significant change in the understanding of nurses' work. Most historical nursing research in the late 20th century will include some kind of reference to issues related to gender, class, race, and politics of professionalism (D'Antonio, 1999). Yuginovich (2000) states, "history is probably a stronger force than language in moulding our social consciousness" (p. 70). Examining nurses' roles as women, caregivers, leaders, administrators, educators, and practitioners in light of a multidisciplinary framework provides the historian with a variety of useful sources, broad interpretations, and necessary tools in which to examine data.

When studying the past, historical researchers use a variety of sources, such as private letters, personal and professional journals, books, magazines, and newspapers. Researchers travel in time and explore these materials, seeking a relationship among ideas, events, institutions, or people. The purpose of a historical study is not to predict but, rather, to understand the past in order to explain present or future relationships. From historical documents, historical researchers derive insight from past lived experiences that they can adapt to generate new ideas (Barzun & Graff, 1985).

Researchers use a historical design if they believe something from the past will explain something in the present or the future. Conflict between what the researcher thinks and what he or she may have read about a particular topic also influences the decision to do historical research. For example, a misconception regarding nurses' participation in the late 19th century women's movement led Lewenson (1990, 1996) to study the relationship between the women's suffrage movement and the four nursing organizations that formed in America between 1893 and 1920. Lewenson conducted a historical inquiry to dispel the tension resulting from a contemporary understanding of the past, also called a present-mindedness, which omitted nursing's political response to the events of the late 19th and early 20th centuries.

Present-mindedness refers to using a contemporary perspective when analyzing data collected from an earlier period. Such data analysis is stigmatized as unhistorical and leads to inaccurate conclusions when ideas and lived experiences of people in the past are compared with later events (Tholfsen, 1977, p. 247). Although Tholfsen warned historians to be careful of absolutes and the dangers of present-mindedness, he has argued that "the best history is rooted in a lively interest in the present" (p. 247). Nevertheless, history refers to constant change, and it is this change that "produces the endless diversity characteristic of the historical world" (p. 248). Researchers must study each period within the context of its age to avoid judging or interpreting the past without respect to changes made over time. Hence, difference found in every age must "be understood in its own terms" (p. 248).

Nursing is a field ripe for historical research. Nurses come from rich, diverse backgrounds that are useful in helping to better understand and explain human behavior. Nurses, who are adept at studying human behavior, are well suited to conduct historical inquiry in which they study human behavior in the context of an event, a place, a person, an institution, or an idea in the past. Like historians, nurses identify and interpret patterns of behavior that occur over time.

HISTORICAL RESEARCH TRADITIONS

M orse and Field (1995) identified two traditions or schools of thought in historical research: the positivistic or neo-positivistic and the idealist schools. In the *neo-positivistic school*, historians take a more quantitative posture. The focus is on "reducing history to universal laws" (p. 33). Historians use data analysis to verify or categorize information. "There is a strong effort to show cause-effect relationships" (p. 33).

In the *idealist school*, historians are most concerned with getting inside an event and trying to understand the thoughts of individuals involved in the event while considering the time, place, and situations (Fitzpatrick, 2001; Morse & Field, 1995). The idealist school is more closely aligned with the values of qualitative research represented in the present text.

Regardless of the tradition observed by historical researchers, the intent is always the "interpretation and narration of past events" (Morse & Field, 1995, p. 33). Historical researchers must clearly identify the focus of the study and then make a commitment to a philosophic position.

Historical research design is being distinguished from other qualitative designs that build on positivistic traditions (D'Antonio, 2005). D'Antonio briefly describes Gaddis's (2002) four methodological practices that structure historical research and separate this design from that of others. Historians look for interactions between and among variables and how these interactions might effect change. The historian plays with the idea of what might have happened if the variables changed. For example, what would have happened if Nightingale did not go the Crimean or if Lavinia Dock did not advocate women's suffrage? This helps historians sharpen their focus on "other events, actors, social themes, or political processes that might otherwise remain hidden" (D'Antonio, 2005, p. 2). Historians look for "contextual specificity" and do so by placing an event within a specific time frame and then examining the time leading up to the event, as well as following the course of the event. Judgments are made about the various factors or variables that contribute to the story. D'Antonio believes that this is where the distinction between historical research and other methods exists. Historians must "consider and assess the significance of the work completed by other historical methods and make judgments" (p. 2).

FUNDAMENTAL CHARACTERISTICS OF HISTORICAL RESEARCH

*A*lthough no single historical method exists, Lynaugh and Reverby (1987) have offered essential guideposts and rules of evidence to ensure the credibility and usefulness of the historian's findings. Lusk (1997) has identified several methodological stages, including selecting "a topic and an appropriate theoretical framework, finding and accessing the resources, and analyzing, synthesizing, interpreting, and reporting the data" (p. 355). In search of an approach, Barzun and Graff (1985) wrote that, "without form in every sense, the facts of the past, like the jumbled visions of a sleeper in a dream, elude us" (p. 271).

The next section offers beginning historical researchers a guide to developing a historical study. As in any process, researchers must allow fluidity between the steps of the guide, that is, they must easily move from one step to another, in both directions. For example, the data collected may direct the literature review, and the literature review, in turn, may determine the thesis.

SELECTION OF HISTORICAL RESEARCH AS METHOD

*T*o understand the wholeness of the past, nurse historians select a framework to guide the study. However, as Lynaugh and Reverby (1987) have warned, no one formula or specific method exists for doing historical research. Tholfsen (1977) contends that "history lacks a coherent theoretical and conceptual structure" (p. 246). No one theoretical framework exists for the study of history. Although there is no "set methodology . . . some methodological consensus exists" (Lusk, 1997, p. 355). History is a discipline with many structures that Cramer (1992) describes as "permanent or semipermanent relations of elements that determine the character of the whole" (p. 6). Superimposed structure enables researchers to organize data. For example, when using geography to frame a study, the researcher may write a regional history, or when using a particular topic to organize a study, the researcher may focus on women's work (Cramer, 1992).

Society asks historians to analyze experiences and use the information gained to explain and prepare society for similar events in the future. For example, historians study the records of war so that society will learn what may help in future wars (Hofstadter, 1959). Writing for a specific purpose creates further tension between the dual natures that exist within the historian's role: the writing of a historical narrative and the writing of a historical monograph. According to Hofstadter, the historical narrative tells a story but often is disappointing in the analysis, and the historical monograph approximates a scientific inquiry but lacks literary style and frequently offers insufficient analytic data. However, both functions are enriched by interrelating social sciences and historical inquiry. Hofstadter believes that a combination of social sciences and historical research produces fresh ideas and new insights into human behavior.

Historians look at other disciplines to help inform and structure their work. To understand the development of nursing education in North America and to provide a theoretical framework, historians might use research from women's and educational history in the United States. Knowledge of U.S. labor history, which is important to nursing history because of nurses' apprenticeship role in hospitals, would also be a useful framework for historiographers to conceptually organize data. To study history using a variety of approaches, such as philosophic, national, psychohistorical, or economic, allows researchers to explore a point in time with a conceptual guide from a particular discipline (Ashley, 1978; Matejski, 1986).

Nurse historians consider different theoretical frameworks to structure their historical studies. They may select from theoretical approaches such as biographical, social, and intellectual histories. A *biographical history*, the study of an individual, opens a wide vista to an entire period (Brown, D'Antonio, & Davis, 1991). Biography uses the story of a person's life to understand "the values, expectations, tensions and the conflicts of the time and culture within which he or she lived" (Brown et al., 1991). Interpretation requires historians to familiarize themselves with a period so that they may derive meanings from within the particular time frame rather than superimpose them from a later, contemporary distance. For example, to understand the life of the early 20th-century nurse and birth control activist Margaret Sanger, it is essential to understand society's attitudes about women's roles and beliefs about procreation. Biographical research lends itself to uncovering stories about nurses who participated in the profession. These studies do not need to be limited to the study of more famous nursing leaders (Grypma, 2005). By studying the lives those who may not have been considered "worthy" of attention in previous periods, historical researchers can enrich and inform the history of nursing.

Social history explores a particular period and attempts to understand the prevailing values and beliefs by examining the everyday events of that period. Connolly (2004) uses a definition of social history that examines the "experience, behavior, and agency of those at society's margins, rather than its elite" (p. 5). Exploration into the lives of women, for example, provides a richer understanding of events than were previously available from a "consensus" framework. Individual stories about those outside of the mainstream of American ideas have not been routinely included in historical accounting of events. Historian Vern Bullough recommended a strategy for doing social history. She suggested including the use of specific quantitative data to understand the life experiences of "'ordinary' men and women" (Brown et al.,

1991, p. 3). An analysis of census data, court records, and municipal surveys, for example, assists historians to go beyond the boundaries of class, ethnicity, economics, and race—hence enabling them to gain a broader understanding of the study subject. In an example of a social history, Melchior (2004) studied the evolution of nursing history in Canada, utilizing nursing and feminist historical research methods. Melchior argued for "new directions" (p. 340) in nursing history that focus attention on the everyday experience of nurses and nursing students.

Intellectual history, in which "*thinking* is the event under analysis," lends itself to several approaches (Brown et al., 1991, p. 2). Historians may explore the ideas of an individual considered to be an intellectual thinker of a period; for example, they might study the ideas of public health nurses such as Lillian Wald. Or, they may explore the history of ideas over time, such as nursing leaders' ideas that influenced the development of nursing education in the United States. Another approach may be to explore the attitudes and ideas of people who are not considered major intellectual thinkers of the period, such as the ideas of practicing nurses (Hamilton, 1991). While conducting their research, historians must be aware that conflict may arise between the ideas and the contextual backgrounds that gave rise to them (Hamilton, 1993).

Historical researchers must be ready to "live in permanent struggle with conceptual ambiguities, missing evidence and conflicting viewpoints" (Lynaugh & Reverby, 1987, p. 4). Historians continually face a methodological polarity whereby tension exists between the "general and the unique, [and] between the particular and the universal" (Tholfsen, 1977, p. 249). However, these tensions and uncertainties are essential to history because they mirror human experience with all of life's contradictions and ambiguities (Tholfsen, 1977). When approaching historical research, researchers must expect ambiguity of design as well as data. Researchers must decide on a particular theoretical framework and understand the conflicting views and ideas regarding the approach. Keeping this information in mind helps historians construct creative designs that address their particular research interest.

DATA GENERATION

Developing a Focus

To apply a historical design, researchers must first define the study topic and prepare a statement of the subject (Kruman, 1985). A clear, concise statement tells readers what researchers have studied and their reasons for selecting particular subjects. Researchers must explain their interest in the topic and justify its relationship to other topics. In addition, researchers establish the purpose and significance of the study to nursing and nursing research in the statement (Rines & Kershner, 1979). According to Lusk (1997), topics "should be significant, with the potential to illuminate or place a new perspective on current questions" (p. 355).

When selecting a topic, Austin (1958) suggests that the subject be "part of a larger whole, and one which can be isolated" (p. 5). Isolating a part of the topic makes the study more manageable. For example, it may be easier to study the curriculum of three nurse training schools in 1897 than to tackle nursing education in the late 19th century.

Because historical study does not predict outcomes, there is no hypothesis. A researcher's interest and hunches about the topic guide the study and move the research toward a particular field or discipline. Researchers base their ideas on background information they have obtained. Patterns that emerge in the initial fact-finding and knowledge-building steps aid in the creative formation of a thesis. For example, instead of predicting the effect of apprenticeship training on the development of nursing education, historians might identify themes or ideas about nursing education and use those themes to relate their findings. An example is Hanson's (1989) study of the emergence of liberal education in nursing education.

To successfully focus the study, researchers must gather information regarding the period to be studied. They must have a working knowledge of the social, cultural, economic, and political climate that prevailed and how these factors influenced the subject. This knowledge helps researchers establish patterns and identify relevant points regarding the subject and justifies the selection of the historical method. Moreover, when selecting a topic, researchers need to be aware of the accessibility of the sources, the relevance of the topic to the audience, and its potential to enhance understanding (Lusk, 1997).

Selecting a Title

Once historians have identified the focus of the study, it is helpful to delimit the project by titling it. The title tells readers what to expect from the study and narrows the topic for the historian. Typically, the title includes the time frame and purpose, for example, A Review of Critical Thinking in Nursing: 1990–2000.

Although the title appears first in a completed study and concisely describes the research topic, it may be the researcher's final step. The advantage of titling a study early in the project is to assist in focusing the work. Historians can always modify the title as the project develops and should be open to change based on newly uncovered data. A well-focused and delimited study will focus the literature search, making it effective and meaningful. It is essential, however, that historians do not prematurely close the literature search because the materials discovered fall outside of the predetermined time frame. Historians should continue their review of materials until they are comfortable that they have fully examined the thesis. It is easier to adjust the title than to risk conducting a poorly developed study.

Conducting a Literature Review

A good starting point for a literature review is to identify major works published on the selected topic. If historians want to study the history of critical thinking, then they must assess what has been written on the subject and identify the themes and inconsistencies related to critical thinking that exist in the literature. Part of the review includes identifying the problems connected with the topic. For example, the ambiguities that have arisen over defining and evaluating critical thinking would be important to the inquiry. A conclusive search of the literature for references from contiguous periods allows for a greater understanding of the subject. Computer databases provide a means by which researchers can obtain data needed in the literature review. Lorentzon (2004) found that the "newly digitalized journal" dating from 1888 until 1956 of the *Nursing Record/British Journal of Nursing* provides an important new avenue for searching topics published in this journal.

A literature review helps researchers formulate questions that need to be addressed, delineate a time frame for the study, and decide on a theoretical framework. In addition, the review affords researchers opportunities to learn what types of materials are available. For example, through the literature review, a researcher will learn whether he or she can obtain primary sources or first-hand accounts of an event, such as the letters written by an individual living during the period of study. The researcher also learns of secondary sources or secondhand accounts of events, such as histories or newspaper articles that have already been written on the particular study subject.

Based on the literature review, historians formulate questions regarding events that influenced the chosen subject. To elucidate the subject, researchers ask questions beginning with "How," "Why," "Who," and "What" in light of the ideas, events, and institutions that existed and individuals who lived during a particular period. If, for example, a researcher narrows a topic such as U.S. public health nursing to the study of public health nurses living at the Henry Street Settlement, then questions such as the following may guide the direction of the literature search: How did the Henry Street Settlement begin? Who began the Henry Street Settlement? What is a settlement house? Why was the settlement located on Henry Street? These questions may prompt the researcher to examine biographies of people who participated in the settlement house movement during the late 19th and early 20th centuries.

Or, to better understand life at that time, the historian might read city records regarding population statistics or examine published materials to comprehend another historian's perception of women's roles, education, work, and life during the study period. Newspaper accounts, written histories, proceedings of minutes, photographs, biographies, letters, diaries, and films may help historians seeking a greater understanding of a particular subject.

During the literature review, historians must develop an organizing strategy that will help them analyze the data. Some facts obtained may seem trivial in the beginning of the project but may become crucial to explaining or connecting events learned later in the study. Thus, careful documentation using an index card filing system or a directory in a word processing program will help researchers retrieve the information at a later time (Austin, 1958; Barzun & Graff, 1985). Bibliographic data should be recorded precisely. The bibliographic entry should include the author, title, and abstract, place of publication, date, and particular archive or library where the researcher found the information. Researchers must include all pertinent information in the notes so that, during data analysis, they will be able to easily retrieve important information or go back to the original source, if necessary.

The literature review will serve as the bibliography for the research. Using historical source materials from libraries, archives, bibliographies, newspapers, reviews, journals, associations, and the Internet, researchers begin to comprehend the extent of the subject under investigation (Matejski, 1986). To accomplish this important step, historians use collections in libraries and archives. Libraries and archives contain different types of reference materials that require different methods of storage and classification. To enable researchers to use each method appropriately, it is necessary to become familiar with both.

Libraries contain published materials that researchers often use as secondary materials. To locate these materials, researchers use a card catalog, computerized catalog system, or computerized database that allows them to locate particular works. A call number, usually given in the catalog, designates the unique location of each volume in the library. Volumes are usually arranged by subject. Libraries purchase books and thus permit the use for them to circulate (Termine, 1992), whereas archival materials remain on-site.

Archives differ from libraries in their holdings, cataloging, and circulation policies. Archives contain unpublished materials that are considered primary source materials, such as the "official records of an organization or persons ... [that] are preserved because of the value of the information they contain" (Termine, 1992). Instead of using a card catalog to find a book, researchers use a *finding aid*, a published book or catalog that lists what is in the archive or repository. The finding aid identifies a collection using a record group, a series, and a subseries. However, instead of material being stored according to these designations, collections are often stored haphazardly within aisles, shelves, and box numbers. Libraries contain a discrete number of volumes, whereas archives contain linear (cubic) feet of records. Archives acquire their material by collections. Many organizations cannot store or maintain their records and transfer this task to archives. For example, a college of nursing may acquire the historical records, including boxes of meeting minutes, curricula, and pictures, of a diploma program that existed in the city before the opening of the collegiate program.

Unlike libraries, where books are circulated, archives require that researchers use the materials on-site. In most archives, researchers may only use pencil and paper to collect data; other archives permit the use of laptop computers. Newer technologic advances have enabled researchers to use handheld scanners in conjunction with their laptop computers. Scanners provide a safe method for copying materials (Lusk, 1997). To gain access to archives, researchers are usually required to make appointments with an archivist to discuss their project. Besides offering researchers primary source references needed in historical research, archives provide materials and memorabilia that researchers may use in exhibitions to illustrate the history of an organization or the life of a person. Because primary source materials may be fragile, archivists will only permit scholars engaged in historical research to use the collections (Termine, 1992). A frequently updated listing of archives containing rich resources for nurse historians can be found on the American Association for the History of Nursing Web site (http://www.aahn.org).

Archivists and librarians assist researchers to access materials, thus rendering an important data gathering service. However, because of the differences between libraries and archives, the work of professional archivists and librarians varies. Whereas archivists work with the records, papers, manuscripts, and nonprinted materials found in the collections, librarians manage books and publications (Termine, 1992). Table 11.1 summarizes the differences between libraries and archives.

The powerful connection between historians and archival materials was part of a discussion during the preconference for the 2004 annual meeting of the American Association for the History of Nursing. Archives provide a setting for nurse historians to relate closely to the subject under study. For historians, the ability to hold the original letters of nursing leaders like Lavinia Dock or Florence Nightingale inspires an almost reverent feeling toward the material and the archives (Rafferty, 2004). Other historians, like Lorentzon (2004) explain that the "musty smell" of paper archives provides the historian with a reassuring sense of ambiance that cannot be replaced by "cold" microfilm readers and computer screens (p. 280). The archives connect historians to vital pieces of data that researchers must read, assess, interpret, and place within the context of the study.

Table 11.1 • Differences Between Libraries and Archives		
	Libraries	*Archives*
Holdings	Published materials	Unpublished materials: records, manuscripts, papers
Locators	Card catalog	Finding aid
	Call number	Record group, series, subseries
	Unique location by subject	Haphazard location of "boxes" by aisle, shelf, box number
Stored	Volumes (titles)	Linear (cubic) feet
Acquired	Purchased by volume or issue	Donated or purchased collections
Use of materials	Circulation	Noncirculation; use of paper and pencil only or laptop computer to collect data

From Termine, J. (1992, March). Paper presented at the State University of New York, Health Science Center at Brooklyn, College of Nursing, Brooklyn, NY. Adapted with permission.

DATA TREATMENT

Identifying Sources

Historians must find some way to understand what actually occurred during a particular period. To research historical antecedents, researchers must identify sources from the period. Primary sources give first-hand accounts of a person's experience, an institution, or an event and may lack critical analysis. However, primary sources, such as personal letters or diaries, may contain the author's interpretation of an event. Thus, researchers must analyze and interpret the meaning of the primary sources.

Ulrich (1990) wrote about Martha Ballard, an 18th-century midwife from Hallowell, Maine. Using Ballard's diary as a primary source, Ulrich wrote a rich biographical account of Ballard, as well as a historical rendering of everyday life during this period. Ballard's diary, which she kept daily for more than 27 years, connected "several prominent themes in the social history of the early Republic" (p. 27). More important, Ulrich explained, "It [the diary] transforms the nature of the evidence upon [which] much of the history of the period has been written" (p. 27). Earlier historians did not consider the potential the diary had for uncovering historical data about this period in the

United States. Rather, they perceived Ballard's daily record as trivial and too filled with daily life to be of any importance—because she documented the births at which she assisted, the travel she endured to reach laboring women, the stories she wrote about other people, and the accounts of her own family. However, on viewing the same diary, Ulrich believed that it reached directly to the "marrow of eighteenth century life" (p. 33). The "trivia that so annoyed earlier readers provides a consistent, daily record of the operation of a female-managed economy" (p. 33).

Unlike primary sources that are written by people directly involved in an event, secondary sources are materials that cite opinions and present interpretations. Newspaper accounts, journal articles, and textbooks from the period being studied are secondary sources that place researchers within the context of a period. For example, newspaper accounts of the 1893 Columbian World Exposition held in Chicago added authenticity to the story about the founding of the American Society of Superintendents of Training Schools for Nurses (known today as the National League for Nursing). However, researchers may use secondary sources as primary sources, depending on the researchers' questions or the purpose of the study (Austin, 1958). For example, although newspaper articles from the late 19th century offered secondary accounts of what happened, they also provided insight into what was considered important during that period. Thus, if researchers are studying the insights of individuals present at a particular point in history, then they may use newspaper accounts as primary as well as secondary sources. Chaney and Folk (1993), for example, used cartoons found in the American Medical Association journal *American Medical News* as a primary source in the study "A Profession in Caricature: The Changing Attitudes Towards Nursing in the *American Medical News*, 1960–1989."

Confirming Source Genuineness and Authenticity

When selecting primary sources, the genuineness and authenticity of those sources becomes an important issue. Barzun and Graff (1985) explained that historians are responsible for verifying documents to ensure they are genuine and authentic. *Genuine* means that a document is not forged; *authentic* means that the document provides the truthful reporting of a subject (Barzun & Graff, 1985). Authenticating sources requires several operations, none of which is fixed in a specific technique. Researchers rely on "attention to detail, on common-sense reasoning, on a 'developed' field for history and chronology, on familiarity with human behavior, and on ever-enlarging stores of information" (p. 112). Authenticity of letters or journals becomes even more important when researchers find them in a nursing school attic or closet. More than likely, primary sources within archival collections have already been found to be genuine and have been authenticated by the institution in which they are housed. Nevertheless, researchers are responsible for the final authenticity of a document. A careful reading of the document, an examination of the type of paper and the condition of the material, and an extensive knowledge of the period can help researchers verify the document as authentic.

The validity of historical research relies on measures that address matters concerning external and internal criticism. *External criticism* questions the genuineness of primary sources and ensures that the document is what it claims. *Internal criticism* of data is concerned with content authenticity or truthfulness. Kerlinger (1986) suggests that internal criticism "seeks the 'true' meaning and value of the content of sources of data" (p. 621). Researchers must ask, Does the content accurately reflect the period in which it is written? Do the facts conflict with historical dates, meanings of words, and social mores from the time?

Spieseke (1953) emphasizes that when determining the reliability of the contents, researchers must evaluate when authors of primary sources wrote their account—whether it was close to the event or 20 years later. Other questions researchers must ask are, Did a trained historian or an observer write the story? Were facts suppressed? If so, why? To ensure the accuracy of the writer, Spieseke suggests that researchers check for corroborating evidence, look for another independent primary source that supports the data, and identify any disagreements between sources. Ulrich (1990), for example, authenticated Ballard's diary by corroborating some of Ballard's entries regarding feed bills with other sources from the town in which she lived.

The data that researchers can validate externally as genuine, however, may be inconsistent when researchers examine the data contents. For example, an individual may have written letters in the 19th century, but the content may conflict with known facts of that period and pose serious questions regarding the truth of the content (Kerlinger, 1986). Nevertheless, external criticism "ultimately . . . leads to content analysis or internal criticism and is indispensable when assessing evidence" (Matejski, 1986, p. 189). Austin (1958) illustrated this point by explaining that learning the date of a source (external criticism) helps researchers determine whether the content reflects the period in which it was written (internal criticism), and vice versa.

In historical studies for which the story can be enhanced or explained by someone who is still alive and who has lived through a period of time, an oral history provides a useful data source. Collecting oral histories provides an important primary source for many historical studies in nursing and adds to the understanding of nursing's history. Kirby (1997/1998) speaks about the use of oral history to illuminate the "hidden worlds" of areas such as nursing, childhood, and family that are often not represented in archival collections. Kirby notes that "oral history offers an alternative form of evidence through which historians can discover the form and structure of these hidden worlds"

(p. 15). For example, a collection of stories told by nurses who have experienced changes in the hospital or the way we care for the terminally ill provides depth and richness to nursing's historical tapestry. "Over the past 20 years, research using oral history method has played a significant role in retrieving and recording historical experiences of 'non-elite' nurses and their patients who have no record of their lives or historical documents" (Biedermann, 2001, p. 61).

To do an oral history, the historian uses many of the same steps used in doing a history. One of the key differences in collecting oral histories is that living subjects are used and thus require consideration afforded to all research using human subjects. The Oral History Association (2000) Web page (http://omega.dickinson.edu/organizations/oha/pub_eg.html) provides detailed explanations of the responsibilities of the interviewer, the interviewee, and the organization sponsoring the oral histories, the archives that stores oral histories, and transcribers. Readers interested in using an oral history method in their study are referred to other sources such as the Oral History Association for a more comprehensive understanding of this method.

DATA ANALYSIS

*D*ata analysis relies on the statement of the subject, including the questions raised, the purpose, and the conceptual framework of the study. The themes developed by researchers direct data analysis. Researchers frame the findings according to research questions generated by the thesis. According to Spieseke (1953), the purpose of the study often directs the data analysis. If researchers want to teach a lesson, answer a question, or support an idea, they organize the selection of relevant data accordingly. How researchers analyze the material depends, in part, on the thematic organization of conceptual frameworks used in the study. Use of social, political, economic, or feminist theory will structure the data and enable researchers to concentrate on particular areas.

In data analysis, researchers must deal with the tension between the conflicting truths so that they may find interpretations or understandings regarding the subject. In some way, researchers must strike a "balance between conflict" (Tholfsen, 1977, p. 246). They need to ask questions such as, Is the content found in the primary and secondary sources congruent with each other, or are there conflicting stories? If a conflict does exist, is there supporting evidence to explain either side of the argument?

Another important aspect of analysis is researcher bias about the subject and the influence of that bias on data interpretation. Awareness of personal bias improves the researcher's ability to provide an accurate interpretation of events. Self-awareness promotes a researcher's honesty in finding the truth and decreases the influence of bias on data interpretation (Austin, 1958; Barzun & Graff, 1985).

Through data analysis, researchers should develop new material and new ideas based on supporting evidence rather than just rehash ideas (Matejski, 1986). Researchers seek to discover new truths from the assembled facts. However, given the same data, individuals will analyze the data differently and thus contribute to the tentative nature of interpretation (Austin, 1958). To interpret the findings and get at a truth, historians must be conscious of the role ideology plays in analysis. Researchers must question how ideology, or any set of ideas, influences the analysis of a particular event. For example, a paternalistic ideological view of the nurse's role in the health care system may starkly contrast with an interpretation of the same data using a feminist lens. Awareness of ideological influence enhances researchers' abilities to study the full effect that ideas have on events and to avoid accepting ideas on face value. Tholfsen (1977) argues that history will suffer if taught from any one ideological stance; instead, its aim should be the "commitment to the disinterested pursuit of truth, accompanied by an openness to continuing debate and discussion" (p. 255). With this understanding, researchers examine and analyze data to try to find alternative truths supported in the available evidence.

Analysis occurs throughout the process of data collection. Historians look for evidence to explain events or ideas. By interpreting primary and secondary documents, researchers form a picture of historical antecedents. However, these documents become part of history only when "they have been subjected to historiography that bridges the gap between lived occurrences and records" (Matejski, 1986, p. 180).

In the search for true meanings and in the attempt to bridge identified gaps, researchers must be aware not only of their own bias and the effect of ideology but also of bias found in the sources themselves that may impede interpretation. For example, in biographical research, the use of both informants through interviews and materials found in archival collections may raise issues regarding the accuracy and validity of the data. Historians doing a biographical study need to be cautious of interviews that often present a biased or one-sided view of the individual being studied. Researchers may also suspect bias in archival holdings of an individual's papers because the individual may have determined what to include in the collection (Brown et al., 1991). Olson's (2000) concern that nurse historians have maintained a "uniform reliance on a narrative approach" and excluded using quantifiable data in their analysis of historical events highlights another type of potential bias in interpreting historical data.

ETHICAL CONSIDERATIONS

*A*n ethical concern regarding the use of an institution or individual's private papers is the right to privacy versus the right to know. Although discussion of this concern is beyond the scope of this chapter, it is important for historical researchers to be aware of this dilemma. Researchers must have a clear idea of the kinds of information they need to obtain from data. If they find the source in an archive, then the archivist is responsible for seeing that "policy, regulations, and rules—governing his action do exist and are effective" (Rosenthal, 1982, p. 4). However, scholars are ultimately responsible for using data appropriately. If historians have as a goal to further the understanding of social, political, or economic relationships among individuals, institutions, events, or ideas, they must question what purpose is served if they expose exploitative or embarrassing details. Historians who misuse data and generate sensationalism by "[presenting] conclusions regarding motives and behavior that transcend the evidence ... [and] turn an ordinary book into a best seller" (Graebner, 1982, p. 23) are discouraging future access and preservation of primary sources. If this type of misuse involves the people or events in the past, then only a historical reputation is damaged; however, if it involves people who are still living or their immediate ancestors, then it places at risk the right to access future contributions of papers from families or institutions. When determining how to use data, Graebner suggests that "decisions, events, and activities which affect the public welfare or embrace qualities of major human interest—and thus add legitimately to the richness of the historical record—set the acceptable boundaries of historical search and analysis" (p. 23).

The confidentiality of source material has become more of an ethical concern for historians as researchers have placed greater emphasis on the lives of ordinary people (Lusk, 1997). Several professional organizations, such as the American Historical Association (1987), the American Association for the History of Medicine (1991), and the Oral History Association (2000), have developed ethical guidelines for historical research. Nurse historians Birnbach, Brown, and Hiestand (1991), members of the American Association for the History of Nursing, have published ethical guidelines as well as professional standards for doing historical inquiry in nursing.

INTERPRETATION OF FINDINGS

*T*he historical narrative is the final stage in the historical research process. During this stage, researchers tell the story that interprets the data and engages readers in the historical debate. Synthesis occurs, and findings are connected, supported, and molded "into a related whole" (Austin, 1958, p. 9).

Decisions regarding what to include and what to emphasize become important. In historical exposition, researchers explain not only what happened but how and why it happened. They explore relationships among events, ideas, people, organizations, and institutions and interpret them within the context of the period being studied. The political, social, and economic factors set a stage or backdrop from which to compare and contrast collected historical data. Historical judgments, based on historical evidence, must pass through the filter of "human understanding of human experience" (Cramer, 1992, p. 7). To accomplish this task, researchers must be sensitive to the material; must show genuine engagement in the subject; and must balance the forces of self, societal, and historical interest. Along with these attributes, researchers need creativity to achieve a coherent, convincing, and meaningful account (Ashley, 1978; Spieseke, 1953).

When writing the narrative, researchers are charged with creatively rendering the events, explaining the findings, and supporting the ideas. Researchers must possess discipline, organization, and imagination to accomplish this Herculean task. Historians must set aside time to write daily, finding a quiet place to concentrate and contemplate the data. They will use a detailed outline to direct the writing of the manuscript, plan the story using a thematic framework established early in the study, and use time and place as landmarks to give balance and direct the flow of the story while critically interpreting the findings (Austin, 1958).

Historians weave historical facts, research findings, and interpretations influenced by the conceptual framework into a coherent story. To guide them in the writing process, researchers may divide the narrative into chronologic periods. Or, they may use geographic places such as regional areas in the United States, thematic relationships, research questions, or political, social, cultural, or economic issues to organize the narrative. These ad hoc inventions are determined by individual researchers and as such are subject to researcher interest, bias, and understanding of the historical method (Cramer, 1992; Fondiller, 1978).

Writers of history who want readers to hear the words spoken during the period studied may use direct quotations. Direct quotations provide corroboration of and credibility to a researcher's interpretation. However, although authentic quotes are a useful narrative tool, researchers must avoid using too many direct quotations. It is better to paraphrase and use limited direct quotes to give the narrative the flavor of a person.

A well-written historical research study illustrates the investigator's creativity and imagination as the story unfolds. Creativity connects thoughts, quotes, and events into a readable story and gives birth to new ideas (Christy, 1978). The interpretations and responses to the themes and questions rely on historians' abilities to go beyond the known facts and develop new ideas and new meanings. No two historians who view the same data will respond in exactly the same way. The human filter through which all information passes will alter researchers' responses to the data and will provide the catalyst for the creation of new ideas (Barzun & Graff, 1985; Christy, 1978).

SUMMARY

*T*he nursing profession needs the infusion of new ideas, new meanings, and new interpretations of its past to explain its place in history and its future direction. Ashley (1978) confirmed this connection when she wrote, "With creativity as our base, and with strong historical knowledge and awareness, nurses can become pioneers in developing new types of inquiry and turn inward toward self-knowledge and self-understanding" (p. 36). The historical method gives researchers tools to explore the past. Even though it is challenging to fully explain and perhaps understand historical methodology, as D'Antonio (2005) notes, it is important to continue to find ways to do so. Using certain guideposts along the way, historical researchers formulate ideas, collect data, validate the genuineness and authenticity of those data, and narrate the story. However, to make the research meaningful, historians must relate the research questions and the findings to the present. Connolly (2004) and other historians in the 21st century ask us to examine our nursing stories so that we can learn about what we do, how we do it, where we do it, and who has done nursing work before us. History, in this way, becomes what D'Antonio (2004) has proclaimed as a "new paradigm for nursing knowledge" (p. 1).

References

American Association for the History of Medicine. (1991). Report of the committee on ethical codes. *Bulletin of the History of Medicine, 65*(4), 565–570.

American Historical Association. (1987). Statement on standards of professional conduct. *History Teacher, 21*(1), 105–109.

Ashley, J. (1978). Foundations for scholarship: Historical research in nursing. *Advances in Nursing Science, 1*(1), 25–36.

Austin, A. (1958). The historical method. *Nursing Research, 7*(1), 4–10.

Barzun, J., & Graff, H. F. (1985). *The modern researcher* (4th ed.) San Diego, CA: Harcourt Brace Jovanovich.

Biedermann, N. (2001). The voices of days gone by: Advocating the use of oral history in nursing. *Nursing Inquiry, 8*, 61–62.

Birnbach, N., Brown, J., & Hiestand, W. (1991). Ethical guidelines for the nurse historian and standards of professional conduct for historical inquiry into nursing. Paper Presentation.

Brown, J., D'Antonio, P., & Davis, S. (1991, April). Report on the Fourth Invitational Nursing History Conference. Unpublished manuscript.

Chaney, J. A., & Folk, P. (1993). A profession in caricature: The changing attitudes towards nursing in the *American Medical News*, 1960-1989. *Nursing History Review*, *1*, 181-201.

Christy, T. (1978). The hope of history. In M. L. Fitzpatrick (Ed.), *Historical studies in nursing* (pp. 3-11). New York: Teachers College Press.

Connolly, C. A. (2004). Beyond social history: New approaches to understanding the state of and the state in nursing history. *Nursing History Review*, *12*, 5-24.

Cramer, S. (1992). The nature of history: Meditations on Clio's Craft. *Nursing Research*, *41*(1), 4-7.

D'Antonio, P. (1999). Rewriting and rethinking the rewriting of nursing history. *Bulletin of the History of Medicine*, *73*, 268-290.

D'Antonio, P. (2004). Editor's note. *Nursing History Review*, *12*, 1-3.

D'Antonio, P. (2005). Editor's note. *Nursing History Review*, *13*, 1-3.

Fitzpatrick, M. L. (2001). Historical research: The method. In P. L. Munhall (Ed), *Nursing research: A qualitative perspective* (3rd ed., pp. 403-414). Boston: Jones and Bartlett.

Fondiller, S. (1978). Writing the report. In M. L. Fitzpatrick (Ed.), *Historical studies in nursing* (pp. 25-27). New York: Teachers College Press.

Gaddis, J. L. (2002). *The landscape of history: How historians map the past.* New York: Oxford Press.

Graebner, N.A. (1982). History, society, and the right to privacy. In *The scholar's right to know versus the individual's right to privacy.* Proceedings of the first Rockefeller Archive Center Conference, December 5, 1975 (pp. 20-24). Pocantico Hills, NY: Rockefeller Archive Center Publication.

Grypma, S. J. (2005). Critical issues in the use of biographic methods in nursing history. *Nursing History Review*, *13*, 171-187.

Hamilton, D. (1991, April). Intellectual history. Paper presented at the meeting of Fourth Invitational Conference on Nursing History: Critical Issues Affecting Research and Researchers. Philadelphia, PA.

Hamilton, D. B. (1993). The idea of history and the history of ideas. *Image*, *25*(1), 45-50.

Hanson, K. S. (1989). The emergence of liberal education in nursing education, 1893 to 1923. *Journal of Professional Nursing*, *5*(2), 83-91.

Hofstadter, R. (1959). History and the social sciences. In F. Stern (Ed.), *The varieties of history* (pp. 359-370). New York: Meridan.

Kirby, S. (1997/1998). The resurgence of oral history and the new issues it raises. *Nurse Researcher*, *5*(2), 45-58.

Kerlinger, F. N. (1986). *Foundations of behavioral research* (3rd ed.). New York: Holt, Rinehart & Winston.

Kruman, M. (1985). Historical method: Implications for nursing research. In M. M. Leininger (Ed.), *Qualitative research methods in nursing* (pp. 109-118). Orlando, FL: Grune & Stratton.

Lewenson, S. B. (1990). The woman's nursing and suffrage movement, 1893-1920. In V. Bullough, B. Bullough, & M. Stanton (Eds.), *Florence Nightingale and her era: A collection of new scholarship* (pp. 117-118), New York: Garland.

Lewenson, S. B. (1996). *Taking charge: Nursing, suffrage and feminism, 1873-1920.* New York: NLN Press.

Lorentzon, M. (2004). Nursing Record/British Journal of Nursing Archives, 1888-1956. *British Journal of Nursing, 13*(5), 280-284.

Lusk, B. (1997). Historical methodology for nursing research. *Image, 29*(4), 355-359.

Lynaugh, J. (1996). Editorial. *Nursing History Review, 4*, 1.

Lynaugh, J., & Reverby, S. (1987). Thoughts on the nature of history. *Nursing Research, 36*(1), 4-69.

Matejski, M. (1986). Historical research: The method. In P. L. Munhall & C. J. Oiler (Eds.), *Nursing research: A qualitative perspective* (pp. 175-193). Norwalk, CT: Appleton-Century-Crofts.

Melchior, F. (2004). Feminist approaches to nursing history. *Western Journal of Nursing Research, 26*(3), 340-355.

Morse, J. M., & Field, P. A. (1995). *Qualitative research methods for health professionals* (2nd ed.). Thousand Oaks, CA: Sage.

Newton, M. (1965). The case for historical research. *Nursing Research, 14*(1), 20-26.

Oral History Association. (2000). Oral history evaluation guidelines (Pamphlet No. 3) [On-line]. Available: http://omega.dickinson.edu/organizations/oha/pub_eg.html.

Olson, T. (2000). Numbers, narratives, and nursing history. *Social Science Journal, 37*(1), 137-144.

Rafferty, A. M. (2004). Pre Conference. Paper presented at the meeting of the American Association for the History of Nursing. Charleston, SC.

Rines, A., & Kershner, F. (1979). Information concerning historical studies. Unpublished manuscript. New York: Teachers College, Columbia University, Department of Nursing.

Rosenthal, R. (1982). Who will be responsible for private papers of private people? Some considerations from the view of the private depository. In *The scholar's right to know versus the individual's right to privacy*. Proceedings of the first Rockefeller Archive Center Conference, December 5, 1975 (pp. 3-6). Pocantico Hills, NY: Rockefeller Archive Center Publication.

Spieseke, A. W. (1953). What is the historical method of research? *Nursing Research, 2*(1), 36-37.

Termine, J. (1992, March). A talk about archives. Paper presented at the State University of New York, Health Science Center at Brooklyn, College of Nursing, Brooklyn, NY.

Tholfsen, T. R. (1977). The ambiguous virtues of the study of history. *Teachers College Record, 79*(2), 245-257.

Ulrich, L. T. (1990). *A midwife's tale: The life of Martha Ballard based on her diary, 1785-1812*. New York: Vintage Books.

Yuginovich, T. (2000). More than time and place: Using historical comparative research as a tool for nursing. *International Journal of Nursing Practice, 6*, 70-75.

12

Historical Research in Practice, Education, and Administration

*U*sing historical research methods to study nursing practice, education, and administration allows us to understand relationships and to view the world from a broader perspective. *Nursing History Review* editor D'Antonio (2003) states that "history matters" (p. 1). History provides an "overarching conceptual framework that allows us to more fully understand the disparate meaning of nursing and the different experiences of nurses" (p. 1). Understanding how nurses practiced, how they educated future generations of nurses, and how they administered hospitals, community agencies, and schools of nursing lends itself to historical inquiry. Historical method provides a way to examine specific periods or events in time and place them within a broader context, giving the researcher insights that numbers alone cannot provide. Self-reflection, imagination, and an awareness of a world beyond oneself are essential tools for the historian to have when looking for relationships between the past and present (Lynaugh, 1996, p. 1). This chapter highlights how historical researchers study and interpret patterns of our past to gain a better understanding of the current and future world. Three critiques of historical research studies in the areas of practice, education, and administration are presented. Based on criteria developed from the material discussed in Chapter 11, guidelines were created for critiquing historical research (Box 12.1). A reprint of the Whelan's 2005 article, "A Necessity in the Nursing World': The Chicago Nurses Professional Registry, 1913-1950," appears at the end of the chapter to help readers understand the critiquing process. Table 12.1 offers a sampling of selected historical research publications.

Guidelines for Critiquing Historical Research

Data Generation

Title

1. How does it concisely reflect the purpose of the study?
2. How does it clearly tell readers what the study is about?
3. How does it delineate the time frame for the study?

Statement of the Subject

1. Is the subject easily researched?
2. What themes and theses are studied?
3. What are the research questions?

Literature Review

1. What are the main works written on the subject?
2. What time period does the literature review cover?
3. What are some of the problems that may arise when studying this subject?
4. What primary sources can be identified?
5. How was the subject narrowed during the literature review?
6. What research questions were raised during the literature review?

Data Treatment

Primary Sources

1. How were primary sources used?
2. Were they genuine and authentic?
3. How was external validity determined?
4. How was internal validity determined?
5. Were there inconsistencies between the external validity and internal validity?
6. Does the content accurately reflect the period of concern?
7. Do the facts conflict with historical dates, meanings of words, and social mores?
8. When did the primary author write the account?
9. Did a trained historian or an observer write the source?
10. Were facts suppressed, and if so, why?
11. Is there corroborating evidence?
12. Identify any disagreements between sources.

Secondary Sources

1. What were the secondary sources used?
2. How were secondary sources used?
3. Do they corroborate the primary source?
4. Can you identify any disagreements between sources?

Data Analysis

Organization

1. What conceptual frameworks were used in the study?
2. How would the study be classified; e.g., intellectual, feminist, social, political, biographical?

Box 12.1 *(Continued)*

3. Were the research questions answered?
4. Was the purpose of the study accomplished?
5. If conflict exists within the findings, was there supporting evidence to justify either side of the argument?

Bias

1. Was the researcher's bias identified?
2. Was analysis influenced by a present-mindedness?
3. What were the ideological biases?
4. How did bias affect data analysis?

Ethical Issues

1. Was there any infringement on a historical reputation?
2. Was there a conflict between the right to privacy and the right to know?
3. Did the research show that decisions, events, and activities of an individual or organization affected the public welfare or embraced qualities of major human interest?

Interpreting the Findings

Narrative

1. Does the story describe what happened, including how and why it happened?
2. Were relationships among events, ideas, people, organizations, and institutions explained, interpreted, and placed within a contextual framework?
3. How were direct quotations used? (Too limited or too long?)
4. Was the narrative clear, concise, and interesting to read?
5. Was the significance to nursing explicit?

CRITIQUE GUIDELINES

*A*s noted in Chapter 11, D'Antonio (2005) reflects on how difficult it is to explain historical research methodology. This difficulty can potentially jeopardize our ability to pass this knowledge onto new historians. There is a certain "inexactness" which historians experience when trying to explain the process of historiography (D'Antonio, 2005). Readers must keep this in mind as they attempt to understand the process of historical research, which is often circuitous in nature. Guidelines are just that—guidelines. They serve as a way to "light the path" and keep the researcher "on track." Historians search for meaning in past events and face the ever present concern that they will not be able to find data to tell "the whole story." Critique guidelines help the historian on this journey of discovery and also help consumers of historical research understand what should be expected from this research approach. This section reviews essential components of historical research methodology

Text continued on page 281.

Table 12.1 • Selective Sampling of Historical Research Studies

Author	Date	Domain	Title	Findings
Ament, L. A.	2004	Education	The evolution of midwifery faculty practice: Impact and outcomes of care.	Midwifery education has undergone changes, and this study examines some of the changes that occurred at the oldest programs of its kind. Yale School of Nursing Nurse-Midwifery program began in 1956 and has adapted more recently to the changes in student enrollment and availability of clinical sites. To understand how this school has adapted over time, this study examines the history of midwifery faculty practices. The outcomes of this historical inquiry are clearly stated and include the need for a "good business infrastructure."
Buck, J.	2004	Administration	Home hospice versus home health: Cooperation, competition, and cooptation.	This study examines attitudes about death and dying in the United States during the later half of the 20th century and how these attitudes influence both the care and cost related to death and dying. The socio-political development of hospice care and the changes in end-of-life care offer a historical perspective on a difficult and often considered "taboo" subject. The study presents the complexities required to negotiate the tensions between the "systems of care and cure" and then balancing this between "a philosophy of care and the realities of sustainability" (p. 41). The study presents the political issues surrounding control of end-of-life care, federal reimbursement for care, and the role nurses played in changing care for the dying. The study raises questions about future health care policy and reform and the need to continue studying in this area.

Author	Year	Category	Title	Description
D'Antonio, P.	2004	Education	Women, nursing and baccalaureate education in 20th-century America.	The purpose of this study was to "analyze the social meaning of the American system of education for nursing practice" (p. 379). Historical analyses of the educational levels of a various groups of American women were compared with current data on educational levels of nurses and women. D'Antonio raises questions about the social class and community status of nurses in relation to their educational levels. Findings revealed that raising the educational level of nurses provided an avenue for upward mobility into middle-class America. The data illustrated that more African-American, Hispanic, and Asian-American nurses hold baccalaureate degrees than their Caucasian counterparts. The study also reveals that during the twentieth century, the level of education decreased among nurses in the United States in comparison to the educational level of all women in the United States. An increase in social and political support for raising the level of nursing education is needed to make changes in that direction. D'Antonio further suggests that the "language of class and community status" be linked with the language of "science, knowledge, and clinical excellence" (p. 384) to gain this support.
Evans, J.	2004	Practice	Men nurses: A historical and feminist perspective.	This study examines the history of men in nursing in Britain, Canada, and the United States using CINAHL, Pubmed, and Sociological Abstracts databases. The findings show that documentation of men's role in nursing has been sparse and incomplete.
Grypma, S.J.	2004	Practice	Neither angels of mercy nor foreign devils: Revisioning	As the title suggests, this study examines the work of Canadian missionary nurses in China prior to and

Table 12.1 • (Continued)

Author	Date	Domain	Title	Findings
			Canadian missionary nurses in China, 1935–1947.	during World War II. The image of the nurse missionary in Western culture as "angel of mercy" did not serve them well in China where they were seen as part of the imperialist West. This study examines the letters of individual nurse missionaries sent to the journal *Canadian Nurse* between 1935 and 1947. The letters illustrate how these women were very professional and interested in the development of nursing in China. They were in China to provide care but still were considered part of the imperialistic force and were sent back to Canada as "Foreign Devils."
Houweling, L.	2004	Practice	Image, function and style: A history of the nursing uniform.	Over time, nursing uniforms underwent change. This study explores changes in nursing uniforms and the way they were perceived. This interesting narrative merges the story of the early nursing uniforms and the changes that occur over time. The uniform was first advocated early in the 1800s by Theodor Fliedner, who opened the Deaconesses Institute in Kaiserwerth, Germany, in 1836, where Florence Nightingale studied. Nightingale promoted the uniform as a way of "enhancing the image and the work of nursing" (p. 41). The nurses at Scutari wore dresses that were modest but contemporary for the period. The uniform underwent several changes throughout the next century but was always connected to the image the public held of nursing. Training schools in the late 19th and early 20th centuries called for a uniformity of dress and

				identification with their school. Popular images of the nurse were also linked to the dress that they wore. Caps, shoes, and style were all part of the image. Uniformity, however, also meant control and thus was often debated and criticized by nurses. For some, uniforms were equated with servitude and thus detracted from the strong independent image some nurses held of themselves. The study follows trends in uniforms into 1970s, charting the changes that occurred and the debate about the image of the nurse.
Lorentzon, M.	2004	Practice	*Nursing Record/British Journal of Nursing* archives, 1888–1956.	The *Nursing Record/British Journal of Nursing,* published between 1888 and 1956, was digitalized, enabling historians to electronically search the database. In this study, Lorentzon explores this database for historical identification of the terms *emotion, feeling, sympathy, comfort,* and *compassion.* The search revealed several "hits" for *sympathy* and *feeling,* however, many of the hits were irrelevant and did not contribute to the historical understanding of these terms. The author expressed that the while the newly digitalized database offered greater access for researchers and protected the loss of fragile documents, the "gold standard" for historical research still remained the slow methodical search of documents by hand.
Reedy, E.A.	2003	Practice	From weakling to fighter: Changing the image of premature infants.	The early incubator shows held at national fairs and exhibitions during the late 19th and 20th centuries featured the premature infant in the incubator as part of the midway entertainment. The fairs and exhibitions, although bizarre events, served as a way

Table 12.1 • (Continued)

Author	Date	Domain	Title	Findings
				to educate the public about the advances made in caring for premature infants. Along with continued scientific advances, these shows played a contributing role in changing public attitudes toward the care of premature infants.
Thomas, K. K.	2004		"Law unto themselves": Black women as patients and practitioners in North Carolina's campaign to reduce maternal and infant mortality, 1935–1953.	This study examines public health initiatives to reduce maternal and infant mortality in North Carolina. It describes the effect that racism, attitudes toward untrained midwives, and poor access to care had on Southern African-American women. Increasing numbers of black women participated in the public health initiative as both patients and caregivers and benefited from these advances. Part of the campaign included the education and training of midwives. As young black women were educated in the caregiver role, they received respect and acceptance from public health professionals as well as maintained their personal connection to the black community.
Wall, B. M	2003		Science and ritual: The hospital as medical and sacred space, 1865–1947	This study looks at three religious nursing orders and their work within hospitals between 1865 and 1947. The focus is on the integration of science and religion in hospitals and what this meant to patients who entered these hospitals. "When patients entered Catholic hospitals and observed the seamless integration of technology and spirituality, they were subtly given assurance that they were not only in the care of skilled professionals but also in the hand of the divine" (p. 63).

Text continued from page 275.

and suggests questions that researchers might ask when using this design. Researchers can use these same questions—which have been applied to the three critiques in this chapter—to evaluate historical research.

The historian searches for facts and evidence that will unveil the nature and relationships of historic events, ideas, institutions, or people. The process of doing historical research, however, is rarely, if ever, completed in a linear fashion. The research will be influenced by the topic selected, the availability of primary and secondary sources, the framework used to review the data, the bias of the researcher, the authenticity of the data, the creativity and originality of the researcher, the organization of the material, the narrative, and even the title itself. Each component of historical research methodology relies on the other, permitting the historian to uncover new meanings and relationships. The availability of primary sources, for example, may lead the historian to rethink the research questions or alter the title to reflect a different time frame.

To accurately assess historical meanings, researchers must assure readers of external validity. Establishing external validity confirms that the source is what it claims it is. Simultaneously, researchers must establish internal validity of the source, verifying the consistency between the genuineness of the primary source and the authenticity of the data. Historical researchers may use a framework that helps to organize ideas and makes connections while simultaneously acknowledging personal and ideological bias. To interpret material and make sense of the data as the story unfolds, the historical researcher must possess excellent narrative and explanatory skills.

Accuracy is extremely important to the historical researcher. The researcher must develop a systematic approach that will help maintain accuracy. How researchers collect data, organize references, and number different drafts of the narrative facilitates an accurate account of the story. Historical researchers must organize data and tell the story in a logical fashion. Furthermore, researchers must honestly address questions that arise from the data, trying to understand and explain what the data are describing. Researchers must be prepared to answer questions such as, Did an event noted in a primary source actually happen? Could it have happened as it was noted in the primary source? Throughout the study, the researcher must be true to the data, allowing the data to unfold and bring a better understanding of the subject under investigation. This process requires researchers to be aware of their own bias and employ honesty in relationship to the findings. Do their own biases hinder discovery of new meanings that may be revealed?

Essential to the historical method is imagination. Imagination lets researchers make connections in the data and create a story that assists in learning more of the truth (Barzun & Graff, 1985). The "truth" varies based on the kind of data used, the organization of these data, the creativity applied to interpreting the data, and other variables that the historian controls.

For example, Connolly (2004) explains how over the past century there has been a shift in the "methodological paradigm" away from a "reconstructed narrative of formal political events to what became known as 'social history,' a broader, more inclusive approach to the past that encouraged scholarship from a panoply of new perspectives" (p. 5). Recognizing the relevance of social history to nursing, Connolly also urges historians to study "nursing's history in the context of our political institutions" (p. 17). This change in methodological approach highlights the need for historians to remain open and aware of a variety of frameworks that can be used in historical research.

To find meaning in the past, historians can re-examine the data used in previous studies as well as look for new types of data that may have not been considered relevant, such as diaries of women or records of nursing students. Historians then need to present the story in a way that will draw the reader in and bring meaning to the interpretation. Lusk (1997) said that "historians must mentally reconstruct an era and the events and the players using primary sources, then interpret the story from this perspective" (p. 5). In a 1953 article published in *Nursing Research*, Spieseke explained that historical researchers must be able to locate and collect data, analyze the reliability of the data, organize and arrange the data into a pattern, and express the data "in meaningful and effective language" (p. 37). The narrative should show the successful attainment of these important skills, thus providing a method to evaluate the process.

Box 12.1 organizes data presented in Chapter 11 and suggests criteria to use when critiquing historical research. The reader will find in the following pages that these criteria were used to critique examples of historical research in the areas of nursing practice, education, and administration. Published historical research should read as an interesting narrative; therefore, analysis using a specific instrument such as Box 12.1 might be inhibiting and suggest a linear model of thinking. Because historical research does not proceed in a linear pattern, neither should the critique. Reviewers need to know that the criteria presented are a guide—not an absolute rule, nor a step-by-step formula. These criteria offer the researcher and critic an approach to examine a study and understand the specificity of the various components. As a result, headings in a published article may not clearly delineate primary or secondary sources or personal bias (as perhaps they might in a historical dissertation or in other forms of reported research). Nevertheless, used as a guide, Box 12.1 highlights important features of historical research and helps consumers critique its worth more effectively.

When starting a research study, the questions to ask are, "What are you studying," and, maybe more importantly, "So what, and who cares?" The answers to these questions will often lead the researcher to determine the study method. For example, when examining the differences between hospice care and hospital care, Buck (2004) used a historical method to understand the variables that influenced the kind of care dying patients receive. The subject of dying is placed within a 20th-century context, and the change in society's attitude toward dying is represented in the place and cost of care. Buck identifies an important subject matter and then explains the rationale for selecting the subject. "Sophisticated palliative care," Buck notes, cannot be found in health care reimbursement or structures. Buck makes the case that the changes in the way we care for the dying patient are essential to document, noting that "few studies [of home care] have delved into the almost invisible realms of nursing care of the dying at home during the latter half of the twentieth century" (p. 30), thus providing the reader the "so what and who cares." The historical approach becomes the method of choice because of the need to understand changes over time in attitudes and beliefs about death and dying, in the way society "pays" for such care, and in how and where this care is delivered. The lack of existing data on this subject makes it essential that it be studied, and in this case, studied using a historical framework that allows for an explication of the sociopolitical context in which this topic is embedded. The subject area, the researcher's interest, and the questions raised determine the selection of method. Armed with the appropriate tools, historical researchers venture into these areas and formulate specific questions. Following selection of the subject, researchers must narrow the topic to enable them to study the area in depth. To build a body of knowledge requires teamwork or the linkage of several historical studies that eventually will fill gaps and offer a fuller understanding of history (Bloch, 1964). Historians probe historical antecedents in broad areas of nursing such as practice, education, and administration to explain relationships, ideas, or events that influenced nursing's professional development. A review of previous studies helps researchers determine their own course of study and stimulates imagination. Thus, in historical research, using studies completed more than 5 years ago is not only appropriate but also essential to better understand the subject under review. Table 12.1 offers a sampling of some of the latest published historical research studies.

APPLICATION TO PRACTICE

*D*uring the early modern nursing movement, nursing education and nursing practice were so closely related that studying one often meant studying the other. During the late 19th century and well into the 20th century, hospitals relied heavily on student nurses to provide patient care. Changes in the traditional apprenticeship educational model and the move to university-based educational settings dramatically and economically altered the delivery of care in hospitals and nursing practice. Before these changes, graduate nurses, after completing their training, were rarely hired to staff hospitals and were forced to look elsewhere for jobs. They worked outside of hospitals as private duty and public health nurses.

In 1928, Wolf (1991) addressed the National League of Nursing Education (now known as the National League for Nursing [NLN]) regarding the transition of graduate nurses employed by hospitals. Wolf explained how graduate nurses who provided patient care—as opposed to student nurses—would be beneficial to hospital administrators, nursing educators, and graduate nurses. Aside from stabilizing nursing service, providing an excellent service, and profiting the employer and employee, Wolf argued that hiring graduate nurses would improve the value society placed on nursing service. Wolf believed that graduate nurses faced undue criticism from hospital administrators, who believed that student nurses were more "buoyant, resilient, and enthusiastic" (Wolf, 1991, p. 140) than graduates. Yet, Wolf argued that "the graduate nurse sees more to be done for a patient than a student, she knows better what to do" (p. 140).

Wolf's (1991) speech provides historians with a perspective of someone personally involved in the changes in nursing practice history that had profound effects on the shape of things to come. Historical research in the development of nursing practice might examine nursing practice in hospitals, private duty, or public health. External factors such as wars, economic depressions, and advances in medicine and science affected the development of the nursing profession and created an infinite number of ways to approach the study of nursing practice. Researchers can find primary and secondary sources in published nursing textbooks, hospital manuals, speeches presented at various professional meetings, minutes of professional meetings, and graduation addresses. Archives of hospitals, schools of nursing, and visiting nurse services contain data that tell the story of early nursing practice.

Discussions in the literature that have defined nurses' roles, specialization, and society's value of care find their origins in history. Bullough (1992) explained that "clinical specialization started in the early 20th century as nurses with advanced knowledge and training were needed to care for groups of patients with special needs" (p. 254). Specialties emerged in nursing such as nurse anesthetist, nurse midwife, public health nurse, and critical care nurse. These specialists required additional education, practical experience, and, in some instances, certification. Unanswered questions about the development of different specialties and the needed qualifications for each invites historical inquiry, such as Ament's (2004), Dawley's (2005), and Thomas's (2004) work on midwifery and Buck's (2004) work on hospice care.

Critique of a Study in Practice

Keeling (2004) argues that "the artificial disciplinary boundaries between medicine and nursing were blurred when nurses assumed the technological skills of cardiac monitoring and cardiac defibrillation in the early coronary care units" (p. 139) in the well-written historical study titled, "Blurring the Boundaries Between Medicine and Nursing: Coronary Care Nursing, Circa the 1960s." The reader of this study is immediately made aware of what the study is about by reading the title and the first paragraph. Keeling lets the reader know that the boundary between medicine and nursing blurred as nurses learned and accepted newly expanded roles in the clinical setting. This marked a change between the way physicians and nurses responded to each other in more typical hospital-based settings. The title also sets the time frame for study, identifying "circa the 1960s." Without giving the exact beginning and end years for the study, the reader is alerted to expect an approximate period rather than exact dates, which may allow the historian greater flexibility in reviewing data. It is often difficult for a historian to know whether something really happened "first," and by broadening the time span and not delineating specific years, the researcher commits to a period of time but not an exact date.

Keeling informs the reader that her work is part of a larger historical project that examines the history of coronary care units in the United States. The study analyzes the pivotal role nurses played in the development of this clinical practice setting during the 1960s, when it emerged as a new specialty. Keeling (2004) captures the major shift in nursing practice as nurses participated in the recognition and treatment of "potentially fatal" arrhythmias by using the complex machinery to correct problems. Nurses assuming these new roles were actually "diagnosing" and "defibrillating" to save patients' lives. These actions contrasted with the traditional caregiver role of the nurses during that time period.

Keeling (2004) provides the reader with historical background beginning in the post–World War II era when so many changes occurred in health care. Although Keeling does not state the framework used, a social framework is evident to the reader. The social framework in which the study is placed allows the reader to "hear" how the postwar era with technological advances in science and medicine changed forever the landscape of nursing practice. Heart disease became a major concern of politicians because of the increasing prevalence of the disease among white middle-class men in America. This segment of the population was important to the economic well-being of the country and as such received greater medical attention as ways to combat heart disease became possible.

Hidden within the narrative, Keeling (2004) provides information about the purpose, themes, research questions, and significance of the study. While each of these questions, and others listed in the Critique Guidelines, are not explicated in a clear fashion, the reader can identify what the researcher expects to find and how she approached the material. Keeling tells the reader how the role of the nurse changed significantly in the 1960s as coronary care units became part of the hospital environment. Whether or not Keeling found the themes difficult to study is not clearly stated; however, the fact that the study was conducted and primary and secondary sources were used indicates that the sources were available. Primary and secondary sources support the narrative throughout the study, and although Keeling does not stop in the narrative to distinguish between the two types, the introduction of direct quotes and other supporting evidence allows the reader to easily identify the two types of sources. Although, for a novice researcher, it may have been easier and clearer if the researcher had delineated the primary and secondary sources. The study is well documented using papers presented at conferences, journal articles, proceedings of various meetings, interviews, federal grants, and unpublished data, which constitute much of the primary source data. Additional sources, mostly secondary in nature, include books about nursing, speeches of political leaders, and other supporting documentation used in the literature review. The use of the *Chicago Manual of Style, 14th edition*, for referencing allows the historian to give more information and explanation about the resources than, for example, the *Publication Manual of the American Psychological Association, 5th edition*, that many nursing journals use for referencing. This allows the reader to look at the notes that Keeling carefully wrote, thus giving the paper greater depth and creditability.

When addressing questions related to whether sources are genuine or authentic, each historian must determine this by drawing on where he or she found the documents and what he or she found within the material examined. Keeling (2004) does not reflect on the methodology used to determine the genuineness or authenticity of the sources. However, the documents that are identified in the references are found in archival collections, governmental records, prestigious journals, and other sources where the nature of the material would have been verified already. However, even when using sources that appear reliable, the researcher must have an understanding of the time period studied. For example, when reading about the role of the nurse and the "blurring" of boundaries between the nurse and physician, the researcher must possess an understanding of the particular time period to determine whether the comment makes "sense." The researcher must also ask, "Do the documents accurately reflect the period?" This is an important question and one that Keeling, by virtue of the use of historical documents, seems to implicitly verify in terms of authenticity. For newcomers to historical research, this is a difficult determination to make and one that would be easier if Keeling had been more explicit.

Keeling (2004) researched this topic almost 30 years after the fact. This can possibly create an interesting ethical dilemma because many of the people who were mentioned in the study may still be alive. People reading the study may have experienced working in the newly opened coronary care units and may have different perspectives on the role of nurses within that particular setting. Ethical issues related to what to publish and how to use the material are considered by historians, but, in this instance, they may not have been considered problematic and as a result not addressed in the text. Little if any personal information about those identified in the study posed an ethical problem. The author did not address ethical concerns in this paper, but, because this paper is part of a larger study, any concerns about using oral histories and use of data in archival collections may have been addressed in the larger project.

Keeling (2004) creatively weaves the narrative together to highlight the story about the changes in emerging technology, scientific discovery, and social need to find ways to improve the care of the patient in need of coronary care. Within the narrative, one can determine whether or not Keeling answered the research question that was posed as a statement in the opening of the paper and that is further reflected in the title. The role of the coronary care nurse in the 1960s and the opening of the two coronary care units are described and interpreted in a way that supports Keeling's purpose. The more traditional nurse's role of caregiver was clearly delineated from the physician's role to provide the cure. Keeling notes that in the 1960s, the boundaries between these two providers "were not always in the best interest of the patient" (p. 143). Nurses needed to do more than just observe to make a difference in patient outcomes. Keeling describes the opening of coronary care units at two different settings in the United States, one at Bethany Hospital in Kansas City and the other at Presbyterian Hospital in Philadelphia. The increasing need for specific knowledge related to the care to be given by coronary care units and the acceptance and training of nurses to assume these roles are juxtaposed with nurses' acceptance and embrace of their new role. Keeling documents the expanding role and how nurses, like Rose Pinneo, developed the skills and shaped the emerging landscape of the coronary care units. The story is told with a number of direct quotes from nurses in the 1960s. This allows the reader to "hear" what was said and how it was said. These quotes assist Keeling with telling the story, interpreting the findings, and placing the events within the context of the period. A concern that historians have is avoiding using current ideas or a state of present-mindedness to critique the past. By allowing the voices of the nurses living in 1960s to be heard and by using several secondary sources to explain the period, the author seems to have avoided the problems related to present-mindedness. For example, Keeling does not compare the work of the coronary care nurses of the 1960s to the expectation we have of nurses today. Keeling compares the coronary care nurses to other nurses of that same era, noting, "these young [coronary care] nurses made independent decisions in emergency situations. They experienced a new level of autonomy and gained a new level of respect" (p. 159). In doing so, Keeling avoided the possibility of interpreting the data using today's standards of practice.

An interesting collection of events and stories presents the reader with a compelling explanation of how the boundaries between the two professions shifted in the 1960s to create a safer environment for patients to recover from life-threatening cardiac conditions. Keeling (2004) offers an interpretation of these events and realistically addresses the changing nursing role. For example, even though nurses were considered more assertive in their new role, had elevated "their status from physicians' handmaidens to emerging nurse specialists" (p. 159), and were now considered part of the scientific team, they still "were not really equals" (p. 159) to their physician colleagues. Keeling weaves the evidence together and brings the reader along so that the interpretation of the events becomes part of the story. Keeling's historical study uncovers important documentation about the 1960s, giving the profession the needed evidence to better understand how nurses have continued to expand and adjust their roles in health care. Keeling (2004) provides an excellent example of historical research even though each of the critique criteria cannot be fully identified. The novice to historical research may find this disconcerting and may find it difficult to identify the quality of the research design. However, as noted earlier in the chapter, historical research is not linear, nor does it fit a specific procedure. The consumer of historical research needs to be able to understand the narrative and make determinations about the quality by sometimes reading between the lines and knowing what goes into the design and raising questions.

APPLICATION TO EDUCATION

*R*esearchers interested in nursing education are concerned with varied aspects of this subject, such as the entry into practice dilemma (D'Antonio, 2004), the move of nursing education into the university (Bartal & Steiner-Freud, 2005), or the biography of an important figure in nursing education (Hawkins & Watson, 2003). By using a historical approach, researchers are able to address topics in nursing education ranging from curriculum design to control of education. This approach not only provides background descriptive information but also answers relevant questions regarding issues that concern nursing today.

Currently, topics such as recruitment of adult learners, critical thinking, and culturally competent care concern nursing educators. However, historians may question whether the concept of recruitment of adult learners is a new idea in nursing education and may attempt to understand this topic by studying nursing students of the past. Historians may examine past records of nurse training schools or professional studies of nursing. For example, the 1923 Goldmark (1984) study *Nursing and Nursing Education in the United States* indicated that, in 1911, about 70% of the training schools required students to be 20 or 21 years old for admission; however, within 7 years, the age requirement had dropped to 18 or 19 years. Given this information, the historian might ask, Why did the admission age drop at that time, and why did training schools initially believe older women would be better training school candidates? What teaching strategies worked better with older women than with younger ones? Both questions address the past and yet relate to current, pertinent issues related to adult learners.

Another contemporary nursing education issue, critical thinking, has its roots in nursing's history. For example, in 1897, Superintendent of Bellevue Training School Agnes Brennan addressed the Superintendent's Society. She stated, "An uneducated woman may become a good nurse, but never an intelligent one; she can obey orders conscientiously and understand thoroughly a sick person's need, but should an emergency arise, where is she? She works through her feelings, and therefore lacks judgment" (Brennan, 1991, p. 23). Was Brennan referring to critical thinking when she reasoned that nurses needed to have the knowledge and theory regarding pathology to understand the appropriate care of sick people? Brennan suggested it was equally important for nurses to spend time in clinical practice learning the "character of the pulse in different patients or finding out just why some nurses can always see at a glance that this patient requires her pillow turned" (p. 24). She firmly believed that a trained nurse required both theoretical and practical knowledge and that, without both, something would be missing in the nursing care provided. As she pointed out, "Theory fortifies the practical, practice strengthens and retains the theoretical" (p. 25). Brennan clearly described her views on the theory–practice dichotomy that still challenges nursing educators today. Brennan firmly believed that nurses must be educated to think so that they can practice.

Historical researchers have addressed the contemporary issue of cultural diversity by studying racial tensions in nursing and in society and offering nurses a better understanding of the inherent conflicts. Questions that might be asked related to the topic include, Was there cultural diversity in nursing or any interest in providing culturally competent care before the current interest in the topic? From where did the nursing student at the beginning of the 19th century come? What socioeconomic-political background did the student bring to nursing? In the book *Black Women in White: Racial Conflict and Cooperation in the Nursing Profession, 1890-1950,* Hine (1989) described the opening of nurse training schools for African Americans who had been excluded from most of the existing U.S. nurse training schools. Of the schools that did not racially discriminate, many admitted African Americans using quotas. The very origin of the National Association of Colored Graduate Nurses (NACGN) in 1908 speaks to the early exclusion of African Americans from the first two national nursing organizations: the American Society of Superintendents of Training Schools for Nurses (renamed the National League of Nursing Education in 1912) and the Associated Alumnae of the United States and Canada (renamed the American Nurses Association [ANA] in 1911).

Young (2005) re-examines the 1925 Johns Report on African-American nurses and adds to the ongoing discussion about how race affected the education and practice of nurses. Historians need to look at what was, as well as what was not, to better understand historic events. For example, How did nursing handle cultural diversity? What was the reaction of nurses to institutional racism? When did the profession welcome people of a different race, color, and religion into the profession? Who were the advocates of an integrated profession?

Historians who search for answers may learn that nursing political activist Lavinia Dock spoke out against prejudicial treatment of any professional nurse. Dock (1910) cited the need for nursing to demonstrate practical ethics and ardently hoped that the nursing association (ANA) would not ever "get to the point where it draws the color line against our negro sister nurses" (p. 902). She believed that the nursing association was one place in the United States where color boundaries were not drawn. As the ANA expanded, however, Dock witnessed evidences that made her remark "that this cruel and unchristian and unethical prejudice might creep in here in our association" (p. 902). Dock said that under no circumstances should nurses emulate the cruel prejudices displayed by "men" and urged nurses to treat each nurse of color "as we would like to be treated ourselves" (p. 902). She supported politically active, black nursing leader Adah Thomas, who became president of the NACGN and who, in 1929, wrote the history of African-American nurses in the book *The Pathfinders* (Davis, 1988).

Questions that arise from conflicting ideas in the existing data and the omission of information in published narrative suggest new areas for historic inquiry. An example is Mosley's (1996) historical study based on examining the influence of four black community health nurses on public health nursing in New York City between 1900 and 1930. Mosley included a discussion specifically addressing institutional racism as it existed in nursing during the first 30 years of the 20th century. To understand the prejudice experienced by African American nurses, Mosley focused on the lives and contributions of four leaders in public health nursing: Jessie Sleet Scales, Mabel Staupers, Elizabeth W. Tyler, and Edith M. Carter.

Critique of a Study in Education

In "Sparks to Wildfires: The Emergence and Impact of Nurse Practitioner Education at Virginia Commonwealth University 1974–1991," Seeger Jablonski (2003) examines the history and impact of nurse practitioner education in the United States using the nurse practitioner program started at Virginia Commonwealth University (VCU) as a case study. The title of the study clearly informs the reader of the time frame, subject, and purpose. By using the term "sparks to wildfires," it quickly alerts the reader to what Seeger Jablonski later explains as the "collision of earlier nurse education pedagogy with the unique clinical path of the nurse practitioner movement" (p. 167). Seeger Jablonski contends that the unique educational experience of nurse practitioner education "collided" with the pedagogy of earlier nurse education programs. Although the author does not state the research question as a question, the reviewer can follow the reasoning the author provides when stating the purpose of the study. Stated as a research question, Did the education of nurse practitioners collide with the more traditional education of nurses?

Seeger Jablonski (2003) gives the rationale for using VCU as a case study, noting three reasons: First, it was one of the first nurse practitioner programs in the United States. Second, it offered both the first family nurse practitioner and obstetric-gynecology nurse practitioner programs in Virginia. Third, faculty members who started the program were influential within the nurse practitioner movement at both the regional and national levels. Thus, the history of the nurse practitioner program at VCU serves as an exemplar in which to examine broader issues related to nurse practitioner education and practice.

The author prepares the reader to expect an overview of the nurse practitioner movement, the history of the nurse practitioner programs at VCU, and, finally, the more general issue of how the nurse practitioner movement affected nursing education in the United States. Seeger Jablonski (2003) provides these three components in an organized and concise manner. The author supports the narrative with numerous references that include the school's accreditation self-study reports, grant applications, interviews with faculty, and various journal articles and books about nurse practitioners. The number of references used speaks to the availability of materials and the ease in which the themes could be studied. The author, however, does not provide the reader with a clearly articulated statement about the primary and secondary sources. Although this is not always necessary, it would help the reader to understand how the author selected the primary sources, including how the author collected the oral histories used. The determination of what is and what is not a primary and secondary source is left up to the reader. The author writes an interesting narrative that illustrates the history of the nurse practitioner movement in the United States. The use of oral histories as part of the evidence in this paper is nicely woven into the fabric of the study and provides primary source data.

A separate literature review section is not included in this article. It is not necessary because the author tells the story by using the literature to support the research. The use of various data sources provides the basis for the literature review and becomes part of the narrative. Seeger Jablonski (2003) also does not clearly identify a framework for the study. The historian appears to use a social history framework because the study examines the history of the nurse practitioner movement by focusing on the specific experience of one school. The school established the program in part because of society's need to establish this independent nursing specialty—nurse practitioners who could provide access to care to traditionally underserved populations.

Whether the author's bias is evident when the data are interpreted is not clear and is not addressed in the paper. The researcher is a Clinical Associate Professor at VCU and a nurse practitioner. Given that the years for the study represent a more recent history, one the researcher may have been part of, it is difficult to assess whether the conclusions drawn by the researcher are partly influenced by her own experience, which may alter her perception of the data. The researcher's "bias" may be assumed to be in support of the nurse practitioner movement, and data may therefore be viewed through a more favorable lens than if someone who may have been politically opposed to the nurse practitioner movement were reporting on the subject. The data presented and the interpretations of the findings are reported in such a way as to provide readers with the opportunity to question and/or accept the findings based on their own critique of the study and further exploration in this area of nursing education and practice.

The ethical issues related to historical studies when subjects are still alive and the history is more recent are not addressed in the study. However, there is no evidence suggesting unethical treatment of those interviewed. It is important to ask whether or not there was an infringement on the historical reputation of those interviewed. Seeger Jablonski (2003) clearly presents the controversy surrounding the nurse practitioner movement. As an example, the historian speaks about the Associate Dean of the Graduate Program at VCU School of Nursing and states that "she was openly antagonistic to the NP programs and faculty, viewing them with suspicion," and making the NP faculty "jump through hoops" (p. 175). The concern that nurses would become "mini-doctors" raised the level of tension among the participants described in this study, as well as among noted nursing leaders at the time. It is not unusual for individuals such as the faculty and deans to prefer that their position, whether in opposition to or in favor of the educational reform, be publicly known. However, the ethical question historians must ask is whether or not the various players had an impact on the public welfare: in this case, they did on nursing education. The use of the various expressed opinions enriches the search for meaning and "truth" regarding the changes in nursing education. Here, the author presents the conflicting views of those involved without seemingly violating their right to privacy.

Seeger Jablonski (2003) discusses the evolution of the nurse practitioner programs at VCU, including the "upheaval" caused when the newly formed nurse practitioner program first met opposition from nursing faculty and how the programs were integrated into the school after faculty and administrators accepted this new educational focus into the mainstream of graduate nursing education. Seeger Jablonski connects the case study at this one particular institution to the larger nurse practitioner movement in the United States. The need to provide primary care in rural and other underserved areas created an "evolutionary" change in nursing education and practice. The story at VCU provides a clear account of the curriculum for the emerging nurse practitioner programs. VCU offered the Family Nurse Practitioner Program beginning in 1973, the Obstetric-Gynecologic Nurse Practitioner Program in 1975, and Pediatric Nurse Practitioner Program in 1976. The curriculum presented for each program highlighted some of the differences between the nurse practitioner programs and other, already established graduate degree programs at the school. The programs at VCU, like at other schools that started nurse practitioner programs, were creating changes in nursing education throughout the United States. The "voices" of those interviewed in this study could be heard in many of the direct quotations used, such as "we took them away from seeing the bright lights of the city and sent them back home to clinical sites that they already had to have" (p. 171), thus giving the reader a feeling of what went on aside from the written record: students were expected to provide their own clinical sites and were expected to use "self-learning modules, teleconferences, and videotapes" (p. 171).

Seeger Jablonski (2003) connects VCU's individual story with the broader nursing community. The issues raised by nursing leaders during that time period could be heard in the ongoing questioning of the rationale for the nurse practitioner role. The argument opposing nurse practitioners changed over time to one of acceptance as more schools began to educate nurses building this new health care. The benefits to schools and the profession became more evident as the evolutionary changes in nursing education and practice took hold. Federal grants supported the nurse practitioner educational programs, enabling nurses and nursing faculty to attend. As promised in the beginning of the paper, Seeger Jablonski addresses how the "sparks from the NP programs rather quickly spread to other aspects of nursing education" (p. 178), thus addressing the purpose of the study and answering the research statement. It is clear that the nurse practitioner movement changed the direction of nursing education and practice.

Seeger Jablonski's (2003) historical study provides nursing with an important story and discussion about the development of this new role and its affect on nursing education and practice. The earlier statements asserting that VCU's program can serve as an exemplar to the larger nursing community is answered by the study. The relationships between the various players in the study and the events surrounding educational reform were all placed within the context of nursing education and practice during this period of time. The significance of the study is that it began the important work of documenting and analyzing important events that were critical to the nurse practitioner movement and nursing education.

APPLICATION TO ADMINISTRATION

*B*y now, it should be clear to readers that doing historical research requires creativity. Researchers may select a topic of interest and study it using different approaches. The history of nursing organizations founded by nursing leaders is an excellent subject for a nursing history. As an example, Birnbach and Lewenson (1991) examined the early speeches presented at the National League for Nursing (NLN), an organization that epitomizes the efforts of nurse administrators to organize and control nursing education and practice. The NLN began in 1893 when a group of nursing superintendents in charge of nurse training schools met in Chicago at the Canada and Columbian Exposition. Superintendents throughout the United States met and founded the American Society of Superintendents of Training Schools for Nurses. In 1912, this organization became the National League of Nursing Education, and, in 1952, became the NLN. Superintendents started this organization so they could collectively address the issues confronting the developing profession. They advocated reforms such as improving educational standards, developing uniform training school curricula, decreasing working hours, and increasing the number of years of training. Through their efforts, the organization developed needed educational reforms in nursing and fostered the control of practice.

To study nursing administration, researchers might use biographies of nursing leaders. A biography offers insight into the characteristics of people as well as their roles. It some cases, it allows the "dots to be connected" and provides insight into broader historical studies. Biographies of leaders before the modern nursing movement, such as the one done by Griffon (1998) on Mary Seacole, give a different perspective on women who contributed to establishing independent practice and setting the stage for future nurses. A biography need not be limited to one person but may compare and contrast the relationships among a group of leaders, such as the study by Poslusny (1989): "Feminist Friendship: Isabel Hampton Robb, Lavinia Lloyd Dock, and Mary Adelaide Nutting." Grypma (2005) believes that biography enables researchers to ask the "newer" questions being asked by historians. Looking at the lives of ordinary nurses, for example, tells a different story than that of more famous nursing leaders who have been captured in biographical sketches. For example, in "Careful Nursing: A Model for Contemporary Nursing Practice," Meehan (2003) presents a "new" model for nursing care that was derived from a historical study of the nursing system developed in Ireland by Catherine McAuley, the founder of the Religious Sisters of Mercy, in the early 19th century.

The following section presents a critique of Whelan's (2005) study that examines the change in employment of nurses from private duty to hospital-based practice. This study highlights the dilemma nurses experience in meeting supply and demand needs caused by economic, social, and political factors. The lessons learned from the decline in the use of private duty nurses following World War II and the inevitable affect on employment practices reverberate today as administrators respond to the continuing concerns produced by the nursing shortage.

Critique of a Study in Nursing Administration

Whelan (2005) writes about the demise of the private duty nursing, challenging the commonly held belief that the economic depression of the 1930s caused the decline in private duty nursing. Instead, Whelan argues in her study "A Necessity in the Nursing World: The Chicago Nurses Professional Registry, 1913-1950" that private duty nursing continued as a specialty into the second half of the 20th century as a result of a variety of factors, including supply and demand issues and changes in hospital hiring practices and in the hospital setting itself. Whelan studies the larger issues related to private duty nursing by focusing on the Chicago Nurses Professional Registry.

The title of the study reflects its purpose and immediately asks the reader to consider the necessity of private duty nursing to the profession. The title also specifically identifies the Chicago Nurses Professional Registry, which draws the reader's attention to this specific registry and its use as an exemplar. The time frame is included in the title and thus the reader knows that the study is about a nursing registry in Chicago between 1913 and 1950.

The opening paragraphs of the study immediately focus the reader's attention to the year 1925 and the importance private duty nursing once held in the nursing profession. Whelan's (2005) use of excerpts from the speech presented by Lucy Van Frank, Head Registrar of the Chicago-based Nurse Professional Registry at the Illinois State Nurses Association, illustrates the phase that appears in the title of the paper. Whelan informs the reader about the once essential nature of private duty nursing and how it was perceived by some of the leaders in the profession at that time. Private duty nurses were considered "as much a necessity in the nursing world as commercial bureaus in the business world, and as essential as a part of the great plan of caring for the sick, as is the system of Training Schools in the hospitals" (Van Frank, 1925, as cited in Whelan, 2005, p. 49). Whelan explains that this once-revered form of hiring practice no longer remained viable by the mid-20th century as changes in hiring practices and hospitals rendered this service "obsolete" (p. 50).

Whelan (2005) explicitly informs the reader of the focus of the study by noting that "this article records the rise and demise of professional private duty registries as demonstrated by the experience of the Chicago Nurses Professional registries during the years 1914-1950" (p. 50). Whelan shares that the purpose of her study is to provide the reader with the origins of the subject, as well as why this particular study presents perspectives that differ from those presented in previously conducted research on this subject. Opening a sentence with "My perspective differs" (p. 50) instantly tells the reader what to expect and why. Whelan also includes a description of the significance of the study and its current relevance to nursing in the following passage:

> the importance of how supply and demand functions in the nurse labor market refines our understanding for the transformation of nurses from independent private practitioners to hospital employees. Examining this intriguing nurse job market offers a unique view of nurses' work and illuminates the foundation on which the contemporary labor market for nurses was formed. (p. 50)

Whelan (2005) provides important historical background that helps the reader understand the perspective presented and uses primary and secondary sources to do so. The literature review on this subject, although not presented in the same way one would expect to see it in a quantitative study, relies extensively on primary and secondary source materials. Although Whelan does not explicitly identify which are primary and secondary sources within the text of the study, the extensive use of documentation evident throughout the paper is explained within the "Notes" section, enabling the reader to obtain a better understanding of the sources used. Whelan includes various nursing journals published during the period under study, such as the *American Journal of Nursing, Trained Nurse*, and *Hospital Review*. According to the researcher, these journals reported on various aspects of private duty registries. Whelan also uses studies that were conducted during the 1920s and does inform the reader of this when introducing the Committee on the Grading of Nursing Schools study published in 1928 as *Nurses, Patients, and Pocketbook*. In addition, Whelan also uses papers housed within the Illinois State Historical Library archival collections, such as "The Problems of a Registrar." This was a paper presented at the annual meeting of the Illinois State Nurses Association in October 1923 and was found in the collection of the Illinois Nurses Association Papers. Secondary sources used and referred to in the "Notes" section include books related to the subject, including Susan Reverby's (1987) *Ordered to Care*, as well as numerous articles by noted historians on this topic. Similar to the critique presented earlier in this chapter by Keeling (2004), the use of the *Chicago Manual of Style, 14th edition*, provides the reader with the additional information on the researcher's choices related to source material. When critiquing historical research studies that use the *Chicago Manual of Style*, the reader may refer to the "Notes" section for additional information. Without completely reading the "Notes" section of a published paper, important information and nuances of the story may be lost to the reader.

The authenticity and genuine nature of the primary sources also can be determined within the "Notes" section. By offering the reader explanations about the subject, such as "For a contemporary description of early 20th century private duty nursing see . . ." (p. 67), Whelan places the citation in context and thus implies its appropriateness to the study. Throughout the "Notes" section, Whelan explains "holes" in data that cannot be found with the source material. For example, Whelan notes that the "exact number of hospital-based registries is indeterminate" (p. 67). She frequently alerts the reader to various histories on the subject of private duty nursing that may offer different perspectives on the same issue. The presentation of various opinions, theses, and ideas about the subject illuminates possible inconsistencies between and among the sources, as well as offers corroboration of certain facts. The numerous articles published during the time frame of the study and used to corroborate facts gives the reader needed information to determine the authenticity and genuine nature of the sources. Whelan does an excellent job of letting the reader know about the sources and offers important evidence that supports the quality and strength of the sources used.

Whelan (2005) implicitly embraces a social and labor history framework to examine how the work and hiring of nurses were influenced by economic fluctuations, wartime economy, and changes in medical technology. Readers are encouraged to look at the demise of the private duty specialization through the lens of nursing shortages during the 20th century. Framing the analysis of this decline enables the researcher and reader to begin to understand the possible consequences that shortages have on individual nurses and on the profession as a whole. The researcher's beliefs about the causes for the decline of private duty nursing were stated in the opening section; however, bias was not addressed, nor were any of the ethical issues that may have surrounded the topic presented. Nevertheless, the study represents an appropriate use of data, and no ethical concern about the people involved is evident.

The narrative in Whelan's (2005) study tells the story of private duty nursing by integrating the social, economic, and political factors that influenced the "story." For example, the unstable nature of private duty nursing within a difficult labor market is noted in the following passage: "The success of the NPR (Nurses Professional Registry) in placing private duty nurses, though impressive, took place in a labor market plagued by serious problems" (p. 56). Making a living based on individual cases meant an inability of nurses to rely on a steady stream of income. Financial viability of private duty nursing was subject to the economy and the larger labor market affecting nursing, hospitals, and health care. Registries opened, and the nature of rightful ownership of these agencies was debated among the early nursing leaders, like Lavinia Dock and Isabel Hampton Robb. Whelan presents these views in the narrative to help the reader understand the relationship among the various events, ideas, people, and organizations involved. By using direct quotes, she adds richness to the narrative. The narrative clearly presented Whelan's ideas and theses. The significance of the study, identified in the beginning of the study, was again explicitly shared with the readers in the concluding section of the paper. The story of the decline of private duty nursing and the change in employment status of nurses serves as a "cautionary tale" as we face current nursing shortages. Whelan ends her compelling narrative with the following warning: "for better or worse, they [nursing shortages] may also carry the potential to change the very structure of nurses' employment and frustrate nurses' attempts to manage their own practice" (p. 65). Whelan's historical study paints an interesting picture of the labor market, specifically supply and demand issues and how these affected the nursing shortage. By her own admission, she offers another view of why the use of private duty nurses changed.

SUMMARY

Grypma (2005) describes the allure of historical research, citing the "thrill of discovery" (p. 171) upon handling papers and materials from noted leaders in the past. Yet Grypma notes that historical research methodology is undergoing changes that require the researcher to question the readership and audience of historical studies. Important information gleaned from the past must be critically examined for themes such as ethics, diversity, technology, and other compelling questions that continue to affect nursing practice, education, and administration. Issues in nursing that are affected by gender, race, and ethnicity lend themselves to study through historical research. D'Antonio's (2005) statement about the lack of specificity surrounding historical research methods does not necessarily alter the quality, importance, or relevance of the historical studies. Nurse researchers must use the appropriate method to gain insights into their practice.

This chapter enables the audience of historical research to better understand the method and provides a guide for critiquing historical studies. The guide should not be considered the only way to understand the historical process, nor is it meant to fit all historians into a single mold. What it is meant to provide is a framework that will allow nurses to assess historical research evidence of a particular nursing technique, an educational reform, or an administrative decision. The reader should ask, Does the study meet the guidelines, and if not, why? What is explicitly stated in the narrative, and what must the audience infer from the work? These questions may be more realistic than expecting historians to fit a proscribed set of criteria. Nursing history, as D'Antonio (2003) noted, "matters." For history to matter, it must first be understood.

References

Ament, L.A. (2004). The evolution of midwifery faculty practice: Impact and outcomes of care. *Nursing Outlook, 52*(4), 203-208.

Bartal, N., & Steiner-Freud, J. (2005). Nursing education moves into the university: The story of the Hadassah School of Nursing in Jerusalem, 1918-1984. *Nursing History Review, 13,* 121-145.

Barzun, J., & Graff, H. F. (1985). *The modern researcher* (4th ed.). San Diego, CA: Harcourt Brace Jovanovich.

Birnbach, N., & Lewenson, S. (Eds.). (1991). *First words: Selected addresses from the National League for Nursing 1894-1933.* New York: National League for Nursing Press.

Brennan, A. (1991). Comparative value of theory and practice in nursing. In N. Birnbach & S. Lewenson (Eds.), *First words: Selected addresses from the National League for Nursing 1894-1933* (pp. 23-25). New York: National League for Nursing Press. (Original speech presented in 1897.)

Bloch, M. (1964). *The historian's craft.* New York: Vantage Books.

Buck, J. (2004). Home hospice versus home health: Cooperation, competition, and cooptation. *Nursing History Review, 12,* 25-46.

Bullough, B. (1992). Alternative models for specialty nursing practice. *Nursing and Health Care, 13*(5), 254-259.

Connolly, C.A. (2004). Beyond social history: New approaches to understanding the state of and the state in nursing history. *Nursing History Review, 12,* 5-24.

D'Antonio, P. (2003). Editor's note. *Nursing History Review, 11,* 1.

D'Antonio, P. (2004). Women, nursing, and baccalaureate education in 20th century America. *Journal of Nursing Scholarship, 36*(4), 379-386.

D'Antonio, P. (2005), Editor's note. *Nursing History Review, 13,* 1-4.

Dawley, K. (2005), American nurse-midwifery: A hyphenated profession with a conflicted identity. *Nursing History Review, 13,* 147-170.

Davis, A. T. (1988). Adah Belle Samuels Thomas. In V. Bullough, O. M. Church, & A. P. Stein (Eds.), *American nursing: A biographical dictionary* (pp. 313-316). New York: Garland.

Dock, L. (1910). Report of the thirteenth annual convention. *American Journal of Nursing, 10*(11), 902.

Evans, J. (2004). Men nurses: A historical and feminist perspective. *Journal of Advanced Nursing, 47*(3), 321-328.

Goldmark, J. (1984). *Nursing and nursing education in the United States.* New York: Garland. (Original work published 1923.)

Griffon, D. P. (1998). A somewhat duskier skin: Mary Seacole in the Crimea. *Nursing History Review, 6,* 115-127.

Grypma, S. J. (2004). Neither angels of mercy nor foreign devils: Revisioning Canadian missionary nurses in China, 1935-1947. *Nursing History Review, 12,* 97-119.

Grypma, S. J. (2005). Critical issues in the use of biographic methods in nursing history. *Nursing History Review, 13,* 171-187.

Hawkins, J. W., & Watson, J. C. (2003). Public health nursing pioneer: Jane Elizabeth Hitchcock 1863-1939. *Public Health Nursing, 20*(3), 167-176.

Hine, D. C. (1989). *Black women in white: Racial conflict and cooperation in the nursing profession, 1890-1950.* Bloomington: Indiana University Press.

Houweling, L. (2004). Image, function, and style: A history of the nursing uniform. *American Journal of Nursing, 104*(4), 40-48.

Keeling, A. W. (2004). Blurring the boundaries between medicine and nursing: Coronary care nursing, circa 1960s. *Nursing History Review, 12*, 139-164.

Lorentzon, M. (2004). Nursing Record/British Journal of Nursing archives, 1888-1956. *British Journal of Nursing, 13*(5), 280-284.

Lynaugh, J. (1996). Editorial. *Nursing History Review, 4*, 1.

Lusk, B. (1997). Historical methodology for nursing research. *Journal of Nursing Scholarship, 29*(4), 355-400. (Retrieved from Gale Group Information Integrity, pp. 1-5).

Meehan, T. C. (2003). Careful nursing: A model for contemporary nursing practice. *Journal of Advanced Nursing, 44*(1), 99-107.

Mosley, M. O. P. (1996). Satisfied to carry the bag: Three black community health nurses' contributions to health care reform, 1900-1937. *Nursing History Review, 4*, 65-82.

Poslusny, S. (1989). Feminist friendship: Isabel Hampton Robb, Lavinia Lloyd Dock, and Mary Adelaide Nutting. *Image, 21*(2), 64-68.

Reedy, E. A. (2003). From weakling to fighter: Changing the image of premature infants. *Nursing History Review, 11*, 109-127.

Reverby, S. M. (1987). *Ordered to care: The dilemma of American nursing, 1850-1945.* New York: Cambridge University Press.

Seeger Jablonski, R. A. (2003). Sparks to wildfires: The emergence and impact of nurse practitioner education at Virginia Commonwealth University 1974-1991. *Nursing History Review, 11*, 167-185.

Spieseke, A. W. (1953). What is the historical method of research? *Nursing Research, 2*(1), 36-37.

Thomas, K. K. (2004). "A law unto themselves": Black women as patients and practitioners in North Carolina's campaign to reduce maternal and infant mortality, 1935-1953. *Nursing History Review, 12*, 47-66.

Wall, B. M. (2003). Science and ritual: The hospital as medical and sacred space, 1865-1920. *Nursing History Review, 11*, 51-68.

Whelan, J. (2005). "A necessity in the nursing world": The Chicago Nurses Professional Registry, 1913-1950. *Nursing History Review, 13*, 49-75.

Wolf, A. (1991). How can general duty be made more attractive to graduate nurses? In N. Birnbach & S. Lewenson (Eds.), *First words: Selected addresses from the National League for Nursing, 1894-1933* (pp. 138-147). New York: National League for Nursing Press. (Original speech presented 1928.)

Young, J. (2005). Revisiting the 1925 Johns Report on African-American nurses. *Nursing History Review, 13*, 77-99.

Research Article

"A Necessity in the Nursing World": The Chicago Nurses Professional Registry, 1913–1950

Jean C. Whelan

University of Pennsylvania

*I*n 1923, Lucy Van Frank, Head Registrar of the Chicago-based Nurses Professional Registry, addressed the annual meeting of the Illinois State Nurses Association (ISNA).[1] The main topic of her talk centered on the problems encountered in administering a private duty registry. However, Van Frank seized the opportunity to emphasize the importance of the establishment of nurse-owned and-operated central registries. Central registries were agencies that placed private duty nurses with patients and provided a source of jobs for nurses in a particular locality. Van Frank's remarks focused specifically on central registries owned and operated either by or in close affiliation with a professional association of nurses, the formation of which was a growing movement among nurses in the early twentieth century.[2] Van Frank's comments left no doubt in the audience's mind of the value she placed on central registries. She declared: "They are now considered as much a necessity in the nursing world as are commercial bureaus in the business world, and as essential a part of the great plan of caring for the sick, as is the system of Training Schools in the hospitals."[3]

Van Frank's position as head of one of the largest and fastest growing central registries in the United States most likely influenced her view of central registries. But many in the professional nursing world of the 1920s agreed absolutely with her assessment.[4] Private duty registries offered early 20th century nurses a convenient means of obtaining work, and professional registries, run specifically by and for nurses, were a vehicle through which nurses could achieve a degree of independent practice and autonomy. Contemporary nursing leaders urged nurses to align with professional registries and forecast the future of nursing as centering around these organizations.

Yet by the mid-twentieth century the vision Van Frank and other nurse leaders held for private duty registries owned and operated by nurses remained unfulfilled. The radical changes in the ways nurses were employed, created by the demands of an acute care-centered modern hospital system, would render professional private duty registries obsolete.

This article records the rise and demise of professional private duty registries as demonstrated by the experience of the Chicago Nurses Professional Registry during the years 1913-1950. I examine the origins of the private duty system, describe how

Nursing History Review 13 (2005): 49-75. A publication of the American Association for the History of Nursing. Copyright © 2005 Springer Publishing Company.

private nurses were distributed to patients, and analyze patterns of supply and demand for nursing services. My perspective differs from previous interpretations, which generally attribute the demise of private duty to the circumstances surrounding the Great Depression.[5] I argue that the private duty nurse market remained viable and very important until sometime after World War II. Private duty nursing declined, not as a direct result of changes taking place in the 1930s, but rather several years later as a consequence of the inability of the labor market to supply sufficient numbers of nurses to meet heightened demand for their services. This examination recognizes the significance of changes during the 1930s, but stresses the importance of fluctuating patterns of supply and demand as a major factor in nurse employment arrangements and how they affected the nurse labor market and created vast changes in the ways nurses were employed.

Highlighting the importance of how supply and demand functions in the nurse labor market refines our understanding of the transformation of nurses from independent private practitioners to hospital employees. Examining this intriguing nurse job market offers a unique view of nurses' work and illuminates the foundations on which the contemporary labor market for nurses was formed.

Beginnings: Businesses Owned and Operated by Nurses

The genesis of private duty nursing lies in the peculiar system of hospital-based nursing education that began in the nineteenth century and combined education with employment in the same body of workers. By 1900, 432 hospital schools of nursing were operating in the United States using what has been called an apprenticeship type of training.[6] Students worked in the hospital, learning whatever nursing procedures the particular institution provided for its patients. After 3 years, they were given a diploma and sent out to find employment.

As hospitals did not hire their own graduates, the majority of nurses sought work in the private duty sector. Private duty nursing meant the direct employment of an individual nurse by a patient. A patient or family hired a nurse either upon the advice of the attending physician or when the family's ability to care for ill members was insufficient. Late nineteenth-century private duty nurses, typically employed for the duration of an illness, generally provided care to patients in their own homes on a 24-hour, 7-day-a-week basis.[7] When middle-class patients began to seek hospital care, private duty nurses followed their patients into the hospital. The setting changed, but the work arrangement remained the same. Nurses were hired by patients, who assumed full responsibility for paying them. The nurse delivered whatever nursing services the patient required.

The success of nursing schools in establishing professional nursing as a necessary requisite for care of the ill ensured a demand for private duty services, and nurses eagerly took on the job of setting up the conventions of the work. How to connect easily with patients, however, was a perplexing problem for early private duty nurses. Chronicles of private duty nursing in the late 19th century indicate that physicians or patients requiring the services of a graduate nurse relied on local knowledge of which nurses were competent and available for taking patients.[8] This word-of-mouth method of securing a nurse was sufficient for rural or low population areas, but large cities or towns required a more systematic method of hiring nurses.

Nurses needed a reliable way to seek cases; patients and physicians needed an easy means of obtaining nurses and verifying their capabilities.

Several options for connecting with patients existed for nurses. For many the most familiar way Involved a private duty registry affiliated with a specific hospital. Hospital-based registries, often operated by alumnae associations of the hospital nursing school, listed nurses, referred to as registrants, who were available for private duty.[9] By 1896, approximately forty alumnae associations existed across the country, several of which operated private duty registries.[10] Persons who wanted a nurse contacted the registry, which then sent out a suitable candidate. By sending only nurses who held a diploma from the specific hospital's school, the registry verified that the nurse met school standards, however high or low those standards might be. The registry thus served as a rudimentary credentialing system.

Hospital-based registries were convenient for nurses who lived close to the hospital from which they graduated. Nurses who moved away from their home hospital, however, lost the benefit of the registry, as these registries usually served only a local area. Furthermore, patients who resided some distance from a hospital and those in hospitals without a school of nursing had difficulty obtaining nurses. The idea that private duty nurse services could be centralized for a locality began to gain favor from nurses in the last decades of the nineteenth century.[11]

Centralized registries were intended to enroll nurses who did not belong to a local hospital-based registry or who were willing to accept cases in a number of different hospitals. Physicians and patients who needed a nurse could contact a central registry, which would assume responsibility for locating the nurse and sending her to the patient. The benefits of a centralized registry seemed obvious. The need for only one contact to one agency meant less time spent trying to locate a nurse. The registry assumed responsibility for checking the credentials of the nurses enrolled on it, lessening the possibility that an unqualified nurse would be sent to a patient. Presumably, a centralized registry serving an entire city or region would receive a greater volume of calls for nurses, thus ensuring steady employment for the nurse registrants.

By the turn of the century, a number of different types of centralized registries existed and were available to nurses seeking work. Commercial employment bureaus often placed nurses with patients, serving as one means through which nurses could obtain patient cases. In Chicago, by 1923, twenty-five commercial registries placing nurses were in business.[12] Contemporary nurse leaders, however, viewed commercial agencies with suspicion. Articles in professional nursing journals frequently referred to commercial agencies in disparaging terms, citing their profit motives, the high fees charged nurses for placement, and their practice of sending out untrained workers as nurses. Nurse leaders, such as Lavinia Dock, cautioned nurses to avoid such agencies when seeking employment. Dock claimed commercial agencies were run by unfit lay people who not only charged nurses a fee for services but took a portion of the their earnings as well.[13]

In some cities, medical societies and libraries operated revenue-generating centralized registries. These registries, many of which were established in the late 19th century, operated as a convenience for physician members and had the added advantage of providing a source of income for the sponsoring organization. In 1879, the Medical Library Association of Boston established the Boston Medical Library

Directory for Nurses, considered to be the first of its kind.[14] Philadelphia physicians, frustrated by difficulties in obtaining the services of trained nurses for their patients, founded the Directory for Nurses of the College of Physicians in 1882. This registry remained in business for 54 years.[15]

As was the case with commercial employment agencies, registries operated by medical groups often came under criticism from nursing groups. Dock, a relentless critic of registries operated by those outside the nursing profession, claimed that medical society registries created local monopolies and often intimidated nurses into accepting physician-set rules.[16] Yet the success of physician-controlled and other commercial nurse placement ventures also convinced nurse leaders that establishing nurse-run centralized registries was an achievable goal. By the end of the 19th century, the idea that centralized registries should be nurse-owned, nurse-operated, and nurse-controlled had become popular in organized nursing.[17] And whereas the convenience of using one agency to provide nursing service was a prime driving force behind the establishment of many of the original registries, the central registry movement was more than just a handy way for nurses to acquire jobs.

The benefits of nurse-owned and-operated private duty registries were evident to early nurse leaders such as Isabel Hampton Robb and Lavinia L. Dock. Both Robb and Dock recognized the potential for nurses to control their own practice via nurse-controlled registries and spoke to the issue in professional meetings. Dock addressed the subject in a paper presented in 1895 at the Second Annual Convention of the American Society of Superintendents of Training Schools for Nurses. She strongly recommended the establishment of nurse-owned and-operated central registries as one means of strengthening a professional spirit among nurses. Robb echoed Dock's remarks, forcefully arguing that nurse-operated central registries were the best mechanism for controlling nursing practice in a city and keeping outside forces from interfering with nurses' work.[18]

Professional nurse leaders did not wish to limit the business of centralized registries to the private duty market. Registries were encouraged to serve as placement agencies for hospitals and other health-related agencies interested in filling positions for nurses.[19] By offering a complete line of nursing services, leaders hoped the central registry would become the prime distributor of nurses to all those who needed nursing services whether at home or in the hospital. Some envisioned statewide networks of central registries with one headquarters connected to smaller centers. Nurses enrolled on the registries could be moved about and distributed throughout the state as local needs required, promoting more efficient use of nursing services and providing greater opportunities for nurses to obtain cases.[20]

To achieve such a wide array of goals was a large undertaking. Nurse leaders believed that objectives could be met more easily by connecting the nurse-run central registry to a local professional nurse association.[21] An already organized nurse association offered a structure for readily establishing a registry. The perceived interest of a local nurse association in wider community affairs was, of course, considered an asset in providing systematic nursing services. Members of professional nurse associations included individuals who could give the benefits of their leadership experience to registry governance. Professional nursing journals in the initial years of the twentieth century reported enthusiastically on the establishment of a number of local nurse association-sponsored central registries.[22]

These formed the nucleus of what would later be known as professional private duty registries, the type of registries to which Lucy Van Frank referred in her 1923 talk to the ISNA.[23] And it was Van Frank's Chicago Nurses Professional Registry that best exemplified the ideals of what a professional nurse registry was meant to be.

Chicago: The Golden Years for Professional Registries

Illinois had possessed all the necessary elements for operating a successful central registry. The ISNA, formed in 1901, was one of the earliest and best organized state nurse associations in the nation. In 1911, the state association, originally composed of nursing school alumnae associations, began a reorganization process that resulted in the establishment of local components called district nurse associations. Shortly thereafter, in 1912, nurses in Cook, DuPage, and Lake Counties formed the Chicago area nurses association, named the First District of the Illinois State Nurses Association. Due to its location in the state's largest city and its ample nurse population, the Chicago district became the center of nursing activity in Illinois.[24]

Members of the new district association quickly went to work on achieving one of the main district objectives: to establish a centralized registry. They were aware that nurse-run central registries flourished in a number of other cities. Chicago offered a promising environment in which to open a registry. At the time, Chicago was the second largest city in the United States and well known for its fast pace and rapid growth.[25] Its large population promised a supply of patients in need of private care. It was home to many of the nation's leading medical facilities, which provided the necessary demand for professional nurse services.[26] By 1913 more than thirty-two schools of nursing were operating within and around the city, guaranteeing a sufficient number of nurses interested in working in the private duty market.[27]

The Central Registry, originally called the Central Directory and later renamed the Nurses Professional Registry (NPR), opened its doors for services in 1913.[28] Under the direction of Van Frank, who would serve as director for its first three decades, the registry was organized along lines similar to other professional registries of the day. Nurses meeting the qualifications of the registry—usually referred to as registrants—paid a fee to enroll as members. In return, they received all the privileges of membership. When a nurse decided she wanted to work, she placed her name on the list of nurses on call. Nurses were assigned to patients as the registry received requests. A nurse not wishing to take on patients simply did not place her name on the list, or removed it.[29]

The new registry met with immediate success in delivering private duty services and experienced tremendous growth in a very short period of time. One month after the NPR opened for business, it claimed 150 members and averaged eight nurse placements a day; it ended its first year of operation with over 500 members.[30] By its 10-year anniversary in 1923, registry membership hovered around 950 and received more than 11,000 yearly requests for nurses, a considerable number by professional registry standards.[31]

What accounted for this rapid expansion? The NPR was quickly able to mobilize and capitalize on considerable financial and moral support from the Chicago nursing community. The city had a well-organized group of active school of nursing alumnae associations, several of which were instrumental in forming the Chicago district and advancing the concept of a central registry. The relationship between these alumnae associations and the NPR was both cooperative and collegial. The associations donated substantial amounts of money to cover the initial expense of launching the NPR. Contributions amounting to $500 were received from the Illinois Training School for Nurses and St. Luke's Hospital alumnae associations. The Michael Reese Hospital alumnae association contributed in excess of $350, and others donated $100 or more each.[32]

In addition to financial support, several area alumnae associations agreed to turn over their own private duty registries to the NPR, thus enlarging its membership. The Illinois Training School for Nurses and Presbyterian Hospital registries were the first to join, bringing in a large number of nurse registrants. By the mid-1930s, twelve alumnae association registries would be listed as NPR members.[33]

The benefits accruing to the NPR from aligning with the alumnae associations were significant. The large number of registrants the alumnae associations brought into the registry, all paying registry fees, ensured financial solvency for the NPR. The arrangement benefited the alumnae associations as well. Joining the NPR spared the associations the expense and effort of running separate registries, while at the same time they received credit for providing means for members to obtain work. Nurses enrolled on the NPR but not aligned with a specific alumnae association (e.g., nurses who had graduated from schools outside the Chicago area) also gained. Tradition required that when an alumnae association registry joined the NPR, the registry would keep a separate list of affiliated alumnae association members. The hospital's own graduates received preference for calls received from the association's home hospital. When such a nurse was unavailable, a non-alumnae association nurse was sent. This improved work opportunities for all registrants, increased the chances of filling a request for a nurse, and resulted in more nurses finding employment.

A Premier Private Duty Registry

By the mid-1920s, the conventions of modern private duty nursing were well established. Nurses cared for patients primarily in acute care hospital settings, generally working twelve-hour shifts.[34] As the NPR entered its second decade of operation, the business affairs of the registry were extremely encouraging. Each year the NPR recorded more success than the year before. From 1923 to 1929, the average number of monthly patient assignments rose 178%, from 919 to 2,555, and membership doubled to almost 2,000 registrants.[35] The NPR's membership represented a significant portion of graduate nurses, not just from Chicago but from Illinois as a whole: 9% of the state nurses and 17 percent of the city area nurses in 1930.[36] The twelve affiliated alumnae associations represented some of the largest hospitals in Chicago and surrounding areas. Presbyterian, Mercy, and St. Luke's had more than 400 beds each; Augustana and West Surburban had more than 300 beds.[37] The NPR provided a stable number of registrants and served as a reliable source of patient calls in the Chicago area. Enough confidence existed in 1927 to permit a private duty fee increase from $6 to $7 for twelve-hour cases.[38] Registry records indicated a financially healthy enterprise. In 1929, the NPR recorded an impressive profit of almost $11,000.[39]

To manage the large numbers of members and patient requests for nurses, the NPR increased its staff, secured larger offices, and installed a switchboard service during the 1920s.[40] By 1930, the staff was composed of a registrar and five assistants, all registered nurses.[41] The NPR developed plans to expand services offered to patients, nurses, and health care agencies by providing hourly nursing services and institutional placement services.[42] First District took pride in the NPR, reporting on tributes it received, such as the warm appreciation expressed by Illinois Central Hospital for the promptness with which NPR nurses responded to and cared for victims of a 1926 train wreck.[43]

Amid the many accomplishments achieved by the NPR it is well to keep in mind one serious limitation. The NPR, which intended to be the main distributor of all nurses for the Chicago area, simply was not. Reflecting the deplorable racist attitudes and common exclusionary practices of the times, the NPR was open to only a select population of nurses—those who were white. This situation did not change until the 1940s, when minority nurses first began appearing on the membership rolls. When asked about the placement of African-American nurses, Minnie Aherns, executive secretary of the Chicago District, justified the segregated policy. Commenting on the reasons African-American nurses were excluded by the registry, Aherns said, "we cannot place them, the social differences are too great."[44]

Private Duty Nursing: A Labor Market in Distress

The success of the NPR in placing private duty nurses, though impressive, took place in a labor market plagued by serious problems. Private duty nursing had always been an unreliable means of making a living, and by the end of the 1920s difficulties that had been identified at the beginning of the century were reaching crisis proportions.

The main issue was a substantial imbalance between supply of and demand for private duty nurse services. There were just too many nurses seeking work in a labor market in which jobs were few and employment uneven. During the 1920s, the number of schools nationwide increased substantially, from around 1,775 in 1920 to 2,286 in 1928, and the number of nurses doubled from 104,000 in 1920 to 214,000 in 1930.[45] Most of these nurses continued to seek work in the private duty field. While the percentage of nurses working as private duty nurses declined from 80% in 1920 to approximately 55% in 1930, the actual number of private duty nurses stabilized at a little over 100,000.[46] This would not have been a major concern except that demand for private duty services remained flat.

Private duty nursing was expensive. By the end of the 1920s, the average fee was around $6-7 dollars for a 12 shift. In a cash-based system, a patient needed to have a ready supply of money to pay the nurse. At a time when the average American could barely afford hospital or medical care, another $80 to $100 dollars a week for private nurses was out of reach for most.[47]

Studies carried out during the late 1920s validated the idea that the nursing education system had produced too many nurses for the amount of work available.

The Committee on the Grading of Nursing Schools' (CGNS) study on private duty nursing, published in 1928 as *Nurses, Patients, and Pocketbooks,* recorded a dismal picture of the field, documenting dangerously low employment levels for private duty nurses and salaries that trailed considerably behind those for nurses employed in other fields.[48] Equally troubling was the revelation that private duty nurses were increasingly disenchanted with their work: 36% of private duty nurses surveyed indicated that they planned to leave the field in the near future.[49]

Private duty nurses were not alone in expressing discontent. Professional nurse leaders began to question the value of private duty nursing as a legitimate occupational field for the majority of nurses. In the early part of the century, it was commonly accepted that most nurses would spend part of their career in private duty. By the late 1920s, however, many saw a different future for nursing, one more closely tied to hospital employment. Private duty was described as an inefficient method of patient care delivery, one that wasted precious nurse resources on a limited number of patients.[50] The CGNS suggested sweeping changes, recommending that, whereas elements of the private system of nurse distribution should remain in place, the majority of nurses should seek employment in hospitals.[51]

Despite dissatisfaction expressed by private duty nurses and a growing consensus among nurse leaders that private duty as an occupational field was in decline, the private duty labor market continued to demonstrate significant resilience. The negative reports on private duty during the 1920s and the conviction of leaders that change was necessary may in fact have overstated nurse unhappiness with the field. If read from the opposite point of view, the CGNS findings reveal that the majority of the nurses surveyed, 55%, intended to remain private duty nurses.[52] Comments from nurses received by the CGNS also indicated that, although private duty nurses identified many areas of complaints, particularly in relation to pay and working conditions, they clearly enjoyed bedside nursing. One nurse from Massachusetts succinctly described her feelings: "Personally, I like private duty even though it is harder; you come in close touch with your patient and see better the results of your work."[53] A New York nurse expressed similar thoughts but added a proviso, "I love my work. I don't regret that I have taken up nursing as a profession, but I do ask for a square deal."[54]

Van Frank observed a high degree of loyalty on the part of nurses to the field, noting that nurses would accept jobs in hospitals in slow periods when calls were scarce, but would leave them as soon as the private duty market picked up.[55] Private duty may well have been a field with significant difficulties, but it was also one in which nurses experienced pride in their work and contentment with their practice.

The Great Depression Years: Beginning the Transformation

The collapse of the economy in 1929 brought havoc and despair to the lives of all Americans. Over twelve million people, about 25% of the workforce, joined the ranks of the unemployed.[56] Workers in all fields searched for ways to endure the lean economic years. By 1930, nurses registered with the NPR were feeling the full effects of the Great Depression. The registry turned its attention to simple survival.

Van Frank reported the unemployment situation among private duty nurses as the worst she had ever encountered.[57] For 3 years, beginning in 1930, the situation deteriorated. The NPR recorded a 30% drop in patient assignments in 1931.[58] By 1932, nurses registered with the NPR averaged 8.75 days of work per month or 80 days a year.[59] The NPR lost more than 700 members in one two-year period; membership dropped from 1,912 in 1929 to 1,149 in 1933.[60] The decline in membership resulted in a drop in registry profits. NPR income over expenses in 1932 was a meager $86.18, a decrease of about $4,000 from 1931.[61]

The NPR instituted a number of actions in an attempt to help its membership. A loan fund was established to provide small amounts of money to those in dire straits.[62] The NPR gave nurses in great need special consideration, calling them out of turn for cases.[63] The registry relaxed policies that required nurses to live in the Chicago area when on call, helping nurses to cut down on living expenses.[64] To preserve their spirits, nurses were encouraged to keep busy by maintaining an interest in professional affairs, studying new methods in medicine, pursuing higher education, and developing recreational interests in areas such as music and art.[65]

More ambitious programs aimed at increasing employment of graduate nurses by hospitals. The ISNA asked hospitals to hire only licensed nursing personnel.[66] In May 1932, the ISNA petitioned hospitals to limit the number of students admitted for the coming year.[67] Several hospitals in the Chicago area complied with this request; others closed their schools altogether.[68] Private duty nurses volunteered a month or more of free service to hospitals that promised to reduce student enrollments, an offer hospitals were quick to accept. Hospitals also offered nurses a variety of schemes that provided small amounts of remuneration, maintenance in the form of room and board, or a combination of both. Some hospitals offered compensation ranging from $1 a day to $20 a month with maintenance for 4 hours of work a day. In other cases, hospitals provided full or partial maintenance with no salary to nurses who were willing to work as staff nurses for a varying number of hours.[69] The NPR sought to decrease the number of nurses seeking private duty work. Nurses graduating from schools outside the Chicago area were first discouraged and then refused membership. Word went out that employment opportunities in Chicago were extremely poor.[70]

Traditionally the Depression years have been characterized as the period of the "Great Transformation" in nursing, the time when large numbers of private duty nurses deserted the field to seek employment as general duty nurses, the predecessors of our contemporary staff nurses.[71] This characterization is only partly true. For a number of reasons, hospitals during the 1930s did begin to turn away from the traditional student nurse-centered care and employ more graduate nurses in staff positions.[72] Technological changes created complex care requirements necessitating practitioners more expert than students. Middle-class patients unable to afford private duty nurses expected hospitals to provide personalized care. Private and semiprivate rooms replaced multiple bed wards, creating a need for more nurses. Finally, the economic effects of the Depression made graduate nurses relatively cheaper workers, increasing their attractiveness as employees.[73] Hospital employment, even at very low wages, often offered nurses the only opportunity for work.

At the same time that hospitals were beginning to value graduate nurses as appropriate patient caregivers, they also demonstrated significant reluctance to employ registered nurses permanently. Rather, significant evidence exists that hospitals resorted to hiring private duty nurses on a per diem basis as temporary staff.[74] Many general duty nurses during this period were actually private duty nurses placed in temporary positions.

Using private duty nurses as general duty nurses, a movement that continued to grow as the 1930s ended, represented a tremendous economic boost for the private duty market. The additional work created an increased demand for private duty nurses that translated into more jobs. As the economy slowly stabilized during the late 1930s, professional nurse registries nationwide reported better employment conditions overall.[75] The NPR documented a steady increase in nurse assignments in the years 1934–1940, recording a rise in average monthly assignments from 1,265 to 2,758, an increase of approximately 1,500 patient cases.[76]

Hospitals found that employing private duty nurses, who could be hired and dismissed as patient occupancy rates rose and fell, was an easy way to temporarily supplement short staffs and save the expense of permanent employees.[77] But the practice was a double-edged sword for private duty nurses and did not enjoy universal appeal. Temporary general duty work did offer nurses a chance to make some money, but problems with determining rates of pay and hours of work and reprisals against private duty nurses who refused to comply with hospitals' requests for temporary help marred the relationship between the parties.[78]

The rate of pay was a major source of contention between hospitals and private duty nurses. Private duty nurses generally received a set fee per shift of work. In the late 1930s, in large cities this may have averaged around $5 a shift.[79] Hospitals hiring per diem nurses generally calculated a daily fee prorated from the monthly salary paid permanent general duty nurses. In most cases this meant that the private duty nurse might be earning a paltry $3–4 a shift.[80] To make matters worse, the nurse was also expected to do a great deal more work.

In Chicago, nurses registered with the NPR reluctantly filled calls for general duty, but complained bitterly over the treatment they received as per diem nurses.[81] They resented the lower fees and the conditions under which they were expected to work.[82] In most instances, when private duty nurses took on a general duty assignment they were required to work split shifts, two 4-hour periods separated by a 4-hour or longer break. In some hospitals nurses were required to give up their position on the registry list when on general duty service. This lessened their chances of obtaining private duty cases. Many NPR nurses reported that hospitals discriminated against them if they refused temporary general duty service. Even in hospitals that did not discriminate, nurses were warned that refusing requests for temporary service would not be regarded in a positive manner by hospital authorities.[83]

At the 1936 ANA national convention, private duty nurses voiced frustration at being asked to fill in as temporary general duty nurses. One Chicago nurse reported that private duty nurses sometimes did not even receive a salary. Some hospitals merely provided room and board and the privilege of taking a private case if one became available. In other instances, the nurse might earn a meager $2 a day. Yet, as this nurse noted, nurses' primary complaint was not their low salaries: "But of all of the nurses I asked why they did not wish to help out in hospitals, not one complained about the money, but she said in every case when she had gone in to do general duty the amount of work required of her was beyond the physical capacity of any person and she just could not go back under those conditions."[84]

Concerns about the use of private duty nurses as temporary general duty nurses emerged as a recurring topic of discussion at the leadership level of the ANA.[85] Acting on reports of trouble among working nurses and the difficulties hospitals encountered in obtaining sufficient numbers of general duty nurses, the ANA launched a study examining the working conditions of nurses. The 1936 *Study of Incomes, Salaries, and Employment Conditions Affecting Nurses* surveyed nurses in three different fields of nursing: private duty nurses, institutional staff, and office nurses.[86] Although the study was based on a small sample (only 11,432 nurses in 23 states participated), the ANA Board of Directors expressed confidence in the accuracy of the results.[87] The study findings confirmed private duty nurses' dissatisfaction with temporary general duty positions and exposed the widespread use of poor labor practices by hospitals. The Board, faced with evidence that nurses were employed under dismal conditions, decided to use the results of the study to achieve reform.

The Board carefully formulated a number of recommendations intended to improve working conditions for private duty nurses engaged in temporary general duty nursing jobs. Hospitals were asked not to require private duty nurses to work as general duty nurses in order to secure work as private duty nurses. The Board recommended that private duty nurses employed as relief general duty nurses be paid based on prevailing private duty rates. Finally, they urged that nurses work straight, not split or broken-hour shifts.[88] Believing that hospitals would seriously consider adopting their recommendations, the Board put significant thought into the ways hospitals would put them into practice, taking into account the feasibility and practicality of each recommendation. Board discussions indicated confidence that the study and its accompanying recommendations would receive careful consideration from hospitals.[89]

Wholesale acceptance of the ANA position on working conditions and action on the study's recommendations by hospital authorities proved to be an elusive goal. To publicize the results of the study among hospital groups, Alma Scott, director of ANA headquarters, presented a paper describing the study, its findings and recommendations to the American Hospital Association (AHA) 1938 annual convention.[90] The paper failed to stimulate discussion. Exactly how many hospitals followed up on the ANA recommendations, or even reflected on the study's implications, is unknown. Continued complaints from private duty nurses indicated that hospitals demonstrated little interest in changing employment practices toward private duty nurses. In reality, the ANA occupied a weak position from which to convince hospital authorities to improve nurses' working conditions. The association had no actual bargaining power and relied primarily on the good intentions of hospitals to act.[91] In the late 1930s, this was an insufficient strategy to effect change.

World War II Years: A Failure of the Market

As the country entered the war years, the nursing profession as a whole and the private duty field in particular faced considerable challenges. Although the future looked bright for the private duty field as the decade began, significant changes in the ways hospitals staffed their institutions disrupted the private system of nurse distribution and led to its eventual demise.

In 1940, the NPR reported its busiest year on record. Twenty-two hospitals used the NPR exclusively for private nursing services; another forty institutions used the registry as needed.[92] NPR finances improved, showing the highest post-depression profit.[93] Reports of registry effectiveness in meeting demand for nurses began to resemble those of the 1920s. The improved outlook for the NPR was directly tied to the changing need for nurses occurring nationwide.

During the 1940s, several factors came together to create an unprecedented demand for nurses. The most immediate need was for nurses to serve in the armed forces. About 70,000 nurses joined military service.[94] The unavailability of approximately 25% of the registered nurse population for civilian needs plunged the country into an immediate critical nurse shortage.[95] At the same time, an increase in hospital use, secondary to the availability of health insurance; a growing population; and wartime activities caused demand for nurses to soar.[96]

By 1942, the NPR was overwhelmed with requests for nurses. For the first time in its history, the registry, which only 10 years before had been unable to supply enough work for its nurses, was unable to supply enough nurses for all the work. Registry statistics documenting the number of calls filled per request reflected the seriousness of the situation. In the late 1930s, the NPR generally had a 98–99% fill rate. Between 1942 and 1945, this rate plummeted to 39%. By the end of the war requests for nurses stabilized somewhat but were still filled only about 50–60% of the time.[97]

As the NPR experienced more and more difficulty filling requests for nurses, a vicious cycle began to play out. Unable to depend on the private duty field for an adequate supply of nurses, hospitals resorted to other means of supplementing short staffs. Hospitals discovered they could easily hire nurses on either a temporary or permanent basis without registry help and started bypassing the registry, choosing to deal directly with nurses when they needed to fill either general or private duty jobs. As nurses found that they could find work through hospitals, they often neglected to place themselves on call with the registry. This further reduced the number of nurses available to the NPR and made it even harder to fill requests. Some nurses most likely left the field of private duty altogether, taking positions as staff nurses instead.[98] As the registry experienced more and more problems filling requests, it came to be viewed as an unreliable source of nurses.

Post–World War II nurses tended to accept hospital employment.[99] New graduates did not consider the private duty field the best venue in which to practice. Other measures instituted by hospitals further endangered the private duty market. Hospitals found that using a differentiated nursing staff composed of several different types of nurse workers met the need for staff and decreased the need for private practitioners.[100] This success allowed them to employ more lesser-trained, cheaper workers and fewer more expensive registered nurses. The cumulative effect of the changes occurring during the 1940s was to marginalize private duty nursing as a viable occupational field.[101] With fewer nurses entering the market, fewer nurses hired for private duty, and hospitals initiating strategies to reduce the need for private nurses and turning away from the private duty market as a source of nurses, the private duty field passed into decline.

A speaker at the 1948 ANA convention summed up the changes in the field and asked poignantly:

> How secure is the future of private duty nursing? . . . The age group of the present membership would indicate that the younger nurse is not interested. Why? Is the answer a question of income, a seven-day week, lack of self-confidence? Does the nurse assume it is her responsibility to remain for staff duty with the hospital from which she is a graduate? Are the rules for accepting calls unsatisfactory? Is the yearly fee unattractive? Are we overlooking opportunities to advance private duty nursing by not promoting good personnel practices? Salary increases in other fields of nursing must be equally balanced by the private duty nurse if we expect to replace the older nurse resigning from our registries.[102]

Despite this nurse's uncertainties over private duty's future, she remained hopeful that the field would continue, concluding, "Collectively, we may establish a satisfactory attractive private duty program that will continue to meet the expected demands of each community for special nursing." Given the contemporary circumstances in the nurse labor market, this nurse's optimism that private duty nursing would survive seemed misplaced.

For the NPR, the downturn in private duty did not result in immediate closure. The registry remained open for another 30 years, but as a greatly reduced business. It did attempt to improve its rate of filling requests for nurses. It also expanded services in the 1950s, when it opened a registry placing private duty practical nurses. But it would never regain its earlier status as the center of nurse distribution for the Chicago area. In 1980, the Chicago Nurses Association, citing financial concerns, closed the 69-year-old NPR.

Conclusion

Providing private nursing services on a one-to-one basis made a great deal of sense to early practitioners of nursing. Late 19th and early 20th century hospitals were not yet interested in hiring the nursing staff necessary to deliver the technical care required by advances in modern medicine. The private duty market bridged the gap in nursing services by supplying professional graduate nurses to hospitals and to those patients fortunate enough to afford private care. Private duty registries functioned as an important source of jobs for the increasing numbers of nurses graduating from schools nationwide.

Analyses of private duty tend to emphasize the system's weaknesses. Private duty was an inefficient, expensive, and unreliable method through which to distribute nurses. Nevertheless, despite its problems, the field operated with a fair degree of success. The private duty market was the largest and most structured job market for nurses in the early years of the profession. The professional registry system offered nurses a unique opportunity to control, organize, and systematize their work. The registries that connected nurses with patients provided not just employment for nurses but also a significant barometer of labor market functioning in supplying enough work for nurses and meeting demands for nurse services. Moreover, when times were bad, such as during the Great Depression, professional private duty registries offered a support system to help nurses survive.

Hospitals used the private duty system to their full benefit. During the first half of the twentieth century, they remained committed to student-centered care, relying on the private duty market to obtain a graduate nursing staff for patients willing and able to pay for private care without the expense and bother of employing nurses. During the 1930s, hospitals became savvy consumers of the registry system, using registries as a source of temporary general duty nurses. This arrangement permitted hospitals to continue avoiding employing permanent staff.

However, it was an arrangement with significant liabilities for both nurses and hospitals. Hiring temporary nurses allowed hospitals to ignore provision of proper working conditions and created considerable dissatisfaction among nurses. Little incentive existed for nurses to remain loyal to hospitals. Speculations only are in order as to the influence of hospital behavior on nurses' decisions to enter, remain in, or leave the labor market. It is unlikely that the treatment hospitals afforded nurses encouraged them to work.

Relying on temporary nurses for delivery of nursing care, whether at a private or institutional level, was a fundamentally flawed system. An increased demand for nurses beginning around World War II demonstrated the precarious nature of their employment situation. As more nurses were required and fewer were available, a crisis atmosphere caused hospitals to take actions that resulted in the marginalization of the private duty market as an employment field. Distributing nurses to patients, one nurse at a time, became an anachronism.

Placing the decline of the private duty market in the context of a nurse shortage has meaning beyond just situating an event in a specific time and place. Analyses of periodic nurse shortages over the century predominantly focus on causative factors and solutions. But shortages create consequences that are important to both recognize and explain. Meeting demand for nurses was a tenacious problem throughout the 20th century. In mid-century, unmet demand resulted in the slow death of the private duty market and the adoption of alternative employment arrangements for nurses. This serves as a cautionary tale as the profession approaches supply and demand issues today. Critical nurse shortages have longstanding effects beyond the very serious and immediate outcomes at the patient's bedside. For better or worse, they may also carry the potential to change the very structure of nurses' employment and frustrate nurses' attempts to manage their own practice.

JEAN C. WHELAN, PHD, RN
University of Pennsylvania
Postdoctoral Fellow
Center for Health Outcomes and Policy Research
School of Nursing
Philadelphia, PA 19104

Acknowledgments

This research was made possible by a National Research Service Award (#NR07270 1997–99) and grants from Sigma Theta Tau Xi Chapter, Sigma Theta Tau International, the American Nurses Foundation Eleanor Lambertson RN Scholar Award, and a Rockefeller Archive Center Grant. Versions of this chapter were presented at the national meeting of the American Association for the History of Nursing, Milwaukee, Wisconsin, September 19, 2003 and at the 37th Biennial Convention of Sigma Theta Tau International, Toronto, Ontario, November, 3 2003. The author gratefully acknowledges the guidance and support of Karen Buhler-Wilkerson, Joan Lynaugh, and Walter Licht in carrying out the original research for this project, to Patricia D'Antonio for her suggestions, to Robin Cheung for her thoughts and comments, and to the NHR reviewers for their useful critiques.

Notes

1. *The name of the association changed several times. Originally known as the Graduate Nurses' Association of the State of Illinois, it became the Illinois State Association of Graduate Nurses in 1902 and the Illinois State Nurses Association in 1929. It acquired its present name, the Illinois Nurses Association, in 1956. See Mary Dunwiddie, A History of the Illinois State Nurses Association, 1910-1935 (Chicago: Illinois State Nurses Association, 1937); Karen J. Egenes and Wendy K. Burgess, Faithfully Yours: A History of Nursing in Illinois (Chicago: Illinois Nurses Association, 2001). I use the contemporary name Illinois State Nurses Association (ISNA) throughout this chapter.*

2. *Terms used to categorize private duty registries for nurses changed over time. "Central registry" was used at the turn of the 20th century for registries in a central location in a city or town. In 1924, as professional nurse groups enlarged their interest in the operations of central registries, private duty nurses at the American Nurses Association (ANA) annual convention recommended adopting the term "official registry" as more fitting. See "Central Registries for Nurses," Trained Nurse and Hospital Review 73 (July 1924): 57. The term "professional registry" came into use during the 1930s to identify a registry approved by a local district nurse association. See "Meetings of the Board of Directors," American Journal of Nursing 38 (March 1938): 329 (hereafter AJN). This paper uses the term "central registry" either in its historic sense to refer to a registry operating in the initial decades of the 20th century or to a specific registry named a central registry. It uses the term "professional registry" as a generic term for registries operated by and for nurses.*

3. *Lucy Van Frank, "The Problems of a Registrar," paper presented at the Annual Meeting of the Illinois State Nurses Association, Peoria, October 10-12, 1923, Illinois Nurses Association Papers, Illinois State Historical Library, Springfield IL, box 2, folder 1 (hereafter INAP).*

4. *See, for example, "Official Registries and Professional Progress," AJN 26 (February 1926): 91-94; Elizabeth Burgess, "The Future of the Central Registry," AJN 15 (August 1915): 1033-35; Editor, "Registries," AJN 26 (March 1926): 206-7.*

5. *Several excellent studies on the change of employment status for nurses from private duty to staff nursing exist. See, for example, Marilyn Flood, "The Troubling Expedient: General Staff Nursing in United States Hospitals in the 1930's: A Means to Institutional, Educational, and Personal Ends" (PhD dissertation, University of California at Berkeley, 1981) and Susan M. Reverby, Ordered to Care: The Dilemma of American Nursing, 1850-1945 (Cambridge: Cambridge University Press, 1987).*

6. *For the number of schools of nursing, see Department of Health and Human Services, Public Health Service, Human Resources Administration, Source Book— Nursing Personnel, DHHS publication (HRA) 81-21 (Hyattsville, MD: U.S. Department of Health and Human Services, Public Health Service, Human Resources Administration, 1981), 83.*

7. *For a contemporary description of early 20th century private duty nursing see Katherine De Witt, Private Duty Nursing, 2nd ed. (Philadelphia: Lippincott, 1917; reprint New York: Garland, 1984). For the best historical analyses of early private duty nursing and nurses, see Susan M. Reverby, "Neither for the Drawing Room Nor for the Kitchen": Private Duty Nursing in Boston, 1873-1920," in Women and Health in America: Historical Readings, ed. Judith Walzer Leavitt (Madison: University of Wisconsin Press, 1984), 454-66; Reverby, Ordered to Care.*

8. *For the ways patients and physicians secured nurses at the turn of the century, see Sister M. Ignatius Feeny, "Central Directories," AJN 4 (July 1904): 796-99; Elizabeth Scovil, "Openings for Nurses," AJN 1 (March 1901): 439.*

9. *Many discussions on the best types and ways to organize hospital-based registries took place in the late 1890s at conventions held by the American Society of Superintendents of Training Schools for Nurses. See, for example, Louise Darche, "Training School Registries," in American Society of Superintendents of Training Schools for Nurses, Annual Conventions 1893-1899 (New York: Garland, 1985), 22-31. For a concise contemporary history of the evolution of hospital-based registries, see Ella Best, "Nursing Supply—How To Balance Supply and Demand," Modern Hospital 39 (August 1932): 97-102.*

10. *The exact number of hospital-based registries is indeterminate. At the Third Annual Convention of the American Society of Superintendents of Training Schools for Nurses, held in 1896, Sophia Palmer reported forty alumnae associations in existence in the United States and Canada. How many of them operated private duty registries was not mentioned. See Sophia Palmer, "Discussion," in Annual Conventions 1893-1899, 63.*

11. *For the evolution of central registries see Best, "Nursing Supply"; Lavinia L. Dock, "Nursing in the United States," in Transactions of the Third International Congress of Nurses in Buffalo, September 18-21, 1901, edited by the Committee on Publication, Isabel Hampton Robb, Lavinia L. Dock, and Maud Banfield (Cleveland: J. B. Savage, 1901), 481-82.*

12. *For the number of commercial employment agencies in Chicago, see Van Frank, "The Problems of a Registrar." Using commercial employment agencies either to obtain work or to hire employees was a common practice for both workers and employers at the turn of the century. For a history of private employment agencies, see Tomás Martinez, The Human Marketplace: An Examination of Private Employment Agencies (New Brunswick, NJ: Transaction Books, 1976).*

13. For negative reports of commercial registries, see Minnie Aherns, "Discussion, 18th Annual Convention, ANA," AJN 15 (August 1915): 1036; Editor, "The Commercial Registry," AJN 14 (February 1914): 329-30; Martha Russell, "Club Houses, Hostelries, and Directories for Nurses," AJN 5 (August 1905): 803. Nurses were particularly critical of agencies that placed them with other domestic workers, such as chambermaids and scrubwomen. See, for example, Editor, "Commercial Directories," AJN 9 (July 1909): 723-24; Mary Thornton to Editor, AJN 3 (December 1903): 243-44. For Lavinia Dock's comments, see Dock, "Nursing in the United States," 481-82.

14. For a discussion of the Boston Medical Library Directory for Nurses, see Reverby, "Neither for the Drawing Room Nor for the Kitchen"; Reverby, Ordered to Care.

15. For a history of the Philadelphia Directory, see Frederick Fraley, "History of the Directory for Nurses of the College of Physicians," Transactions and Studies of the College of Physicians of Philadelphia 4, 1 (1936): xi-xvi.

16. Dock, "Nursing in the United States," 482.

17. See, for example, Helen MacMillan, "Central Registration," AJN 4 (July 1904): 791-94; Mary Thornton, "The Organization and Management of Clubs and Homes for Graduate Nurses," AJN 1 (February 1901): 378-80.

18. Lavinia L. Dock, "Directories for Nurses," in Annual Conventions 1893-1899. 57-60; Isabel Hampton Robb, "Discussion," in Annual Conventions 1893-1899, 63.

19. See Elizabeth Burgess, "The Future of the Central Registry," AJN 15 (August 1915): 1033-35; Editor, "Central Registries and the Idle Nurse," AJN 9 (December 1909): 145-47; Marion Mead, "Registry from the Point of View of the Registrar," AJN 14 (July 1914): 827-29. Early 20th century nurse-run central registries were also often associated with club houses or living quarters for nurses and provided a spectrum of services, including meals, recreation, and educational opportunities. See MacMillan, "Central Registration"; Sister Ignatius Feeny, "Central Directories." Some believed a nurse registry should offer a variety of services to patients, in effect serving as a one-stop nursing shopping center for the community. Paying individuals could use the registry not just for nursing services when ill but also for purchasing special diets and sickroom supplies. See, for example, Sophia Rutley, "Private Duty Nurses and Their Relationship to the Directory," AJN 15 (August 1915): 939-43.

20. Editor, "Central Registries and the Idle Nurse."

21. The establishment of central registries often paralleled the organization of state and local nurse associations. State nurse associations began forming in the early years of the 20th century, many with the specific purpose of passing nurse practice acts. Although variation existed in the ways in which each state association organized, eventually state associations included smaller, locally based units called district associations. District associations were considered to be the best sponsor of a central registry. For discussions regarding the organization and ownership of central registries, see Katherine De Witt, "The County Association and Its Relationship to the State," AJN 9 (August 1909): 809-15; Janette Peterson, "Central Directories—The Nurse's Obligation to Support Them," Nurses' Journal of the Pacific Coast 7 (October 1911): 441-49. In 1911, the conglomeration of state, district, and alumnae associations became the American Nurses Association. For the organization of the ANA and its constituent state associations, see Lyndia Flanagan, One Strong Voice: The Story of the American Nurses Association (Kansas City: American Nurses Association, 1976).

22. *Nurse association-run central registries were reported in Boston, Denver, Washington, D. C., Minneapolis, Philadelphia, Oklahoma City, and Kansas City. See Editor, "Central Registries," AJN 12 (January 1912): 281-282; Reba Thelin Foster, "The Organization of Nurses Clubs and Directories Under State Association," AJN 9 (January 1909): 247-52; Grace Holmes, "An Ideal Central Directory," AJN 6 (June 1906): 606-8; Susan Bard Johnson, "The Boston Nurses Club," AJN 9 (April 1909): 662-63; Lily Kanely, "A Successful Central Registry," AJN 9 (April 1909): 496-98; Sarah F. Martin, "Central Directories," AJN 10 (December 1910): 162-67; Marion Mead, "Registry System of the Hennepin County Graduate Nurses Association, Minneapolis, Minn.," AJN 10 (August 1910): 819-24.*

23. *Exact estimates of how many professional central registries existed prior to the mid-1930s are difficult to obtain. In 1915, the Special Registry Committee of the ANA located more than forty central registries; see "Report of the Special Registry Committee," AJN 15 (September 1915): 1121-22. A 1924 ANA survey reported on seventy-five professional registries; see "Official Registries and Professional Progress," AJN 26 (February 1926): 92. In the mid-1930s the ANA began compiling statistics on professional registries, providing a more accurate estimate of the number of such agencies. Prior to World War II, the ANA recorded as many as 145 professional registries in business. The number fluctuated during the 1940s but began rising steadily after the war until 1956, when 176 registries were in operation. After 1956, the number of professional registries fell, but as late as 1965 there were 153 professional registries listed with the ANA. For numbers of professional registries, see the ANA annual publication Facts About Nursing: A Statistical Summary (New York: American Nurses Association, 1935-): 1939, 43; 1953, 80; 1957, 109; 1966, 116.*

24. *For the organization of nursing in Illinois, see Dunwiddie, A History of the Illinois State Nurses' Association; Egenes and Burgess, Faithfully Yours.*

25. *In the first decades of the 20th century, Chicago was the second largest city in the nation in population, with 2,701,705 inhabitants in 1920. See U.S. Department of Commerce, Fifteenth Census of the United States: 1930, vol. 1, Population (Washington, DC: U.S. Government Printing Office, 1930), 18.*

26. *For a history of the Chicago medical world, see Thomas Neville Bonner, Medicine in Chicago, 1850-1950, 2nd ed. (Urbana: University of Illinois Press, 1991).*

27. *Egenes and Burgess, Faithfully Yours, 23.*

28. *The registry took on many names during its years of operation. For the first 30 years, Central Directory, Registry, or Official Registry were names commonly used. Sometime in the 1940s the name was changed permanently to Nurses Professional Registry (NPR), the name I use throughout this article.*

29. *For rules and regulations, see "Regulations," undated, most likely 1935, Chicago Nurses Registry Collection, Midwest Nursing History Center, College of Nursing, University of Illinois, Chicago, box 1 (hereafter CNRC).*

30. Dunwiddie, A History of the Illinois State Nurses Association, 94; Minnie Aherns, "Discussion, 18th Annual Convention," 1035-36.

31. "Nurses Professional Registry, Average Number of Registrants and Average Monthly Number of Private Duty Assignments, 1917-1946," 26 July, 1947, CNRC, box 1.

32. For the amounts of contributions made by area alumnae association see Dunwiddie, A History of the Illinois State Nurses Association, 163-65.

33. The twelve alumnae associations were those of the Illinois Training School, Presbyterian, Augustana, Chicago Memorial, Mercy, Mt. Sinai, St. Elizabeth's, St. Joseph's, St. Luke's, Washington Boulevard, Wesley Memorial, and West Suburban Schools of Nursing. See Dunwiddie, A History of the Illinois State Nurses Association, 94; "Annual Report Club and Registry, 1926," First District Bulletin 24 (February 1927): 10-11, INAP, box 3, folder 10.

34. Exact statistics are not available on the number of patients NPR nurses cared for in the home versus in the hospital. In 1929, Van Frank reported that the majority of cases were in the hospital and that nurses clearly preferred hospital to home care. See Lucy Van Frank, "The Private Duty Nurse," paper presented at the Annual Meeting of the Illinois State Nurses Association, Moline, October, 10 1929, INAP, box 4, folder 12. The Committee on the Grading of Nursing Schools (CGNS), which carried out a study of private duty nursing in 1928, estimated that about 79% of private duty cases were in the hospital. See May Ayres Burgess, ed., Nurses, Patients, and Pocketbooks: A Study of the Economics of Nursing (New York: Committee on the Grading of Nursing Schools, 1928; reprint New York: Garland, 1984), 74.

35. "Nurses Professional Registry, Average Number of Registrants and Average Monthly Number of Private Duty Assignments, 1917-1946."

36. For the number of graduate nurses in Illinois and Chicago, see U.S. Department of Commerce, Fifteenth Census of the United States: 1930, vol. 4, Occupations, 428.

37. For the number of beds in Chicago hospitals, see "Hospital Service in the United States," Journal of the American Medical Association 94 (29 March 1930): 941-43 (hereafter JAMA).

38. "Nurses Fees, 1913-1980," April, 7 1976, CNRC, box 1; "Annual Report, Private Duty Section, Illinois State Nurses Association, 1926-1927," INAP, box 3, folder 10.

39. "Income over Expenses," undated, most likely 1947, CNRC, box 1. As a nonprofit agency the NPR did not make profits in a commercial sense. I use the term profit to indicate income over expenses.

40. "Annual Report, First District, 1924," INAP, box 2, folder 2; "Annual Report Club and Registry Committee, 1926," 11.

41. "Report of the Registry Committee," June, 7 1930, INAP, box 4, folder 13.

42. Hourly nursing services were private nursing services paid for by the hour, as opposed to the patient hiring a nurse for a designated shift. For a description of the NPR's hourly nursing program, see Jean C. Whelan, "Smaller and Cheaper: The Chicago Hourly Nursing Service 1926-1950," NHR 10 (2002): 83-108. Institutional placement services offered registered nurses a means to obtain permanent or temporary positions in hospitals and other health care agencies. The NPR's attempts to expand the institutional placement service were never very successful. For a contemporary discussion of institutional placement services in the Chicago area and the efforts of the Chicago Nurses Association to enter this market, see "The Registry as Placement Bureau," First District Bulletin 24 (August 1927): 4, INAP, box 3.

43. *"Registry," First District Bulletin 23 (March 1926): 3, INAP, box 3, folder 8.*

44. *Ethel Johns, "A Study of the Present Status of the Negro Woman in Nursing, 1925," unpublished report, Exhibit B-2, folder 1507, box 122, series 200 United States, Record Group 1.1 Projects, Rockefeller Foundation Archives, Rockefeller Archives Center, North Tarrytown, NY Darlene Clark Hine recorded the difficulties African-American nurses experienced because of exclusionary, segregated policies; see Darlene Clark Hine, Black Women in White: Racial Conflict and Cooperation in the Nursing Profession, 1890-1950 (Bloomington: Indiana University Press, 1989).*

45. *I have used Mary Roberts's estimate of the number of schools for the 1920s; see Mary Roberts, American Nursing: History and Interpretation (New York: Macmillan, 1954), 110. According to Roberts, the number of schools of nursing peaked in 1927 at 2,286 and by 1930 had declined to 1,844. See Department of Health and Human Services, Source Book—Nursing Personnel, 83; for the number of nurses, see p. 26.*

46. *Estimating the number of nurses working as private duty nurses is problematic. The best contemporary estimate is from the CGNS; see Burgess, Nurses, Patients, and Pocketbooks, 249. The Committee surveyed 24,389 nurses from ten states selected by the CGNS on a nonrandom basis; the results indicated that 54% of the nurses worked as private duty nurses. This statistic has been generally accepted as reflecting the size of the private duty market in the late 1930s. It is also the statistic frequently compared to figures cited by the 1923 Rockefeller study on nursing (which estimated that 80% of all nurses were in the private duty field) as indicative of a movement of nurses out of private duty. For the Rockefeller study, see Josephine Goldmark, Nursing and Nursing Education in the United States (New York: Macmillan, 1923; reprint New York: Garland, 1984). Caution needs to be exercised when using these percentages. First, the nonrandom nature of the sample used by the CGNS might or might not reflect an accurate measure of the population. Second, percentages can be indicative of different phenomena. For example, a declining percentage might reflect a decrease in the total number of private duty nurses or a stable or even increasing number of private duty nurses in an increasing population.*

47. *For a discussion of the cost of private duty nursing, see Elizabeth Gordon Fox, "The Economics of Nursing," AJN 29 (September 1929): 1037-44. Fox estimated that only about 1.5 to 2% of the population could afford private duty nurses. The CGNS also addressed the cost of private duty, concluding that many patients needed nursing care but failed to receive it because of high cost. See Committee on the Grading of Nursing Schools, Nursing Schools Today and Tomorrow (New York: the Committee, 1934), 237-38.*

48. See Burgess, *Nurses, Patients, and Pocketbooks*, 83-85, 304-9. *Another study on private duty nursing, completed in 1926 in New York state, found results similar to those of the CGNS; see Janet Geister, "Hearsay and Facts in Private Duty," AJN 26 (July 1926): 515-28.*

49. Burgess, *Nurses, Patients, and Pocketbooks*, 311.

50. *See, for example, Geister, "Hearsay and Facts in Private Duty"; Janet Geister, "The Economics of Nursing," Bulletin of the American College of Surgeons 13 (December 1929): 14-17.*

51. Burgess, *Nurses, Patients, and Pocketbooks*, 500-551; *Committee on the Grading of Nursing Schools, Nursing Schools Today and Tomorrow*, 233-49.

52. Burgess, *Nurses, Patients, and Pocketbooks*, 311. *The study found that 9% of private duty nurses were hesitant about whether to stay in or leave the field.*

53. *Ibid.*, 318.

54. *Ibid.*, 320.

55. Van Frank, "The Private Duty Nurse."

56. *For an analysis of the Great Depression, see William Leuchtenberg, Franklin D. Roosevelt and the New Deal, 1932-1940 (New York: Harper & Row, 1963). Leuchtenberg estimated that the number of unemployed was as high as fifteen million.*

57. "Report to the State Private Duty Section, Annual Business Session," ISNA, 16 October 1930," *INAP*, box 4, folder 13.

58. "Report of the State Private Duty Section, Regular Meeting, Board of Directors," ISNA, 13 October 1931," *INAP*, box 4, folder 14.

59. "Registry," *ISNA Bulletin* 30 (April 1933): 6, *INAP*, box 5, folder 16.

60. "Nurses Professional Registry, Average Number of Registrants and Average Monthly Number of Private Duty Assignments, 1917-1946."

61. "Income over Expenses."

62. "Unemployment and Relief," *ISNA Bulletin* 30 (April 1933): 7-8, *INAP*, box 5, folder 16.

63. "Annual Report, Private Duty Section, First District, 1933," *INAP*, box 5, folder 20.

64. "Registry," *ISNA Bulletin* 30 (April 1933): 6.

65. "Objectives of the Private Duty Section for the Coming Year," *ISNA Bulletin* 29 (March 1932): 7-8, *INAP*, box 5, folder 16.

66. "Minutes, Annual Meeting, Private Duty Section, ISNA, 13 October 1933," *INAP*, box 5, folder 20.

67. "Education and Distribution of Nursing Services." *ISNA Bulletin* 29 (December 1932): 6, *INAP*, box 5, folder 16.

68. "Annual Report, Private Duty Section, First District, ISNA, 1933."

69. "Education and Distribution of Nursing Service," 6; "Report of Illinois Committee on the Distribution of Nursing Service Organization, Questionnaire No II, 1933,"

INAP, box 5, folder 20; "Report of Committee on Distribution of Nursing Service, ISNA, 11 October, 1933," INAP, box 5, folder 20.

70. "Annual Report, Private Duty Section, First District, ISNA, 1933." See also Egenes and Burgess, Faithfully Yours, 77.

71. For the best discussions of this period, see Flood, "The Troubling Expedient"; Susan M. Reverby, 'Something Besides Waiting': The Politics of Private Duty Reform in the Depression," in Nursing History: New Perspectives, New Possibilities, ed. Ellen Conlife Lagerman (New York: Teachers College Press, 1983), 133-56. The various terms used to identify nurses employed by hospitals for bedside patient care included general duty nurse, floor duty nurse, institutional nurse, and staff nurse. This paper uses the term general duty nurse.

72. Estimates of how many general duty or staff nurses existed during this time period are difficult to make. Contemporaries generally cited statistics generated from CGNS studies in the late 1920s as a base from which to measure the growth of staff nursing during this time period. See, for example, Roberts, American Nursing, 286; "Did You Ever See a Nurse Nursing?" AJN 38 (April 1938): 30(s). The CGNS found approximately 4,000 nurses employed as floor duty nurses (general duty or staff nurses) in a survey of 1,397 hospitals affiliated with schools of nursing in 1929. See Committee on the Grading of Nursing Schools, Results of the First Grading Study of Nursing Schools, Section III—-Who Controls the Schools (New York: the Committee, 1930), 24. At the time of this survey, there were 6,665 hospitals in the country, leaving a significant number of hospitals unaccounted for in the estimate. For numbers of hospitals, see "Hospital Service in the United States," 921. It is possible to track the growth of staff nursing in hospitals associated with schools of nursing. In 1937 the National League for Nursing surveyed 1,259 schools of nursing, finding that in hospitals associated with schools, 27,000 general staff nurses were employed. This represented a sevenfold increase in the number of staff nurses from 1929 levels, at least in hospitals associated with a school of nursing. See "More General Staff Nurses," AJN 38 (February 1938): 186. Whatever the exact figures, it was accepted at the time that the growth in the number of general duty nurses was remarkable.

73. For an analysis of the factors leading to the employment of staff nurses, see Flood, "The Troubling Expedient"; Reverby, Ordered to Care, 180-98. Contemporaries attributed the rise of staff nursing to a decrease in the number of student nurses, a growing awareness that a graduate nursing staff was essential, an increase in the number and occupancy rates of hospital beds, and the growth of hospital insurance plans that contributed to increased hospital usage. See "Did You Ever See a Nurse Nursing?" 17(s)—34(s).

74. This statement is based on a number of indicators. Professional nurse registries nationwide began reporting an increase in the number of calls received for private duty nurses to fill temporary staff nurse positions. Between 1937 and 1940, professional nurse registries recorded an increase of 10,000 calls received for temporary staff positions. See "What Registries Did in 1937," AJN 38 (October 1938): 1115-23; "What Registries Did in 1938," AJN 39 (September 1939): 998-1006; "What Registries Are Doing," AJN 41 (August 1941): 902-8. The 1936 ANA study of working conditions of nurses highlighted the widespread practice of using private duty

nurses as temporary staff nurses. See American Nurses Association, Study of Incomes, Salaries and Employment Conditions Affecting Nurses (New York: ANA, 1938). See also "The American Nurses Association and the Eight-Hour Schedule for Nurses," AJN 36 (October 1936): 979–83; Barbara Hunter, "An All Graduate Staff and the Eight-Hour Day," AJN 37 (May 1937): 473; Margaret Tracy, "The Eight-Hour Day for Special Nurses: At the University of California Hospital," AJN 35 (January 1935): 29–32.

75. See, for example, reports from professional nurse registries as published in the AJN: "What Registries Did in 1937"; What Registries Did in 1938"; "What Registries Are Doing."

76. See "Nurses Professional Registry, Average Number of Registrants and Average Monthly Number of Private Duty Assignments, 1917–1946." This is not to suggest that the private duty market had completely recovered from the economic effects of the Great Depression. Despite the improved overall conditions, other indices reveal a less positive picture. Although the number of requests for nurses rose, the NPR continued to record large numbers of nurses as on call and without patient assignments. See "Annual Report, Executive Committee, Board of Directors, ISNA, 1936," INAP, box 6, folder 26. In 1938, bad economic conditions caused the NPR to limit its membership to graduates of hospitals affiliated with the registry. See "Annual Report, First District, ISNA, 1938," INAP, box 7, folder 28.

77. For the use of private duty nurses as temporary general duty nurses, see "The American Nurses Association and the Eight-Hour Schedule for Nurses"; Hunter, "An All-Graduate Staff and the Eight-Hour Day"; Tracy, "The Eight-Hour Day for Special Nurses."

78. For the problems private duty nurses experienced with temporary general duty, see "The American Nurses Association and the Eight-Hour Schedule for Nurses."

79. Fees paid by patients for private duty nurses dropped during the Great Depression and did not return to pre-Depression levels for several years. By 1936, the fee charged by NPR nurses for an 8-hour shift was $5. Nurses working 12-hour shifts received $6. See Retta Gasteyer, Secretary, First District, ISNA, to Directors of Nursing, January, 23 1936, CNRC, box 1.

80. ANA, Study of Incomes, Salaries and Employment Conditions, 509.

81. Complete statistics on how many calls for temporary general duty were received and filled by the NPR are lacking. In 1936, the NPR filled 448 calls for temporary general duty; see "Annual Report, First District, ISNA, 1936," INAP, box 6, folder 26. Reports for later years mention filling calls for general duty nurses but do not estimate the numbers of calls fitting this category; see, for example, "Annual Report, First District, ISNA, 1940," INAP, box 7, folder 33. By the early 1940s, filling calls for general duty nurses seems to have increased as noted in discussions on the matter; see "Annual Report, Private Duty Section, ISNA, 1942," INAP, box 8, folder labeled "Minutes, Board of Directors and Annual Meeting, 1942; "Annual Report, First District, ISNA, 1942," INAP, box 8, folder 37.

82. "Report of the Private Duty Round Table, 1940," INAP, box 246, folder 1.

83. "Annual Report, Private Duty Section, ISNA, 1942."

84. *"Proceedings, Round Table for General Staff Nurses, American Nurses Association," June 23, 1936," American Nurses Association Papers, Mugar Library, Special Collections, Boston University, Boston, box 87 (hereafter ANAP).*

85. *See, for example, "Board of Directors Meeting, American Nurses Association," January, 28-31, 1936; June, 20-26, 1936, ANAP, box 18; "Board of Directors Meeting, American Nurses Association," January, 25-29, 1937, ANAP, box 19.*

86. *See ANA, Study of Incomes, Salaries and Employment Conditions.*

87. *"Board of Directors Meeting, American Nurses Association," January, 25-29, 1937, ANAP, box 19.*

88. *ANA, Study of Incomes, Salaries and Employment Conditions, 499-512.*

89. *"Board of Directors Meeting, American Nurses Association," January, 24-28, 1938, ANAP, box 20.*

90. *Alma Scott, "Status of Graduate Nurse Service as Indicated by Recent Studies Conducted Through the American Nurses Association Headquarters," Transactions of the American Hospital Association 60 (1938): 410-17.*

91. *This era, from the late 1930s to the early 1940s, a time when nurses became more vocal regarding their working conditions and the ANA began to take very tentative steps in addressing the needs of working nurses, is worthy of further investigation by historians.*

92. *"Annual Report, First District, ISNA, 1940."*

93. *"Income over Expenses."*

94. *Roberts, American Nursing, 343.*

95. *This estimate of the percentage of nurses serving in the military is based on dividing the 70,000 nurses in the armed services as reported by Roberts by the total number of nurses as enumerated by the 1940 U.S. census. For the number of nurses in 1940, see Source Book—Nursing Personnel, 26.*

96. *Numerous contemporary articles appeared in professional journals describing and analyzing the increased demand for nurses. See, for example, "Why America Needs More Nurses," AJN 43 (February 1943): 132-33; "Wartime Nursing Is Different," AJN 43 (September 1943): 835-38; Joseph Mountin, "Nursing—A Critical Analyis," AJN 43 (January 1943): 29-34.*

97. *"Annual Report, Private Duty Section, ISNA, 1942"; "Annual Report, First District, 1944," INAP, box 9, folder labeled "Minutes, Board of Directors and Annual Meeting; "Annual Report, First District, 1945," INAP, box 9, folder labeled "Proceedings House of Delegates 20 October, 1945." Nationally as well, professional registries experienced low rates of filling calls. Between 1946 and 1950, professional registries reporting to the ANA recorded unfilled calls ranging from 29 to 46%. See Facts About Nursing: A Statistical Summary (New York: ANA, 1963), 126.*

98. *For the difficulties the NPR experienced in filling calls, see "Annual Report, First District, 1942"; "Summary of Activities, First District, 1942," INAP, box 313; "Annual Report, First District, 1945," INAP, box 9.*

99. *The number of nurses employed in hospitals increased considerably in the 1940s. The 1941 National Inventory of Registered Nurses listed 81,708 nurses as*

employed in hospitals, 47% of the active employed registered nurses surveyed. See Pearl McIver, "Registered Nurses in the United States," AJN 42 (July 1942): 769-73. No indication is given in what positions these nurses were employed, so it cannot be determined how many were general duty or staff nurses. The 1944 annual survey of hospital data carried out by the Council on Medical Education and Hospitals of the American Medical Association listed 64,741 nurses employed as general duty nurses (56,766 full-time and 7,975 part-time); see "Hospital Service in the United States," JAMA 127 (31 March 1945): 780. Four years later, in 1948, this figure had almost doubled to 121,318 general duty nurses (104,041 full-time and 17,277 part-time); see "Hospital Service in the United States," JAMA 140 (7 May 1949): 34. It is also likely that in different parts of the country staff nursing became the norm at different points in time. For example, Flood notes that hospitals in California may have instituted staff nursing earlier than did other parts of the country. See Flood, "The Troubling Expedient."

100. As with registered nurses, obtaining accurate counts of nursing assistive personnel is problematic. In many cases, different names and categories were used when estimating the number of assistive personnel, making an exact count difficult. The 1943 American Medical Association annual survey of hospital data listed 175,677 individuals in the categories of practical nurse, nurse's aide, attendant, and orderly. In 1949 there were 225,001 persons listed in similar categories. See "Hospital Service in the United States," JAMA 124 (25 March 1944): 848; "Hospital Service in the United States," JAMA 140 (7 May 1949): 34.

101. For a discussion of the post-World War II health care environment and the many problems facing nursing during this time period see Joan E. Lynaugh and Barbara L. Brush, American Nursing From Hospitals to Health Systems (Malden, MA: Blackwell, 1996), 1-15.

102. "ANA, Proceedings, Private Duty Section," May, 31-June, 4 1948, ANAP, box 89.

Action Research Method

*N*urses in recent years have been challenged to provide documentation to support how what they do makes a difference in peoples' lives. Although it would seem obvious that improving outcomes based on nursing practice would necessarily involve those who are the recipients of care in an active way, this is not often the case. Traditional research methods value objectivity. Consequently, much of nursing research focuses on measuring the effect of what we do to our patients rather than working with them to discover what creates the overall best outcomes. Action research offers nurse researchers the opportunity to work *with* their patients to discover what make the greatest difference in their lives. Letts (2003) states that "participants are involved in planning and evaluating actions to address issues of importance to them, so that knowledge is gained through the process of acting to improve or address issues" (p. 78). Action research method is participatory. It is based on democratic principles. According to Stringer (1999),

> The desire to give voice to people is derived not from an abstract ideological or theoretical imperative but from the pragmatic focus of action research. Its intent is to provide a place for the perspectives of people who have previously been marginalized from opportunities to develop and operate policies, programs, and services—perspectives often concealed by the products of a typical research process. (p. 207)

Action research seeks to empower those who are part of the process to act on their own behalf to solve *real world problems*.

Nurses conducting research in the United States have been slow to embrace action research. This is despite the fact that it is a research method that has demonstrated great success in the areas of social research. It is particularly interesting, given federal support for this type of research. Recently, the Centers for Disease Control and Prevention (CDC) has funded 25 community-based prevention research grants totaling $13 million; these 3-year grants are intended to fund multidisciplinary, multilevel, participatory research with the goal of enhancing capacity of communities and population groups to address health promotion and prevention of disease, disability, and injury. (Minkler, Blackwell, Thompson, & Tamir, 2003, p. 1211)

It is the intent of this chapter to help the reader understand the collaborative, emancipatory process that is known as action research. The goal will be to share important insights about action research development, its fundamental roots, characteristics of the method, and information on how to generate, analyze, and utilize the findings of an action research study. Once knowledge of the method is acquired, it is hoped that it will be incorporated more often by nurse researchers because of its significant utility in offering an action-based, emancipatory approach to problem solving for nurses and those they serve.

ACTION RESEARCH DEFINED

*A*ction research is known by various names, including *cooperative inquiry, action inquiry, participatory action research, community-based action research, collaborative research*, and *participative inquiry* (Reason, 1994; Stringer, 1999; Tetley & Hanson, 2001). The various terms make using one definition difficult, although the definition of this approach may not be as important as its assumptions. It is the assumptions of the action research process that can better assist the nurse researcher in deciding whether action research is a useful research approach for the problem to be studied.

Greenwood and Levin (1998) define action research as "social research carried out by a team encompassing a professional action researcher and members of an organization or community seeking to improve their situation" (p. 4). According to Winter and Munn-Giddings (2001), action research "is a form of social research which involves people in a process of change, which is based on professional, organizational or community action" (p. 5). "Action research is first and foremost a group activity" (Bennett, 2000, p. 1). Bradbury and Reason (2003) offer a particularly inclusive definition of action research:

a participatory, democratic process concerned with developing practical knowing in pursuit of worthwhile human purposes, grounded in a participatory world-view. It seeks to reconnect action and reflection, theory and practice, in participation with others, in pursuit of practical solutions to issues of pressing concern to people. More generally it grows out of a concern for the flourishing of individuals in their communities. (Reason & Bradbury, 2001, p. 156)

Some action researchers have suggested that rather than offering a single definition, action research should be seen as a continuum of methods, with the ends of the continuum being both insider and outsider models (Badger, 2000; Rolfe, 1996; Tichen & Binnie, 1993).

> At the outsider end [is] the sociological approach of testing out theory in a real situation and Lewin's (1946) traditional approach of the researcher as professional expert entering the situation to facilitate and evaluate change. At the continuum's other end, termed endogenous research by DePoy & Gitlin (1994), lie those approaches where practitioner and researcher collaborate loosely, or are even the same person. (Badger, 2000, p. 202)

Coghlan and Casey (2001) share that the insider is sometimes the nurse working in his or her own situation: "Rarely is there much consideration of action by the permanent insider" (p. 675).

To assist in understanding the action research method, four specific approaches will be described. These are cooperative inquiry, community-based action research, participatory action research, and action science or action inquiry.

Cooperative inquiry is a type of action research that values above all else the notion that the individual is self-determining, and as such, cannot be researched without full participation. John Heron first advanced the ideas related to cooperative inquiry (Brown, 2001; Reason, 1998). According to Reason (1998),

> one can only do research on persons in the full and proper sense of the term only if one addresses them as self-determining, which means that what they do and what they experience as part of the research must be to some significant degree determined by them. (p. 264)

Therefore the implementation of cooperative inquiry requires that both researchers and informants cooperate to derive new knowledge.

As suggested earlier, the definitions/descriptions of the approaches presented here are not fundamentally different. The emphases in all action research studies are the reciprocity between researchers and informants and empowerment of those who have not traditionally had a voice. Participatory action research (PAR), as described by William Foote Whyte (1984), is a type of action research that is best known because of its interdisciplinary focus. Also, it is recognized for its political aspects (Reason, 1998). In more recent years, researchers have sought to remove the strong political overtones that characterize the method. According to Tetley and Hanson (2001), "it is these issues of knowledge creation, control and power that makes participatory research distinctly different from other types of social research" (p. 71). In PAR, the emphasis is on relinquishing control, learning through mutual interactions between researchers and participants, and giving voice to those who would otherwise not be heard.

Community-based action research represents the ideas advanced by Stringer (1999). Like PAR, community-based action research has faced some difficult times because of its association with radical political activism.

> It has reemerged in response to both pragmatic and philosophical pressures and is now more broadly understood as "disciplined inquiry (research) which seeks focused efforts to improve the quality of people's organizational, community and family lives" (Calhoun, 1993, p. 62). Community-based action research is also allied to recent emergence of practitioner research (e.g., Anderson et al., 1994), new paradigm research (Reason, 1988), and teacher-as-researcher. (Kincheloe, 1991; Stringer, 1999, p. 9)

As a research method, its most frequent application has been in problem solving by practitioners such as educators, occupational therapists, social workers, nurses, organizational leaders, and human service workers. According to Stringer (1999), researchers "engage 'subjects' as equal and full partners" (p. 9). The method can be used to improve work activities, resolve problems or crises, and develop special projects. The overall goal is to deal with the problems that practitioners face in their everyday lives.

Action science or action inquiry is described by Reason (1998) as "forms of inquiry into practice" (p. 273) with the greatest emphasis being on developing action that will lead to systemic change within organizations, ultimately leading to "greater effectiveness and greater justice" (p. 273). The emphasis is on identifying theories of action that guide behavior (Reason, 1998). According to Argyris, Putnam, and Smith as cited in Reason (1998), theories-in-use are rendered explicit by reflection on action. Therefore, action science concerns "itself with situations of uniqueness, uncertainty, and instability which do not lend themselves to the mode of technical rationality. It would aim at the development of themes from which ... practitioners may construct theories and methods of their own" (Schon, 1983, p. 319). Ultimately, the reflection in action that is part of the action science process leads to a fuller understanding of how theory guides practice.

Holter and Schwartz-Barcott (1993) offer three classifications of action research. These are technical collaboration, mutual collaboration, and enhancement. In the technical collaboration approach, the researcher has a predetermined agenda that often involves intervention or theory testing; in the mutual collaboration approach, the researcher and participants identify the focus of the research together and decide together how to study and ultimately manage the problem; finally, in the enhancement approach, the researcher and participants work together but move beyond the collaborative approach to engage in critical dialogue to raise group consciousness

(Sturt, 1999, p. 1059). According to Holter and Schwartz-Barcott (1993) and Kendall and Sturt (1996), most reported nursing action research studies use the technical collaboration approach.

Given a basic understanding of the multiple definitions and descriptions of action research, it is important to examine the historical roots of this important research methodology. It is only through understanding of the method that nurse researchers will have an appropriate framework to determine its applicability to problems faced in practice.

ACTION RESEARCH ROOTS

*A*ction research is a method that might well be described as a research method that has gone through several phases. The early work is attributed to Kurt Lewin. Lewin, a social psychologist, is cited frequently as the first person who coined the term *action research*. Most nurses know Lewin as the person who described change theory. Lewin's theoretical ideas about change were very basic. Simplistically, Lewin said that for a change to occur, individuals would need to unfreeze—give up their ideas about something or give up the dominant structure. They would then need to change. The change would require the acceptance of new ideas or a new structure. Finally, once the new ideas were formally in place, the individuals involved in the change would refreeze, or hold the new ideas or structure as permanent. Lewin's change theory remains an influential model for social change up to the present (Greenwood & Levin, 1998).

Lewin, based on his ideas about change, saw action research as a process by which a researcher could achieve a goal by constructing a social experiment (Greenwood & Levin, 1998). "This research approach . . . fell very much within the bounds of conventional applied social science with its patterns of authoritarian control, but it was aimed at producing a specific, desired social outcome" (p. 17). As action research has developed, there is less emphasis on the stagnant manner of change than on being a process with a definitive ending point. Current action researchers believe the process is open with ongoing dialogue and that the refreezing described by Lewin is not a permanent condition.

A group of individuals who worked on the ideas of action research in its early development is the Tavistock group. This group advanced Lewin's ideas in the post–World War II period. Following the war, when the English were rebuilding their industrial base, they found that traditional methods were not effective (Greenwood & Levin, 1998). To help with the understanding of why prewar strategies no longer worked, the British government called on the Tavistock Institute of Human Relations to study the problem. "Tavistock brought Lewin's work on the concept of natural experiments and [action research]

(Gustavsen, 1992) back to the United States, and committed itself to doing direct experiments in work life" (Greenwood & Levin, 1998, p. 20). The works of Tavistock led to additional exploration of the work environment and change process in Norway. The Norwegian Industrial Democracy Project used the ideas of Lewin and further developed by Tavistock to advance understanding of the work environment. For a complete description of this period, the reader is directed to Greenwood and Levin (1998).

The expansions of Lewin's work in Norway led to yet other modification in Sweden. The term used to describe the application of action research in the work environment is *socio-technical thinking* (Greenwood & Levin, 1998). This type of organizational thinking and action spread to the United States. Trist (1981) identified the new paradigm of socio-technical design for organizations as follows: person was complementary to machine, people were resources to be developed, people should have broad skills and be grouped by tasks, people were internally motivated, organizations should be flat and represent participative models of functioning, activity should be collaborative and collegial, people in the organization should be supported in their commitment to the organization, and individuals should be rewarded for innovation. Ultimately, it was discovered that if individuals were part of identifying and creating their work environments, then based on the interaction among all concerned parties, positive action and direction for the organization would be achieved.

Brown (2001) states that Argyris and Schon represent the present-day transformation based on their conceptualization of action research as action science. Both Argyris and Schon are most interested in theory in action as described earlier in this section.

It should be obvious that action research has experienced a number of permutations. Despite its development, the most important facets of the design remain its focus on emancipation of others and the collaborative nature of the research process. In the next section, the fundamental characteristics of the method will be explored.

FUNDAMENTAL CHARACTERISTICS OF THE METHOD

Similar to the definitions of action research, there is no one method of doing action research. According to Whitehead, Taket, and Smith (2003), "action research is methodologically flexible to the point that it encourages methodological triangulation/pluralism approaches (p. 8). Despite the flexibility of the approach, there are some fundamental characteristics about the method and the way that it is executed. Common to all descriptions is the fact that the research is context bound. Second, the process seeks to have full engagement by researchers and participants. The process is truly collaborative. Third, those engaged pay regular attention to the process and how it affects the lives of others. Fourth, an action or change is the focal point of the process. And finally, the decision to implement the action or change is in the hands of the stakeholders.

Like other types of qualitative research, the purpose is to produce not a generalizable study but rather one that is locally important. When initiating an action research study, the researcher would ideally become engaged in the process after a local group found a problem that they wanted to solve and when they sought the insights of an individual with research expertise. Because the problem is local and the planned change is practical, the findings will most likely be local. This is not to suggest that a local problem may not develop ideas or theories that can be applied in other situations but rather to state that the purpose of an action research study is to create a real change for the stakeholders involved in the situation.

The collaboration that is identified as fundamental is at the root of this emancipatory research process. Those engaged must be *equal* members of the research team. The use of a truly democratic process to create new knowledge is potentially liberating for those involved (Greenwood & Levin, 1998).

> The logic of inquiry is linked to the inquiry process itself; in the struggle to make an indeterminate situation into a more positively controlled one through an inquiry process where action and reflection are directly linked. The outside researcher inevitably becomes a participant in collaboration with the insiders. (p. 78)

For example, if a group of disabled individuals who require power chairs to participate in activities of daily living discover that the chairs do not give them the flexibility to function independently in their homes, they might enlist the help of local health care providers or researchers to help them determine the best way to influence the health care system to meet their needs. To do so, it would be necessary to bring all the stakeholders to the table to examine the problem rather than the power group (therapists, insurers, manufacturers) deciding the best way to handle the situation. If all stakeholders work together to develop a practical solution to the problem, then the needs of all should be met. The researcher facilitates the process but does not control it. "The emphasis [in action research] is on a critical approach to social problems and practices which arise from and are embedded in social context" (Bellman, Bywood, & Dale, 2003, p. 187).

Those involved in the research process must be aware of the impact participation in the process will have on their lives. Those involved must agree to be constantly aware of the differences in beliefs, values, needs, and objectives of those involved to support an effective process. Using the example above, if the most powerful stakeholders come to the table with preconceived ideas based on their beliefs, cultural values, and class and are not attentive to those who require the power chair to live independently, then the process will not yield an outcome that is in the best interest of all concerned. Similarly, if those needing the power chairs are unwilling to collaborate with the researcher, therapists, manufacturers, and insurers because of preconceived notions about power, class, and existing systems, then again what is best for all concerned will not emerge. Once there is commitment on the part of all concerned to stay attuned to the needs of each person, then the process can proceed, ultimately leading to an effective change.

Implementation of an action or change is the fourth fundamental characteristic of the action research process. The purpose of the process is not to describe an existing situation but rather to construct new knowledge, a new way to deal with a practical problem (Winter & Munn-Giddings, 2001). "Participants are empowered to define their world in the service of what they see as worthwhile interests, and as a consequence they change their world in significant ways, through action" (Reason, 1998, p. 279). The action is developed based on what is discovered through the process of dismantling the problem. For example, in work completed by Crist and Escandon-Dominguez (2003), a process was developed to eliminate health and use disparities among Mexican-American elders living in Arizona.

The last characteristic of action research is that the power to act is always in the hands of the stakeholders. If the process works as it should, the action determined through collaboration results in an outcome that is acceptable and can be implemented by those involved. The action is part of the continuing process of emancipation and democracy. No one outsider or no one insider can determine the action that needs to be taken. The conclusion and subsequent action must reflect the collective thinking of the group.

SELECTION OF ACTION RESEARCH AS METHOD

Nurses who choose to use action research as an approach to solve a particular practice problem should have a clear understanding of what the purpose of their research is. As described earlier, action research is specifically designed as a research method whose outcome is the implementation of an action or change. The types of action that can be considered include bringing about a change in behavior, developing a plan of action to deal with resistance to change, implementing new nursing practices, or empowering providers or those for whom they care (Hart & Bond, 1996; Jenks, 1999). In addition to dedication to action or change, the nurse interested in using action research must be committed to the development of local theory. The outcomes of an action research study will not be generalizable and will usually not have broad reaching application outside of the context in which the study occurs.

Second, the nurse researcher must be committed to collaboration. The collaboration in action research is different from that which generally occurs among researchers in a typical nursing research study. In action research, the collaboration is not between colleagues with equivalent knowledge and power but rather among individuals who may have little or no understanding of research. The participants usually are members of groups who come from backgrounds that are different from the researcher's. For example, the women living in a low-income housing development may be interested in improving the quality of care provided to their children in a neighborhood clinic. In this case, the women interested in solving the problem most likely come from a different socioeconomic background than the nurse. As a result, the nurse researcher will need to take his or her lead from what the women living in the community think the problem is, rather than the nurse researcher determining what the problem is and moving forward to solve it. There may be any number of differences between the participants and researchers. What is most important in the collaboration is that nurse researchers *must* view those with whom they engage in the research process as *equal* partners. Without this commitment, another method of inquiry will be most helpful.

Another important consideration in the selection of action research is the value placed on empowerment and voice. Nurse researchers interested in engaging in action research must be comfortable with self-reflection relative to the issues of process, power, and control. "The process of reflection is used to understand the power relationships and imbalances in the experiences of the participants" (Koch, Selim, & Kralik, 2002, p. 111). One of the fundamental characteristics of action research is the empowerment of others. That empowerment can only occur honestly when the researcher constantly attends to the issues of power and control in the research process and the setting in which the research takes place. For instance, if the nurse researcher is interested in studying student nurses and their difficulty in being part of the clinical education setting, then the researcher must be ready to listen carefully to what is said, help the participants find their voice, and assist them in the development of a process that will empower them to take action.

The final consideration in choosing action research is the realization that in action research, the power to act resides exclusively with those who engaged in the process. "Change may come in the form of individual or group empowerment, greater community capacity to solve shared problems, or transformed organizational structures" (Cockburn & Trentham, 2002, pp. 21–22). No amount of external pressure can force the participants to carry out the change or action that becomes apparent during the conduct of the study. The nurse researcher who chooses action research has to be comfortable with "others" making the decision about what is best for them.

Once the nurse researcher is comfortable with the fundamental characteristics, understands the outcome of the method, and is willing to share the power and control, which is ordinarily the purview of the principal investigator, then and only then should action research be selected. Action research has the potential to dramatically change the life experiences of many individuals. However, the study must be conducted with attention to the fundamental issues of empowerment and action.

ELEMENTS AND INTERPRETATIONS OF THE METHOD

*A*ction researchers have many interpretations of method. This can be seen from the information provided earlier regarding the many terms and descriptions given to the process. There are, however, some basic elements to which most researchers engaged in action research subscribe. These will be shared in the hope that they give the nurse researcher who is interested in the methodology enough information to determine whether the approach will be useful in dealing with a specific problem. Once the decision is made to conduct an action research study, the researcher is encouraged to read primary sources on the method and engage a research mentor.

Data Generation

Data generation begins as soon as the problem becomes apparent. Ideally, this occurs when a community recognizes it has a problem and enlists the consultation of trained researchers to help them deal with it. The initial discussions about the problem will become an important part of data analysis, as will all of the other information collected in the course of the study.

Defining the Problem

"An initial and large aspect of the process of participatory action research involves the careful documentation of the concrete and specific ways that people view a problem affecting their lives" (Taylor, Braveman, & Hammel, 2004, p. 75). For example, a group of young women who are pressured by some of their peers in the community to become gang members might discuss this with the nurse practitioner who runs the local clinic. Using the knowledge and skills of the nurse practitioner, these young women can work to understand the dynamics of their environment and move to change the variables within their social group that value gang membership over employment or academic success. Generally, this is not how action research problems in nursing are identified. More often, nurses see a problem in practice or a problem in the lives of those with whom they work and propose an action research approach to study and act on the problem. Regardless of who identifies the problem, it is likely that the stakeholders in an action research study will be more committed to an action or a change if they believe that the situation is important to them and that they can bring about a change in the situation.

It is important to recognize that there are two perspectives in any action research study. These are the insider, or emic, view and the outsider, or etic, view. This dichotomy exists because the insiders are living the problem and have a unique understanding of it. The outsider, the researcher, is the person who comes to the situation with the intention to assist those involved but who usually is unable to internalize the situation because he or she does not live it. It is also important to remember that insiders are the ones who will implement the change and thus have to live with the outcome. As can be seen, the insider's stake is much higher than the outsider's. The earlier discussion made it clear that collaboration is essential. Thus, there may be two views on the problem, but both views are equally valuable because of the partnership that must be developed to fully understand the problem and create the change.

To fully define the problem and begin to understand it, the insiders will need to bring their personal knowledge of the problem to the researcher. The researcher will bring theoretical and practical information relative to the change process, and the ability to act as a liaison between those in power and those who have been marginalized. Together, the participants and the researcher will work to identify the problem. Ideally, the problem can be identified clearly. From a practical standpoint, clearly defining the problem will be an evolving process.

Planning

One of the important initial stages of an action research study is to identify all the stakeholders. It is essential to bring as many of the stakeholders as possible forward for initial conversations about the existing problem. All who may be affected in any way by the problem or the desired change need to be part of the early conversations.

Once the stakeholders are identified, it is important to determine how the investigation will proceed. Taylor and colleagues (2004) suggest that choosing an action-oriented solution and designing research methods and assessment procedures that will be used to solve the problem are important steps. To move these processes forward, a model advocated by Greenwood and Levin (1998), called the Cogenerative Action Research Model, might be useful. In the description of the model, Greenwood and Levin recommend that communication arenas be developed. Communication arenas are spaces where participants and researchers can come together for mutual learning. Developing these spaces will be one of the most important aspects of engaging all the stakeholders. "Arenas must be designed to match the needs of the issue" (p. 117). Therefore, there may be a need for large group, small group, and one-on-one meetings. There may be a need for specific arenas for explicit purposes, such as information sharing or team building. There also will be the need to develop spaces for reflection. Ground rules for participation will be essential. It is also important that all parties clearly understand how the feedback loop for communication will work. As an example, the researcher or a member of the community group may record minutes. When the minutes become available, it is important that an appropriate forum be created to discuss the recording.

As part of designing the study, it is important to decide how information will be collected. Will interviews, observations, focus groups, and printed material comprise the major data collection strategies, or will survey and questionnaires be the tactics of choice? Who will be responsible for collecting data? These decisions must be made by all members of the research team. It will be the responsibility of the trained researchers to bring as much information as possible forward so that the members of the team who are not skilled in the strategies for data collection or the research process are provided with the opportunity to learn about the various data collection strategies and the method so that they can make informed decisions about how to proceed.

Bradbury and Reason (2003) describe the importance of being attuned to how individuals/researchers interact with community partners throughout the research activity. These action researchers discuss the importance of understanding the researcher as instrument, specifically how essential it is to consider how the researcher's ideas influence the framing and implementation of the study. One of the ways for the researcher to remain attuned to his or her actions throughout the study is to consider using some form of reflection. One of the better ways to encourage reflection is to include journaling or keeping a diary as one of the data collection strategies. Using a self-reflective mechanism can help sort out some of the important issues that may arise throughout the study. It is equally important that time and space be created for all members of the research team to reflect on their planning and implementation strategies. The opportunity for group members to consider their actions in a more formal reflection helps to manage differences in opinions about the way the research progresses.

Different from other qualitative methods, the participants in an action research study are not separate from the research process. Those who are the stakeholders are often the ones who can most effectively inform the study. However, there will be times when data need to be collected to reflect the experience of members of affected groups who are not intimately involved with the study. For example, using the teen gang scenario presented earlier, all of the teens being pressured to join gangs in the community may not be part of the research team, but from time to time, it will be essential to collect information from as many of those teens as possible to fully understand the problem. When individuals are deliberately selected to inform the study, the sampling is called purposive. Depending on which data collection strategies are used, a decision will need to be made regarding who will conduct the interviews, do the observations, or collect survey or questionnaire data. It is important to consider whether data collectors should be from within or outside the group. Using outsiders to collect these data may provide a potentially more open-minded and detached view of the situation. However, using insiders may reduce potential barriers that may arise when data collectors are not part of the group. There may be very intentional reasons for choosing insiders or outsiders to collect data. As long as the research team agrees on who the data collectors are and why they have been selected, data collection will move forward in a productive manner.

Jenks (1999) recommends that at least three strategies of data collection be utilized to ensure that there is cross-validation of information. All strategies will not need to be identified before the study begins. Because the question may not be clearly defined, data collection strategies not originally identified may need to be added in light of evolving data. For instance, using the situation described earlier of the teenagers and gang membership, a survey may have been selected as one of the data collection strategies. However, as the study progresses, it is discovered that there is information that the survey is not capturing. Focus group interviews or other data collection strategies then may be recommended.

The preparations that have been described represent the planning phase of the action research study. Stringer (1999) calls this developmental phase "setting the stage" (p. 43). Regardless of the name given to the initial planning phase, all participants need to agree on how best to proceed.

Once the decisions are made regarding how best to collect data, data collection should commence. As stated earlier, the process of planning, collecting data, and analyzing data does not proceed in a linear manner. The process is dynamic and as such needs to respond to the changing needs of all involved.

Data Treatment and Analysis

As data are collected, they will be analyzed using the appropriate methodology for the strategy selected. For instance, if interviews were used, analysis can proceed using the constant comparative method. Jenks (1999) states that this method is useful in analysis of action research data. For a complete description of the constant comparative method, the reader is directed to Chapter 7.

The analysis phase of the study should include all stakeholders. Interpretations and explanations cannot be offered unless the context is fully understood. The participants in the study will be the individuals who can most accurately determine whether the findings are appropriate within context. By doing analysis as a joint activity, the entire research team can bring its perspectives to the discussion, providing the opportunity for dialogue and debate about the findings and their respective meanings. As stated earlier, it is appropriate to use a group reflection activity to make clear the possible influences on the interpretations.

The researcher will have primary responsibility for leading the data analysis phase based on knowledge of the process and experience. However, it will be the team that will draw the final conclusions.

Action

Unlike some of the other types of qualitative research, action research does not end with documentation of the findings. When data analysis is completed, the team decides on an action or a change that they want to occur. The change is a result of and based on the findings. The outsiders take no active role in the change. They may remain part of the team by contributing to guiding the process or assisting with reflection, but they have no formal role in the change (Jenks, 1999).

In some instances, the action research process may start with the action or change, in which case the study is conducted to assess the change as it is implemented. When the study is implemented in this way, it is conducted as an evaluation study, with all members of the research team contributing. Modifications in implementation of the change can take place as the research team deems appropriate.

An important part of the change or action phase of the research process is reflection. Reflection is used in this stage of the process as a way of gaining insights about the change and its impact on those who are part of it. Reflection can be conducted as a one-on-one activity, in a group, or in a personal diary. "Data recorded during reflection are important contributions to the theory that emerges from the action research study" (Jenks, 1999, p. 260). Winter and Munn-Giddings (2001) speak to the cycle of action and reflection that is based on the work of Lewin. This spiral cycle includes planning, action, and fact finding. The cycle repeats itself to more effectively understand some aspect of the research process.

According to Jenks (1999), reflective critique can be used to facilitate reflection.

Reflective critique is based on an understanding that all statements made during data generation—including participants' and researchers' written and verbal language—are subject to reflexivity. Reflexivity describes the belief that the language individuals use to describe an experience reflects that particular experience and also all other experiences in each individual's life. Knowing that observations and interpretations are reflexive creates two assumptions for action researchers: (1) a rejection of the idea of a single or ultimate explanation for an event and (2) the belief that offering various explanations for an experience explicitly increases understanding of the experiences. (p. 260)

Another process that can be used to assist in reflection is dialectical critique. In contrast to reflective critique, dialectical critique "probes data to make explicit their internal contradictions rather than complementary explanations" (Jenks, 1999, p. 261). The ultimate goals of each process are to ask important questions and reveal biases about data as they are revealed.

Evaluation

Evaluation of the action research process takes place throughout the study and at its end. A timeline for evaluation should be established during the planning phase. The timeline gives specific direction to keep evaluation in front of all members of the team. During evaluation, the process is assessed, and questions such as these can be asked: Are we using the correct instruments? Are we getting the data we need? Who else do we need to interview? Is the process working? These questions and others developed by the research team will keep the project focused.

Researchers have the responsibility to guide the evaluation process. This should not be done without consultation or the consent of the entire research team (Jenks, 1999). The evaluation process will be most effective if co-facilitated by members of the community and the trained researchers.

Writing the Report

The report that results from the study will be a document prepared by the team. Information to be included and excluded should be agreed on by all members of the team. The report is not necessarily the end of the action or change, but it does represent the end of the formal study. Hopefully, if the action is effective, the change will be evaluated for its long-term impact on the individuals involved and be part of the formal report.

One important feature of the report is the recommendations section. The recommendations are meant to be helpful and give direction for long-term implementation of the change. The recommendations should be determined collaboratively and should be based on a solid understanding of the problem, careful data collection, and analysis and review of appropriate literature. Review of the literature is an activity that takes place throughout the study. It should be part of informing the planned change or action in concert with the data that are collected. Conducting the literature review at the end of the study can place the findings in the context of what is already known. Because action research focuses on local problems, the literature review most likely will not yield directly applicable information. However, the researcher may find conceptual connections that can help make sense of the action or provide support for the local theory.

As part of the study process, the team should decide before initiation of data collection with whom the study report will be shared. This can be a very emotional conversation; therefore, the earlier the discussion takes place, the better. It is important to know who the primary recipient of the report will be for it to be written in a meaningful style for the intended audience. For example, writing the report for a city council will take a very different format than writing the report for the community at large.

Rigor

All research should be evaluated for its rigor. Action research is no exception. Stringer (1999) suggests that action researchers establish the rigor of their research by utilizing the trustworthiness criteria recommended by Lincoln and Guba (1985). These include credibility, transferability, dependability, and confirmability.

According to Stringer (1999),

> credibility is established by *prolonged engagement* with participants; *triangulation* of information from multiple data sources; *member checking* procedures that allow participants to check and verify the accuracy of the information recorded; and *peer debriefing* processes that enable research facilitators to articulate and reflect on research procedures with a colleague or informed associate. (p. 176)

Transferability is established by creating thick descriptions that, when read by another researcher, can be applied in other contexts. It is the researcher's responsibility to describe as fully as possible the potential for applying the information in other contexts (Stringer, 1999).

Dependability and confirmability are established through an audit trail. The researcher is responsible for providing enough information so that another researcher reading the study would reach similar conclusions.

Waterman (1998) recommends that action researchers focus on the validity of their research. She offers three types of validity: dialectical, critical, and reflexive.

Dialectical validity "refers to the constant analysis and report of movement between theory, research and practice in examining the tensions, contradictions and complexities of the situation" (Badger, 2000, p. 204).

Critical validity involves analyzing the process of change. "The measure of validity is not the change effected but rather the analysis of intentions and actions, their ethical implications and consequences" (Badger, 2000, p. 204). "Action researchers tend to demonstrate a sense of timing or sensitivity to the situation which has been cultivated through an intimate understanding of the context and the people involved" (Waterman, 1998, p. 103).

Reflexive validity is the attempt by the researcher to constantly be examining the biases, suppositions, and presuppositions of the research. It is only through constant attention to the researcher's view that a true understanding can result. The researcher must be certain that in the end he or she has told the story of the insider.

The very real concern in any qualitative research study is that the story that emerges is the story of the people. Action research is no exception. Action research is useful because of its fundamental characteristics. It would be inadvisable to apply criteria for rigor that subtract from the value of the fundamental characteristics. The rigor of an action research study should be measured by how well the researcher has attended to the fundamental characteristics of the method.

Ethical Considerations

Action research studies have inherent ethical dilemmas that may not be seen in most other types of research. For example, one of the characteristics of an action research study is the focus on cooperation and collaborative decision making among stakeholders with the goal of carrying out a change or action project. Individuals from the marginalized group may become involved in the study without being aware of the potential tensions inherent in group process. For instance, individuals who share contrasting opinions from those in the dominant membership may find that although a consent form clearly stated the option to withdraw from the study at any time, pressure from within the group may be such that this is impossible to do so. The action researcher should try to identify as many of these tensions as possible. It may not be possible, however, to identify them all. The best that the researcher may be able to guarantee is a regular review of what the participants have agreed to. Munhall (2001) refers to this as process consent. Process consent is a procedure that allows the researcher and participants to renegotiate aspects of informed consent based on the changing nature of the inquiry.

Kelly and Simpson (2001) offer another ethical dilemma that may occur— the feelings of vulnerability felt by those who are invested in making a change.

There are always those who are invested in maintaining the status quo who will work relentlessly to maintain their position. To limit the potential for oppression, Kelly and Simpson recommend that action researchers seek as much consultation as necessary with relevant authorities and provide for close inclusion of all participants throughout the process.

Williamson and Prosser (2002) speak specifically about the ethical dilemmas that may arise as part of conducting an action research study within one's own organization. Some of the areas of concern include difficulty guaranteeing confidentiality and anonymity, complexity of obtaining informed consent, and difficulty protecting subjects from harm. As these authors share, when involved in a study in one's own organization, it may be impossible not to be in a position of conflict with one's supervisors if the recommended action requires an organizational change. Similarly, when an organization grants permission for a study to be conducted, it is unlikely that those in power would not be aware of who the participants are. This limits one's anonymity. Finally, it is very difficult to completely protect research participants from harm should they engage in debates with institutional administrators about how the organization functions or needs to be changed. Although these may appear to be insurmountable problems when conducting research in the parent organization, Williamson and Prosser suggest that using a steering group to convey information to the administration may be one way of limiting the ethical concerns raised here. If the steering group shares the problems and proposed actions, as well as assumes responsibility for conducting face-to-face confrontation, then those who are in less powerful positions in the organization may experience less of the anxiety and distress that may be an outcome of an organizational change.

Ethical issues can arise despite the most meticulous planning. Action researchers need to be cognizant of all the potential problems that may arise and inform their co-researchers of as many of them as can be identified before and during the study.

SUMMARY

Action research is a dynamic approach to inquiry. The researcher who opts to adopt the approach as a way to study a problem and assist in making a change in the lives of those who live in a particular situation must be willing to accept the important characteristics of this method. An attitude of collaboration, a commitment to cooperation, and an obligation to democracy and empowerment will be essential for the researcher who chooses the method. If the nurse researcher understands the possibilities that exist when adopting the method and is willing to participate in research that is locally meaningful, then action research can be an invigorating process that can create *real* change. According to Jenks (1999), "when used appropriately, action research can result in lasting change that creates a more meaningful nursing practice" (p. 263).

References

Anderson, G., Herr, K., & Nihlen, A. (1994). *Studying your own school: An educator's guide to qualitative practitioner research.* Thousand Oaks, CA: Corwin.

Badger, T. G. (2000). Action research, change and methodological rigor. *Journal of Nursing Management, 8*, 201-207.

Bellman, L., Bywood, C., & Dale, S. (2003). Advancing working and learning through critical action research: Creativity and constraints. *Nursing Education in Practice, 3*(4), 186-194.

Bennett, O. M. (2000). Action research: Reflective practice in occupational therapy education. *Education: Special Interest Section Quarterly, 19*(4), 1-2.

Bradbury, H., & Reason, P. (2003). Action research: An opportunity for revitalizing research purposes and practices. *Qualitative Social Work, 2*(2), 155-175.

Brown, C. L. (2001). Action research: The method. In C. L. Munhall (Ed.), *Nursing research: A qualitative perspective* (3rd ed., pp. 503-522). Sudbury, MA: Jones and Bartlett.

Calhoun, E. (1993). Action research: Three approaches. *Educational Leadership, 51*(2), 62-65.

Cockburn, L., & Trentham, B. (2002). Participatory action research: Integrating community occupational therapy practice and research. *Canadian Journal of Occupational Therapy, 69*(1), 20-30.

Coghlan, D., & Casey, M. (2001). Action research from the inside: Issues and challenges in doing action research in your own hospital. *Journal of Advanced Nursing, 35*(5), 674-682.

Crist, J. D., & Escandon-Dominguez, S. (2003). Identifying and recruiting Mexican partners and sustaining community partnerships. *Journal of Transcultural Nursing, 14*(3), 266-271.

DePoy, E., & Gitlin, L. N. (1994). *Introduction to research: Multiple strategies for health and human services.* St. Louis: Mosby.

Gustavsen, B. (1992). *Dialogue and development.* Assen-Maastricht: Van Gorcum.

Greenwood, D. J., & Levin, M. (1998). *Introduction to action research: Social research for social change.* London: Sage.

Hart, E., & Bond, M. (1996). Making sense of action research through the use of a typology. *Journal of Advanced Nursing, 23*, 152-159.

Holter, I. M., & Schwartz-Barcott, D. (1993). Action research: What is it? How has it been used and how can it be used in nursing? *Journal of Advanced Nursing, 18*, 298-304.

Jenks, J. (1999). Action research method. In H. J. Streubert & D. R. Carpenter (Eds.), *Qualitative research in nursing: Advancing the humanistic imperative* (2nd ed., pp. 251-264). Philadelphia: Lippincott Williams & Wilkins.

Kelly, K., & Simpson, S. (2001). Action research in action: Reflections on a project to introduce clinical practice facilitators to an acute hospital setting. *Journal of Advanced Nursing, 33*(5), 652-659.

Kendall, S. A., & Sturt, J. A. (1996). Negotiation access into primary health care: Insights from critical theory. *Social Sciences in Health, 2*(2), 107-120.

Kincheloe, J. (1991). *Teachers are researchers: Qualitative inquiry as a path to empowerment.* London: Falmer.

Koch, T., Selim, P. & Kralik, D. (2002). Enhancing lives through the development of community-based action research programme. *Journal of Clinical Nursing, 11,* 109-117.

Letts, L. (2003). Occupational therapy and participatory research: A partnership worth pursuing. *American Journal of Occupational Therapy, 57*(1), 77-87.

Lewin, K. (1946). Action research and minority problems. *Journal of Social Issues, 2,* 34-46.

Lincoln, Y. S., & Guba, E. G. (1985). *Naturalistic inquiry.* Beverly Hills, CA: Sage.

Minkler, M., Blackell, A. G., Thompson, M. & Tamir, H. (2003). Community-based participatory research: Implications for public health funding. *American Journal of Public Health, 93*(8), 1210-1214.

Munhall, P. L. (2001). *Nursing research: A qualitative perspective* (3rd ed.). Sudbury, MA: Jones and Barlett.

Reason, P. (1994). *Participation in human inquiry.* London: Sage.

Reason, P. (1988). *Human inquiry in action: Developments in new paradigm research.* New York: Wiley.

Reason, P. (1998). Three approaches to participative inquiry. In N. K. Denzin & Y. S. Lincoln (Eds.), *Strategies of qualitative inquiry* (pp. 261-291). Thousand Oaks, CA: Sage.

Reason, P. & Bradbury, H. (2001). Introduction: Inquiry and participation in search of a world worthy of human aspiration. In P. Reason & H. Bradbury (Eds.), *The Handbook of Action Research* (pp. 179-188). London/Thousand Oaks, CA: Sage.

Rolfe, G. (1996). Going to extremes: Action research, grounded practice and the theory-practice gap in nursing. *Journal of Advanced Nursing, 24,* 1315-1320.

Schon, D. (1983). *The reflective practitioner: How professionals think in action.* New York: Basic Books.

Stringer, E. T. (1999). *Action research* (2nd ed.). Thousand Oaks, CA: Sage.

Sturt, J. (1999). Placing empowerment research with an action research typology. *Journal of Advanced Nursing, 30*(5), 1057-1063.

Taylor, R. R., Braveman, B., & Hammel, J. (2004). Developing and evaluating community-based services through participatory action research: Two case examples. *American Journal of Occupational Therapy, 58*(1), 73-82.

Tetley, J., & Hanson, L. (2001). Participatory research. *Nurse Researcher, 8*(1), 69-88.

Tichen, A., & Binnie, A. (1993). Research partnerships: Collaborative action research in nursing. *Journal of Advanced Nursing, 18,* 858-865.

Trist, E. (1981). *The evolution of socio-technical systems* (Occasional Paper No. 2). Toronto: Ontario Quality of Work Life Council.

Waterman, H. (1998). Embracing ambiguities and valuing ourselves: Issues of validity in action research. *Journal of Advanced Nursing, 28*(1), 101-105.

Whitehead, D., Taket, A., & Smith, P. (2003). Action research in health promotion. *Health Education Journal, 62*(1), 5-22.

Williamson, G., & Prosser, S. (2002). Illustrating the ethical dimensions of action research. *Nurse Researcher, 10*(2), 38-49.

Winter, R., & Munn-Giddings, C. (2001). *A handbook for action research in health and social care.* London: Routledge.

Whyte, W. F. (1984). *Learning from the field: A guide from experience.* Beverly Hills, CA: Sage.

14

Action Research in Practice, Education, and Administration

*A*ction research is an exciting research methodology that "changes the relationship between theory and practice by producing knowledge not only for its own sake but also to produce change" (Kelly, 2005, p. 66). Nurses are uniquely positioned to support community-based research. Minkler and Wallerstein (2003) offer that outside experts' perspectives have not been effective and more importantly are not well suited to addressing health needs of individuals from different ethnic or racial groups or those who experience health disparities. Nurses frequently find themselves caring for individuals from diverse backgrounds who have unmet health needs. Working *with* individuals who have been marginalized by the current health care system in a systematic way can lead to improved outcomes. Action research can also be used to create change in nursing education and nursing administration. This chapter presents examples of nurse researchers who have used the method to solve local problems. More important, it demonstrates how collaborative research can empower individuals to make effective changes that improve their lives. Table 14.1 offers a summary of recent action research studies to educate the reader about the ways action research has been used to solve nursing practice, education, and administration problems. In addition, a critical review of three studies is shared to give the reader a perspective on what is important in reporting action research. Box 14.1 provides a list of questions that is used for reviewing the articles presnted. The intent is to provide direction for critical review of action research studies and specifically to determine the merits of the study and the overall utility and practical application of the findings. A reprint of Joyce's (2005) article is offered at the end of the chapter to facilitate the reader's understanding of the critique process.

Text continued on page 355.

Table 14.1 • Selective Sampling of Action Research Studies

Author(s)	Domain	Purpose	Co-researchers	Data Generation	Findings
Averill (2003)	Practice	To determine community attributes and strengths for the purpose of contributing to positive change	Community-dwelling elders, family members, care providers, and key informants from the community and researcher	Interviews/dialectic, participant observation, photography, archival data, analysis of contextual information	The community faces significant challenges, including rising prescription costs, reduced access to care, isolation, and loneliness. They also have assets, including knowledge of how to remain healthy and manage health care on limited resources, and nurses and community members who will advocate for them.
Joyce (2005)	Education	To discover needed revisions in content and	Nursing students in the program and researcher	Focus groups, interviews, questionnaires, document	Nurses participating in a nursing education

		delivery of a nursing management program		analysis, and reflective journals	program may not have a full understanding of what they need to know in light of external changes in nursing management. Personal development planning as a learning strategy may be helpful in providing a framework for examining practice and one's professional goals.
Koch, Jenkin, & Kralik (2004)	Practice	To explore self-management of asthma by elders	Asthmatic elders and their family members and researchers	Interviews, questionnaire, and focus groups	Three asthma models of self-management were described: medical, collaborative, and self.

Table 14.1 • (Continued)

Author(s)	Domain	Purpose	Co-researchers	Data Generation	Findings
Lee-Hsieh, Kuo, & Ysai (2004)	Education	"To plan, develop, implement and evaluate the effectiveness of the first year course of a 5-year nursing caring curriculum" (p. 391)	Nursing instructors and nursing education administrator researchers	Interviews, observations, and questionnaires	By using "an appropriate curriculum and learning strategies, caring capacity can be taught" (p. 399). Instructors need to be taught how to role-model and teach caring.
Smith, Bailey, Hydo, Leep, Mews, Timm, & Zorn (2004)	Education	To link the humanities with the teaching and learning processes in a graduate nursing education course	Graduate nursing students and their teachers/researchers	Writing samples, group discussion, reflection	Including the humanities in a graduate nursing education course helps students to see the connections in their learning experiences and provides a deeper level of learning about self and others.

Author	Focus	Purpose	Sample	Methods	Findings
Spirig, Nicca, Voggensperger, Unger, Werder, & Niepmann (2004)	Practice/Administration	To improve care for patients and families experiencing an HIV/AIDS diagnosis	Nurses in an outpatient clinic and University nursing faculty researchers	Group discussion, interview, observation	Implementing an advanced practice team model for the care of HIV/AIDS patients improves patient outcomes and increases clinical expertise of staff.
Williamson, Webb, & Abelson-Mitchell (2004)	Education	To develop a lecturer/practitioner role, examine its implementation, and quantify burnout and stress experienced by those in the role	Lecturer/practitioners, researchers, university "stakeholders," and "local trusts"	Focus groups, meetings, feedback, reflective journals	"Five themes emerged… personal motivation, workload pressures, role clarity, preparation and support and gains in roles" (p. 153). Burnout and stress were no greater in this group than in similar occupational groups.

Box 14.1

Critiquing Guidelines for Action Research

Planning

1. Does the researcher justify the use of action research?
2. Does the study begin with an analysis of the situation, or does it begin with implementation of the action?
3. Who initiated the study? The community? The researcher?
4. Does the research team demonstrate a commitment to mutual goal setting, sharing resources and action?
5. Analysis of the situation
   a. Is the setting described in sufficient detail?
   b. What methods of data generation are used to describe the practice situation? Are qualitative and qualitative techniques used appropriately?
   c. Are procedures for selecting participants described? Are they the appropriate participants?
   d. What is the extent of collaboration between researchers and participants during the analysis of phase of the study?
   e. Is protection of human subjects documented?
   f. Are strategies for data analysis described? Are they used appropriately?
   g. Are participants involved in the interpretation?
   h. Does the description reflect understanding of the situation?
6. Action planning
   a. Is the planned change described in detail?
   b. Are methods of implementing the planned change described?
   c. Are methods for evaluating the planned change described?
   d. Are participants included in action planning?

Acting

1. Is the planned change implemented in the setting where the problem occurred?
2. Is the period for implementation specified?

Reflecting

1. Are methods for facilitating reflection specified?
2. Are the results of reflection described?

Evaluating

1. Are strategies for evaluating the change described?
2. Are the processes for implementing the change and the outcomes of the change evaluated?
3. Are data evaluation methods appropriate to factors evaluated?
   a. Are qualitative and quantitative techniques used appropriately?
4. Are participants included in the evaluation?
5. Are appropriate methods used to analyze evaluation data?
6. Does the research address validity and reliability of quantitative findings and trustworthiness of qualitative findings?

Conclusions, Implications, and Recommendations
1. Do the conclusions reflect the findings?
2. Is a local theory formulated from the findings?
3. Are implications described in sufficient detail?
4. Has the researcher discussed ethical and moral implications of the study?
5. Are recommendations for research and/or practice included?
6. Does the researcher describe the benefits participants gained from the study?

Text continued from page 349.

APPLICATION TO PRACTICE

*I*n recent years, health disparities among marginalized groups have grown. This is evident in the development of a goal to eliminate health disparities (Healthy People 2010). As Minkler and Wallerstein (2005) suggest, action research provides an effective way of helping to meet the health care needs of those who are marginalized in our society. If, as a researcher, you are committed to empowerment of others; understanding health problems through the eyes of stakeholders; sharing power, information, and resources; and co-creating an action or change, then action research may provide the key to effectively managing local health problems.

Clinical nursing practice is considered by some to be the place where nurse researchers should focus their resources. The problems in the clinical practice area deal specifically with the focus of nursing care: individuals, families, groups, or communities who need health promotion, health maintenance, disease prevention, or treatment to manage health deviations. In the article entitled "Chronic Illness Self-Management: Locating the 'Self'," Koch, Jenkin, and Kralik (2004) share how they used action research to gain a better understanding of self-management by asthmatic elderly. This article will be critically reviewed using the questions in Box 14.1 to demonstrate the quality of the work.

Koch and colleagues (2004) begin their report by sharing the problem with self-management programs for chronic disease. They move from a general review of the literature to a description of what is known about self-management programs for asthmatics. They conclude their literature review by sharing with the reader that collaboration models are preferred over strong medically directed programs for individuals with asthma, thus substantiating the value of utilizing an action research approach.

The researchers report that the aim of their study is to understand how asthma affects the lives of elderly and the context, barriers, and issues that are important to them through utilization of a collaborative research model (Koch et al., 2004). Although the researchers initially approached the elderly, the willingness of the elderly to participate in prolonged data collection and work with the researchers to solve the problem demonstrated their commitment and set the stage to empower them to act on their own behalf.

In action research, data can be collected first, which informs the choice of action, or it can begin with an action that is then evaluated based on the data collected. Following institutional ethics approval, the researchers opted to begin with data collection rather than action. Those who participated responded to advertisements or were referred by asthma educators. They were individuals who were medically diagnosed with asthma and were either using or had been prescribed daily medication to treat the disease. Initially, the researchers conducted 24 one-on-one in-depth interviews. The guide questions included the following:

> How has asthma affected your life? Give an example of an incident or episode with asthma that really affected your life. What has changed in your life since you were diagnosed with asthma? What strategies do you employ to manage your asthma? Where and how did you learn about these strategies? Is there anything that would help you in the future to manage your asthma that is not available now? (Koch et al., 2004, p. 486)

Koch and colleagues tell the reader that these questions were selected because they are part of developing the story that, according to Stringer (1999), includes three types of questions: look, think, and act.

In addition to using one-on-one interviews, the researchers also employed focus group methodology, which they labeled participatory action research (PAR) groups. The stimulus for the conversations in the focus groups was sharing the results of the one-on-one interviews conducted with the initial 24 informants. Because of the large number of elderly people and their family members who wanted to be included in the focus group, the researchers conducted two meetings. Participants in the first group were asked to take home a questionnaire, which included two questions related to their understanding of asthma and self-management. Koch and colleagues (2004) reported that they used data analysis strategies described by Colaizzi. Although not specifically stated, it appears that the second focus group was provided with the one-on-one interview data, the responses to the questionnaires, and the findings from the data analysis of the first focus group. The authors do not report collaborative data analysis. They do, however, report that "analysis of the PAR group data was also concurrent to ensure prompt feedback of issues to participants, thus creating the opportunity to build our (participants' and facilitators') understandings collaboratively" (p. 487). This activity demonstrates the willingness of the researchers to involve participants in the interpretation of the data phase of the study.

The researchers conclude the work by identifying three models of self-management: medical, collaborative, and self-agency. The first two have been discussed in the literature, but the authors claim that the third, self-agency, is new.

Koch and co-researchers (2004) do not discuss the action planning or a specific action that is the part of this study. They do report that focus group participants are asked to reflect on information provided. In addition to a lack of information on the action phase of the study, there is also no report of evaluation. The reader might assume that the action step will be taken by providers who will use the information generated from this study to provide more informed health care of elderly asthmatic patients. However, without a statement from the researchers, the reader is left without a clear understanding of what the action step is.

The conclusions, the three models of asthma self-management, do reflect the personal statements by participants included in the report. The "theory" that is developed relates to the models that are identified from data analysis. These may well have application beyond the local group. Testing will be needed, but ultimately the findings may be very beneficial to those who care for elderly asthmatic patients.

The researchers do not describe specific ethical or moral implications of the study. The report would be stronger if it included a description of the benefits gained by participation. It is difficult to identify how the empowerment aspect of the research was achieved.

The study completed by Koch and colleagues (2004) adds to the literature on self-management of asthma in the elderly. It also provides a substantial description of data collection strategies useful in action research. The identification of a new category of self-management of asthma adds to the literature and clearly has the potential to affect nursing practice.

APPLICATION TO EDUCATION

Since the completion of the last edition of this book, more studies have been published using action research in nursing education. For example, action research has been shown to be useful in developing a caring curriculum in Taiwan (Lee-Hsieh, Kuo, & Ysai, 2004), developing lecturer practitioner roles (Williamson, Webb, & Abelson-Mitchell, 2004), integrating the humanities into graduate nursing education (Smith, Bailey, Hydo, Lepp, Mews, Timm, & Zorn, 2004), and developing a nursing management degree program to meet the needs of Irish nurse managers (Joyce, 2005). These examples illustrate that sharing power, giving voice to those who would otherwise not be heard, and developing collaborative action plans lead to effective nursing education outcomes. In this section, an article by Joyce

(2005) entitled "Developing a Nursing Management Degree Programme to Meet the Needs of Irish Nurse Managers" is reviewed using the critiquing criteria found in Box 14.1. A complete reprint of this study can be found at the conclusion of the chapter.

Joyce (2005) begins her report by placing the study in context for the reader. She tells us that Ireland has seen major changes in recent years in its health care system, resulting in an increased need for highly qualified nurse managers. She also tells the reader that nursing education for managers is in need of a change. Information on the state of management and nursing management specifically is provided. Joyce also shares that it is her belief that if the program is to be changed, it is important to work collaboratively with students to change it. The problem is identified, and Joyce indicates that a solution is needed. In this case, the students do not approach the researcher to solve the problem but believe that participating in the process will benefit them by allowing them to participate in the identification of gaps in the current program and by getting first-hand nursing research experience (Joyce, 2005).

Specifically, the aim of the study is "to explore nurses' expectations of the content and delivery of a nursing management degree programme" (Joyce, 2005, p. 76). To address the aim of the study, Joyce states that action research is the appropriate method of study and that she will employ both qualitative and quantitative data collection strategies. The sample selected for the study is identified as purposive. More than 117 students in the program provided data for the study. There is no mention of protection of human subjects review. However, Joyce does state that she was careful to adhere to ethical principles throughout the study.

The study began with an examination of the current curriculum. The literature related to nursing management also was examined. The researcher conducted an analysis of the curriculum in light of the literature review and existing professional and governmental recommendations for nursing management curricula. Joyce (2005) does provide a fairly comprehensive overview of the information collected.

In the second phase, data were collected using focus groups, interviews, and questionnaires. Thematic analysis was used to analyze the qualitative data. SPSS was used to analyze quantitative data from the questionnaire. Students participated in data analysis. A cyclic process of data collection and data analysis was applied to gain agreement on a variety of topics related to the curriculum. After data analysis, proposed changes to the curriculum were discussed with the students, and a plan for implementation was jointly developed. In addition, Joyce (2005) reports that an action plan for the changes with specific timeframes and evaluation points was created with input from all participants. The cyclic nature of collecting and analyzing data based on new information and the active participation of researcher and members of the group—in this case, students—are hallmarks of action research.

Input from the students and researcher informed the planning and implementation of the change. When the new students who would be affected by the change in curriculum were admitted, the researcher reports that they too were included in data collection and analysis. The newly revised curriculum was evaluated by the students and judged favorably.

Joyce (2005) reports that evaluation is ongoing throughout the implementation phase. Students are part of the ongoing evaluation, and questionnaires are used to assess different aspects of the curriculum as it is implemented. The author does not report whether the questionnaires are open ended, which would provide an opportunity for reflection. However, she does indicate that she encouraged self-reflection on the part of the participants throughout the study.

Joyce (2005) does use data collection triangulation to strengthen the validity of her findings. She also reports that she engaged in multiple and repetitious action research cycles to strengthen the credibility of her findings. The current status of the curriculum implementation is unclear based on this report.

Joyce's (2005) conclusions related to the current state of the project support data presented. It is obvious that she is developing a change that will improve nursing management as judged by her participants. Her recommendations for the future focus on the need for nurse educators to be cognizant of the importance of research in curriculum planning and revision. She does share that the students have demonstrated a willingness to be open in sharing what they think is working and what is not in the curriculum. She believes that true emancipation will be evidenced by practitioners/graduates who critically reflect on their practice and bring forward norms and conflicts that are at the heart of problems identified in their places of employment (p. 81).

The study by Joyce (2005) is an excellent example of action research. It is obvious from the report that she has a clear understanding of action research and the assumptions that underlie implementation of the method. The study offers an excellent approach to curriculum planning and revision. The contributions of the study are obvious. She has contributed to the literature on action research, nursing education generally, and curriculum planning specifically. In addition, the study adds to the nursing administration literature.

APPLICATION TO ADMINISTRATION

*T*he roots of action research are in organizational change.

Issues of organizational concern such as quality patient care, systems improvement, organizational learning and the management of change are suitable subjects for action research, as (a) they are real events, which must be managed in real time, (b) they provide opportunities for both effective action and learning and (c) can contribute to the development of theory of what really goes on in hospitals and to the development of nursing knowledge. (Coghlan & Casey, 2001, p. 676)

Despite the opportunities that exist to conduct organizational studies in nursing, a current review of the literature reveals few action research studies that focus on organizational change. One example is an article published by Bryant-Lukosius and DiCenso (2004), in which they illustrate how they created a framework for introducing and evaluating advanced practice nursing roles. Their article clearly outlines the steps required to implement an organizational change, such as the introduction of the advanced practice nurse from a nursing administration vantage point using an action research approach. The nurse interested in this specific type of institutional change is encouraged to read this article.

In this section, a publication by Spirig, Nicca, Voggensperger, Unger, Werder, and Niepmann (2004) entitled "The Advanced Nursing Practice Team as a Model for HIV/AIDS Caregiving in Switzerland" is critiqued using the criteria found in Box 14.1. This article gives the reader an understanding of how action research can be used to develop a new approach to patient care.

Spirig and associates (2004) begin their report by sharing some insights on the current state of HIV/AIDS care at an outpatient clinic in Basel, Switzerland. In addition, they offer a larger picture of HIV/AIDS care by explaining the current situation in Switzerland. This provides a context for their report. To help the reader understand the work environment, the authors relate that the clinic employs individuals with different educational backgrounds to care for HIV/AIDS patients. Despite their educational difference, they shared a common vision, to provide high-quality care. To ensure the level of care, the nursing team chose to use participatory action research to "enhance nursing care in the clinic" (p. 48).

According to the authors, a collaborative relationship was established between the clinic staff and the Institute of Nursing Science at the University of Basel. The goal of the collaboration was "to offer competent and effective long-term nursing care to patients and families" (Spirig et al., 2004, p. 49). The university's staff was engaged to support the implementation of an action research study. The selection of action research was based on the researchers' belief in the value of continuous learning and their understanding of organizational change. They report that they enlisted the support of supervisors and physicians. This is important because these are individuals who potentially can influence the success of the action research study. Spirig and co-researchers do not report how they maintained human subjects' protection.

The setting of the study is described to help the reader place the study in context. Before the initiation of this research, the first author previously conducted studies focusing on the illness experience of patients and the caring experiences of those living with HIV/AIDS and their families. The focus of this inquiry is to view HIV/AIDS care from the perspective of health care providers.

The first step in implementing the research included a careful analysis of nursing care in the clinic. According to Spirig and associates (2004), group discussions, observation, and interviews with nurses and physicians provided a view of the care that individuals and their families received. These are appropriate methods for data gathering.

The study informants are appropriate given that the focus of the study was understanding health care providers' perspectives of care. At the conclusion of the first step, an analysis was completed. This analysis led the researchers to move to the action phase of the study. Spirig and colleagues (2004) report that participants were involved in data analysis and in direction setting.

Initially, the action phase included defining practice. The collaborators chose to use an advanced practice model; therefore, a definition of advanced nursing practice (ANP) was determined to be an important first step. The definition chosen required the development of a highly skilled and competent team of professionals. According to Spirig and associates (2004), "the nurses started to develop their clinical knowledge and skills by attending continuing education programs to obtain specialist or public health certificates" (p. 50).

The authors reported that there was ongoing reflection "that helped to bridge their experiences with the theory they learned in their courses" (p. 50). Reflection is an essential part of the action research process and is used appropriately in this study.

With their practice model defined and formal education started, the advanced practice team focused on several new action areas. These included "understanding the culture and organization of the ANP in the outpatient department, developing clinical leadership and interdisciplinary collaboration, and implementing and evaluating new nursing services" (Spirig et al., p. 50).

Although there is little description of how data gathering and analysis continued throughout the first 30 months of the study, the authors do share that reflection was used at various points throughout the research process to fully understand the care needs of HIV/AIDS-infected clients and their families. Clear understanding of the care needs enabled nurses to move from a position of routine care based on tradition to a model that enabled more effective health care for clients and families experiencing HIV/AIDS.

Spirig and co-researchers (2004) report that evaluation interviews were conducted with nurses. They do not report the specific type of interview, qualitative or quantitative, nor do they report the method of analysis. The researchers do not report how they maintained methodological rigor. Describing how trustworthiness was ensured would strengthen the report.

The findings are provided in narrative format without supporting data, making it difficult to determine whether they reflect data collected throughout the study. However, it is apparent from the report that action research contributed to a shift in the practice paradigm in this clinic and that those working there reported that the change was an improvement. From a research reporting perspective, the report would be enhanced by including subjective statements and quantitative data supporting practice developments. Spirig and colleagues (2004) do provide some insight into the value of the methodology in creating change and report that it will continue to be used as implementation of the advanced practice model continues.

This study represents a very good example of how to use action research to implement an organizational change. The researchers contribute to nursing knowledge in nursing practice and administration and provide valuable insights into the utility of action research in nursing.

SUMMARY

*I*n 1999, Jenks reported, "nurse researchers in the United States rarely use action research because they do not regard it as a rigorous form of research" (p. 263). In this chapter, each of the studies offered demonstrates that when action research is implemented appropriately, it is a rigorous methodology that can be useful in creating change. Increasing numbers of nurses in the United States are utilizing action research based on its collaborative, emancipatory framework for understand the events and circumstances that shape the lives of those with whom nurses work. As nursing continues to build its knowledge base, nurse researchers should consider the value of the method in developing more humanistic practice environments. Learning more about the method, understanding its assumptions and characteristics, and applying its framework will not only build the body of nursing knowledge but it will also create practice opportunities for sharing power and knowledge, which will lead to more holistic understanding and care of individuals.

In this chapter, critique has been the focus. Through rigorous review of published studies and careful implementation of the critique process, those unfamiliar with the method will gain an understanding and appreciation of the method as a valuable approach to nursing research.

References

Averill, J. (2003). Keys to the puzzle: Recognizing strengths in a rural community. *Public Health Nursing, 20*(6), 449–455.

Bryant-Lukosius, D., & DiCenso, A. (2004). A framework for the introduction and evaluation of advanced practice nursing roles. *Journal of Advanced Nursing, 48*(5), 530–540.

Coghlan, D., & Casey, M. (2001). Action research from the inside: Issues and challenges in doing action research in your own hospital. *Journal of Advanced Nursing*, *35*(5), 674–682.

Healthy People 2010 (n.d.). Retrieved January 29, 2005, from http://www.healthypeople. gov/About/goals.htm

Holkup, P. S., Tripp-Reimer, T., Salois, E. M., & Weinert, C. (2004). Community-based participatory research: An approach to intervention with a Native American community. *Advances in Nursing Science*, *27*(3), 162–175.

Lee-Hsieh, J., Kuo, C., & Ysai, Y. (2004). An action research on the development of a caring curriculum in Taiwan. *Journal of Nursing Education*, *43*(9), 391–400.

Jenks, J. (1999). Action research method. In H. J. Streubert & D. R. Carpenter (Eds.), *Qualitative research in nursing: Advancing the humanistic imperative* (2nd ed., pp. 251–264). Philadelphia: Lippincott Williams & Wilkins.

Joyce, P. (2005). Developing a nursing management degree programme to meet the needs of Irish nurse managers. *Journal of Nursing Management*, *13*(1), 74–82.

Kelly, P. J. (2005). Practical suggestions for community interventions using participatory action research. *Public Health Nursing*, *22*(1), 65–73.

Koch, T., Jenkin, P., & Kralik, D. (2004). Chronic illness self-management: Locating the 'self.' *Journal of Advanced Nursing*, *4*(5), 484–492.

Minkler, M., & Wallerstein, N. (2003). Introduction to community-based participatory research. In Minkler, M., & Wallerstein, N. (Ed.), *Community-based participatory research for health* (pp. 3–26). San Francisco: Jossey-Bass.

Smith, R. L., Bailey, M., Hydo, S. K., Lepp, M., Mews, S., Timm, S., & Zorn, C. (2004). All the voices in one room: Integrating humanities in nursing education. *Nursing Education Perspectives*, *25*(6), 278–283.

Spirig, R., Nicca, D., Voggensperger, J., Unger, M., Werder, V., & Niepmann, S. (2004). The advanced nursing practice team as a model for HIV/AIDS caregiving in Switzerland. *Journal of the Association of Nurses in AIDS Care*, *15*(3), 47–55.

Stringer, E. T. (1999). *Action research* (2nd ed.). Thousand Oaks, CA: Sage.

Williamson, G. R., Webb, C., & Abelson-Mitchell, N. (2004). Developing lecturer practitioner roles using action research. *Journal of Advanced Nursing*, *47*(2), 153–164.

Research Article

Developing a nursing management degree programme to meet the needs of Irish nurse managers

PAULINE JOYCE MSc, RGN, RM, BNS, RNT, FFNMRCSI

Lecturer, Faculty of Nursing and Midwifery, Royal College of Surgeons in Ireland, Dublin, Ireland

JOYCE P. (2005) Journal of Nursing Management 13, 74–82

Developing a nursing management degree programme to meet the needs of Irish nurse managers

Background *The study is placed within the context of the Irish health care system, which has undergone tremendous change, at the dawn of the new millennium, in particular from the nursing management and leadership viewpoint.*

Aim of the study *The aim of this study is to explore nurses' expectations of the content and delivery of a nursing management degree programme.*

Methods *This is an on-going action research study. Data has been collected using a focus group interview, questionnaire, document analysis and a reflective diary. Data was analysed using thematic analysis and SPSS as appropriate to qualitative and quantitative data respectively. To date two action research cycles are near completion and a total sample of 117 students have taken part in the study.*

Findings *Nurses commencing the programme were unsure of their education and training needs, as they had not yet taken on board the recommendations of the Irish Commission on Nursing (Government of Ireland 1998). The findings suggest that nurse managers may not know what they need to know in light of the many current changes taking place in the Irish health systm. The introduction of personal development planning (PDP) is among new strategies taking place as part of the second action research cycle. PDP can help nurse managers to reflect on their current responsibilities and plan for their future career pathways.*

Conclusions *The findings are presented in the context of one institution. Action research, which nests comfortably with certain management styles, has proved suitable as a tool for developing and changing this programme. The need for university teachers to focus on management development skills as well as the transmission of management theory is supported.*

Keywords: *action learning, action research, change, management learning, personal development planning*

Accepted for publication: *17 December 2003*

Introduction

Educational providers of nurse management programmes are faced with the critical task of designing curricula that will address present and future health care needs of nurse managers. It is suggested that existing management courses, in the Irish setting, have not met these needs. Nevertheless, current nurse managers are expected to move confidently into their roles, within the current climate of change (Joyce 2002a). In order to meet the requirements of consumers of care and of health care organizations, Flanagan (1998) emphasizes the importance of nursing education and nursing management working in partnership. This study attempts to make these links by using an action research approach to develop a nursing management degree programme.

Self-reflection and learning of action researcher

This project set out in a technical orientation, with me as the main researcher realizing before approaching the students that there were some problems with the content of the BSc Nursing Management programme. Carr and Kemmis (1986) identify three orientations of action research: technical, practical and emancipatory. The technical orientation is similar to what Schon (1983) has described as technical-rational. It assumes a position in which problems are defined at the outset and solutions sought. As the educational researcher, I set out to improve the effectiveness of educational practice, coopting the students, as co-researchers in the study. If change was to be successfully implemented it required that the students had some ownership of these developments. They were keen to become involved in the study as they hoped it would benefit them from two perspectives; firstly, in identifying any training and education gaps in the current programme; secondly, by their participation they would also appreciate first-hand the research process.

It was recognized that the students in year 1 of the programme were not sure of their education and training needs emanating from the recommendations of the Commission on Nursing (The Commission) (Government of Ireland 1998) which was established by the Minister for Health in 1997. In relation to the management of the health services, in particular, concerns brought to the Commission related to a sense of exclusion from the strategic planning process, communication with nurses within organizations and the development of management potential within nursing. The students in the second year of the programme verbalized difficulties with particular content in the programme. Some modules were viewed as being at MSc level, e.g. Health Economics and there was some repetition between modules (Table 1). Students emphasized their needs for specific skills training, in for example, devising service plans and budgeting. These reflections lead me to the literature on management learning.

Management learning

As far back as Mintzberg (1975, p. 61) suggested that '...cognitive learning no more makes a manager than it does a swimmer'. According to Fox (1997) management education, largely provided by university schools, tends to be mainly theoretical. Management development mainly provided by the Human Resources department of an organization focuses on the practical aspects of skills development. The skills of management learning emerged in an effort to bridge the gap between management education and development. Fox (1997) suggests that although the worlds of management education and development are overlapping there is some distinct differences. In content, management development focuses on developing personal knowledge and skills (time management, assertiveness etc.) while management education focuses more on acquiring analytical and critical skills in the academic skills relevant to management (finance, research etc.). In teaching methods, management education is delivered by and large by traditional methods (lecture, tutorial and seminar) while management development uses a muchvaried range of methods. The Council for Excellence in Management and Leadership (2002) found

Table 1 • BSc nursing management modules	
Modules 1999/2001	*Modules 2002/2003*
Year 1	*Access to diploma level for all BSc degree programmes (nursing, management, practice development)*
Management theory and practice	Personal and professional development in nursing
Legal and ethical issues	Teaching and assessing in clinical practice
Research appreciation	Research appreciation
Employee relations	Communication and interpersonal skills
Health financing and financial management	Understanding the environment of care
Quality improvement	
Year 2	*BSc management pathway*
Managerial psychology	Nursing management and leadership
Health comparative analysis	Quality improvement
Information technology	Research methods
Health economics	Employee relations
Human resources management	Health financing and financial management
Research methods	Human resources management

little evidence of innovation in management teaching practices, suggesting that universities resist shifts in teaching methods. The council recommends more research into management to improve the process.

According to Zuber-Skerritt (1992, p. 219) management development for the future needs to be process-oriented as opposed to merely content oriented. She suggests that

> 'Academics are also managers (of learning, teaching, self-development, curriculum, administration, committees, budgets etc.) and facilitators of learning process rather than mere transmitters of content and subject knowledge'.

According to Williams (2002) the possession of qualifications at higher levels cannot be assumed to be strongly related to skill for managers. In fact Eraut (1994, p. 82) would propose that much management learning is 'haphazard and semiconscious'. Zuber-Skerritt (1992) proposes that the increasing importance of responding to the fast-changing environment is the reason for this shift from content to process. General competencies and methods to acquire new knowledge and skills rather than specific knowledge and skills, per se, are required to solve completely new problems.

Likewise, McNiff (2000) believes that learning is a creative process and it should enable people to learn to do things for themselves and take responsibility for potential implications of their own practice. Managers need to find ways to ensure that individual and organizational growth will be aided by the quality of their relationships with others. Through the individual's collective learning such relationships should sustain the process of organizational change. She believes that management schools should encourage participants not to accept theory or practice that are unsuitable for their practical everyday needs. They should facilitate them to question such systems.

Context

The context in which practice occurs has an impact on professional and organizational outcomes. It is important then, according to McCormack et al. (2002), to make explicit the focus of this context, either as a presentation of the complexity of factors that enable effective practice or the way in which organizational systems and structures interact with each other.

As Irish nurse managers welcomed the third millennium a number of transitions were taking place both in nursing and in nursing management. Some of these transitions include a move from a predominately nursing workforce to the introduction of non-nursing personnel, diploma to degree level education for nurses, the introduction of three grades of first line nurse managers, strengthening of nurse managers roles, and a move from transactional to transformational leadership styles. These transitions have come about following a number of documents published by the Irish Nursing Board (An Bord Altranais) and the Irish Government. In particular, the Commission on Nursing (Government of Ireland 1998) has been instrumental in these changes.

This study is taking place in a university setting where a nursing management programme has been delivered from certificate to diploma level since the early 1980s. The BSc in Nursing Management commenced as a 2-year part-time degree programme, in the academic year 1999. I, as researcher was also the lecturer/coordinator of the programme, at the commencement of this study and joined the staff in the department in 2000. As an 'insider' action researcher there are two main challenges. According to Coghlan and Casey (2001) being close to the data there is a danger of not probing as much in interviews as an outsider might. Secondly, there may be role conflicts within the organization.

Beginning the post in the second semester of the programme brought its own difficulties. The students were dealing with a new lecturer/coordinator half way through year 1 of their programme. Gaining the trust and support of the students took time, as did getting to know each student on a one-to-one basis. There were 20 students in this first group. Having a special interest in action research I introduced the students to this approach in their research module.

The study

The aim of this study was to explore nurses' expectations of the content and delivery of a nursing management degree programme.

The objectives were:

- To explore nurses' expectations of how a nursing management programme enables them to meet their leadership and management needs in the context of their practice settings.
- To explore nurses' expectations of a nursing management programme in terms of meeting their personal and professional development.
- To identify any education and training gaps in the current nursing management degree programme.
- To develop a programme which could address the needs identified.

Design and sample

An action research approach using both quantitative and qualitative data collection methods were employed. Action research has been described as

> '...a participatory, democratic process concerned with developing practical knowledge in the pursuit of worthwhile human purposes... It seeks to bring together action and reflection, theory and practice, in participation with others, in the pursuit of practical solutions to issues of pressing concern to people, and more generally the flourishing of individual persons and their communities (Reason & Bradbury 2001, p. 1)'.

The main benefits of action research are the improvement and understanding of practice by its practitioners, and the improvement of the situation in which the practice takes place (Zuber-Skerritt 1992).

A purposive method of sampling was chosen as most appropriate for the study. Four groups of students have participated on the programme to date, bringing the

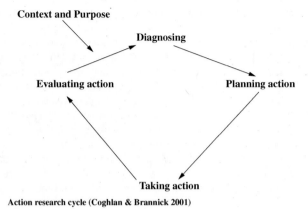

Action research cycle (Coghlan & Brannick 2001)

Figure 1. **Action research cycle.**

total sample to 117. These groups come from diverse backgrounds. The majority of the students were in managements posts and some of them moved into promotional posts during the programme. They worked in both rural- and urban-based organizations, which vary in size and in their management structures.

Demographics of the second year participants were profiled in terms of the management course they had already completed, the title of their current position, the level of management that best described their position, and the number of years in this position. Data was collected through interviews and questionnaries. The story and outcomes of the project are outlined in Figure 1.

Initial groundwork—first action research cycle

This involved examining the content of the curriculum document in light of the changing role of the Clinical Nurse Manager (ward sister) in the recommendations of the Commission on Nursing (Government of Ireland 1998). The Commission identified education, together with a range of other issues such as greater budgetary control as needing more attention in the development of nurse managers. The motives for undertaking a management course in the Irish setting were investigated by Jennings (1996). The prime motive for attending management courses was that nurses foresaw these courses offering a route towards promotion. Howley (1997) conducted another Irish study to examine the continuing education needs of ward sisters and nurse managers relevant to the existing needs of the service and their own future development. Budgeting was identified as a top training need. Other management topics identified as necessary in management positions included legal issues, counselling and communication skills, research, time management, new technology and clinical update. In addition, nurse managers identified leadership as a training necessity.

A training needs analysis of all nursing personnel working in the Eastern Health Board (EHB), the largest health board in Ireland, was carried out in 1997. Management was reported as one of the seven courses most often taken yet the majority of respondents who had completed these courses listed management subjects as required by them to improve practice (Nursing Research and Development, Eastern Health Board 1997). The studies by Jennings (1996), Howley (1997), and the Nursing Research and Development, Eastern Health Board (1997) highlight that although nurses are taking management courses for promotional and achievement reasons, they still identify a need for more professional development in this area. An Bord Altranais (1997) in their framework document on continuing professional education for nurses in Ireland also identified a need for appropriate management courses to be provided to meet the needs of nurses functioning at all levels of administration and of those remaining in clinical practice.

In relation to education and preparation of first line managers Duffield (1991) found that methods suggested to improve this preparation vary considerably. These include group problem solving, workshops, journal clubs and the use of leadership self-assessment tools. Davidhizar (1995) suggests that 'shadowing' a successful nurse leader is a highly valuable way to learn management skills. Topics identified as important for nursing managers in Davidhizar's (1995) study included budgeting and resource allocation, conflict resolution and the management of change. An education needs assessment conducted by Sullivan et al. (1994) indicated that motivating others, managing change, developing leadership and mentoring/coaching staff were among top priorities. These findings are in keeping with a later Irish survey (Office for Health Management 1998) exploring the managerial skills identified by those working in the health care sector.

The content of the modules in the BSc programmes were examined in the light of the recommendations of the Commission (Government of Ireland 1998). It was suggested that expanding practice, accountability, clinical governance and ethics were not fairly represented in the programme, at that time (Table 1).

Data collection—diagnosing

Data was initially collected via a focus group interview with seven students. These students were all working in management posts. The interview was guided by the study objectives. Following analysis of the interview a questionnaire was designed and distributed to a wider sample of 40 students in their second year of the programme. Both open-ended and closed-ended questions were incorporated. The questionnaire included Likert, ranking and visual analogue scales. Following questions about demographics of participants they were asked to rank, in order of importance (1–8) the teaching/learning approaches identified in the literature, as appropriate to a nursing management programme.

Results—data interpretation

Data from the focus group interview and from the openended questions of the questionnaire was analysed by thematic analysis. This analysis included the participation of the students and met a dual purpose of involvement and in experiencing research. Themes were allowed to emerge capturing the spirit of the respondents' own words. Three main themes emerged, professional and personal development, providing an evidence-base, and communication. The following are examples of comments from participants:

'It changes your whole way of thinking and exposes you to an amount of different situations...' (Std D)'.
'...I feel I owe it to myself... (Std G)'.
'It is really to give myself the knowledge to back up things that I am trying to change and implement in the hospital (Std G)'.
'I want to back my practice with theory (Std B)'. the programme ...will help to define our roles (Std F)'.
'...it gives us the language to put forward a particular point... we don't have the language to articulate whatever we want (Std D)'.
'Student A stressed the importance of "...getting the language to deal with them (other professions) more confidently"'.

Quantitative data from the questionnaire was analysed using SPSS statistical analysis. These results suggested that the majority of the 40 students (response rate 75%) had completed a diploma level programme in nursing management. Seventy-three percent were at Clinical Nurse Manager (ward sister) level while 6% were at Director of Nursing level. In addition, 80% of the group were 0-5 years in their current position. On identifying the approaches to teaching/learning as appropriate to nursing management programmes the majority of respondents agreed that group discussions, problem-centred learning and lectures were of greatest importance. Reflective diaries were seen as having lesser importance (Table 2). These findings are in keeping with French *et al.* (1996) who explored similarities and differences between nursing degree programmes internationally where the lecture method was the most used. French *et al.* (1996), in their study, also found that there appeared to be little relationship between course content and reflective learning across nursing degree courses.

Topics identified as having some importance on nursing management degree programmes were scored on a 7-point visual analogue scale. Such topics included negotiation skills, change management, budgeting, coaching and mentoring. These findings are similar to findings in a recent evaluation of a Leading an Empowered Organization programme in Ireland (Centre for the Development of Nursing Policy and Practice 2003). Coaching and mentoring has been addressed at a theoretical level on the BSc nursing management programme. It has been

Table 2 • Teaching/learning approaches	
Teaching/learning approaches	*Order of importance*
Lectures	1
Group discussions	2
Problem-centred learning	3
Experiential learning	4
Practical sessions	5
Reflective practice workshops	6
Reflective practice diaries	7
Role play	8

recognized that there needs to be practical application of these supports. The majority of topics were deemed to be of a level of importance at 5 or greater on the scale.

A 5-point Likert scale was used to assess the participants' level of agreement or disagreement with programme outcomes. The outcomes of the programme listed included: 'gives me the language to articulate my point of view with other professionals', 'gives me the practical tools to deal with situations at work', 'helps me define my role in the context of current health care changes', 'addresses relevant professional issues as they relate to nursing management'. Some participants disagreed with the latter statement, which is in keeping with the data from the focus group interview. The final question was an open one regarding any gaps in education and training needs of the nurse managers not addressed in the current programme. Only one student suggested that more time to be spent on communication and resolving conflict. Participants in Cooper's (2003) study also identified skills for handling conflict as necessary for their roles as leaders. In addition, a recent Irish study (Department of Health and Children/Dublin City University 2003) points to examples of conflict between nurse and managers. The need for improved communication in the health service was highlighted in the Commission on Nursing (Government of Ireland 1998).

Planning action

Following data analysis there were proposed changes discussed with the groups of students and with the external examiner at programme team meetings. The proposed changes were accepted and it was suggested that these changes be implemented in the next academic year. An action plan for the proposed changes, setting timeframes and evaluation checks was drawn up with the participants.

Taking action

These changes were introduced, on a phased basis, at the commencement of the academic year 2001/2002. As there was a new group of students ($n = 40$) joining the nursing management degree programme they were also introduced to these changes and became part of the action research study. The students were enthusiastic about the changes.

Evaluating action

These changes were evaluated positively via questionnaires to students. The concept of one access to diploma level year for all nursing degree programmes was viewed favourably. This diploma year for all programmes was in keeping with the concept of the curriculum principle of flexibility (Joyce 2002b). The students then had the choice of selecting a pathway to BSc in Nursing (which primarily focuses on clinical practice), BSc in Nursing Management or BSc in Nursing Practice Development. The change was accepted as a much needed one. In order that change is managed effectively, Coghlan and McAuliffe (2003) believes that there must be a sense of commitment, which is built through communication. This must involve hearing the responses from those working in the organization, so that the change process may be altered in the light of that feedback. The importance of communication was explicit in following the action research approach.

Having the potential for changing practice, action research can also be ethically problematic. Williamson and Prosser (2002) suggest that, given the political nature of action research, it is very difficult to guarantee confidentiality and anonymity. Secondly informed consent is more difficult than in other research projects. As an insider researcher I tried to address these ethical issues by ensuring participant feedback or member checking. The participants got the opportunity to comment on and add to my interpretations. I, as principal researcher was also aware of adhering to the ethical principles of research throughout the study.

Second cycle—diagnosing

The diagnosing part of the second action research cycle involved the evaluation of the first cycle. It also took cognisance of the recommended guidelines for the future development of nursing management programmes, as outlined by the Office for Health Management (2002). It was reassuring to note that the content of the nursing management degree programme was developing in line with these recommendations. However, there are some teaching/learning strategies yet to be implemented. These include the use of action learning sets, action plans, mentoring and personal development planning (PDP). These strategies have been suggested as appropriate for the clinical setting also and greater usage of PDP, in particular, should help meet the needs of nurses who want to become more empowered (Department of Health and Children/Dublin City University 2003). My role has now changed from a coordinator of the nursing management programme in its totality, to coordinating and facilitating the nursing management and leadership module only. To date, I have introduced these strategies to the students in the current academic year. The concept of action learning has been introduced.

Action learning

The concept of action learning has been promoted in the literature as a powerful tool for individual and organizational change (Margerison 1988, Neubauer 1995, Bouldon 2002). Revans (1980) originally used action learning in his approach to management training. He focused on developing managerial skills rather than just increasing knowledge. According to Revans (1980) the learning and development of management skills are directly linked to the learner's real needs based on actual experience. Action learning is based on the concept of learning being comprised of programmed knowledge (things that people have been taught or have been learned through experience) plus questioning skills (the ability/willingness to challenge this knowledge). Revans (1980) believes that, in addition to knowledge gained over the years, managers need to constructively question themselves and those around them in order to successfully adapt to the changing environment. According to the Action Learning Associates (2002, p. 1) website there is a need to move away from the boss who 'gives the orders' towards the boss who 'helps people work things out for themselves'. To achieve this people need to have good questioning and problem-solving skills and employees at every level in the organization must be empowered to act to solve the problems they face. The action learning set brings participants together to question, challenge and support each other. Sets are formed of people who have the same learning goals focusing on new knowledge coupled with personal learning (Pedlar 1996). The use of action learning sets and leadership networks for future nurse managers has been proposed by Malby (1997).

Second cycle—planning action

Because of the large number of students ($n = 156$) undertaking the management/leadership module it was not feasible to use action learning sets with the group. The benefits of action learning were discussed with the students as a challenging approach, which they themselves may be able to introduce in their place of work. The use of action plans, however, was successfully introduced in the assignment for the module. Here, the students were asked to plan a change initiative in their workplace. They were guided to develop action plans using the Force Field Analysis of change (Lewin 1946). These plans have been analysed. The initiatives will be followed up to ascertain how many of them are implemented in practice. Hopefully this exercise will impact on fostering a culture of changing practice.

Second cycle—taking action

I have been influenced by the evaluation of the module and by a document from the Office for Health Management (2002) on the development of nursing management programmes. In addition, the literature on management learning has also been influential in developing the focus of the management and leadership module. The changes, acted on, included more emphasis on skills training and less on management theory. Teaching/learning strategies include more group discussion, student participation, and the introduction of an action plan as part of an assessment. Providing the students with a framework for PDP at the beginning of the module has also been initiated.

Second cycle—evaluating action

It is hoped to evaluate these new teaching/learning strategies by using questionnaires and interviews. I have recently introduced action learning into a practice-based module of the masters in nursing programme which I now coordinate. There are smaller numbers of students on this programme. The assignment for the module is a portfolio. This initiative is currently being evaluated.

Discussion and conclusion

The findings of this study to date suggest that the action research approach was a suitable means of developing a nursing management degree programme. This approach is a powerful tool for change and improvement at a local level. I have tried to ensure credibility of the study by engaging in multiple and repetitious action research cycles. It is hoped that the action research has moved on to the practical kind focusing on the practitioners' understanding and professional development.

I have attempted to achieve this move by encouraging self-reflection on the part of the participants of the study. Ideally, it is envisaged that the study will finally move to being emancipatory which will prompt practitioners to reflect critically on their practice, bringing to the fore norms and conflicts which may be at the core of the problems identified.

The study highlights the need for university teachers to engage in ongoing research of their programmes. Rather than being mere transmitters of knowledge we can be facilitators of the learning process (Zuber-Skerritt 1992). Rather than instilling a culture of acceptance of theory, university teachers should encourage a critical thinking atmosphere among students, facilitating them to question systems. According to French et al. (1996) although critical thinking and personal development are explicit in the aims of curricula developed for nursing degrees, this may not be achieved via content, teaching/learning methods or assessment. The introduction of PDP may encourage such personal development and critical thinking and encourage the linking of education to management. Students using PDP can be encouraged to discuss their plans with their line managers at the commencement of the programme.

Limitations of the study to date include the small sample size and the research being confined to one setting. As principal researcher, I was also coordinator and facilitator of the programme, which could have influenced the findings. My relationship with the students was good but this may have led them to feeling compelled to take part in the study. To date, the study results have suggested the need for constant updating and changing of the curriculum to meet service needs. According to recent Irish documents (Office for Health Management 2002, Department of Health and Children/Dublin City University 2003), the emphasis should be on management development in the first place which can later be underpinned by theoretical principles. Although, this study did not involve the other lecturers in the department as co-researchers their support was sought. I was fortunate to have had autonomy in decision-making for the change planned. According to Cohen et al. (2000) action research nests comfortably within certain management styles. I believe that there is evidence of a participatory and transformational style of leading and managing in this study setting and this aided the satisfactory implementation of the change process to date.

The focus for educational providers should be to create nurse managers who can operate independently with confidence in today's health service environment. According to the Office for Health Management (2002) in developing nursing management programmes it is vital to centre on the value of people, inter-professional collaboration, team working, quality and continuous improvement. These are all characteristics that are consistent with the principles of the most recent Irish Health Strategy (Department of Health and Children 2001). The next step in the development of this management programme is to introduce inter-professional learning and collaboration. This is the way forward for management programmes and is in keeping with all recent Irish government documents. A strategy for education and development of nurse managers at all levels should be supportive in their quest to face a turbulent and uncertain future with confidence in themselves and their values.

References

Action Learning Associates (ALA) International Ltd (2002) *Introduction to Action Learning*. Available at: http://www. alaint.demon.co.uk/actionlearning.htm, accessed on 06/12/2002.

An Bord Altranais (1997) *Continuing Professional Education for Nurses in Ireland: a Framework*. An Bord Altranais, Dublin.

Bouldon G. (2002) Action learning. In *Business, the Ultimate Resource* (L. Carden ed.), pp. 12–13. Bloomsbury, London.

Carr W. & Kemmis S. (1986) *Becoming Critical: Education, Knowledge and Action Research*. Falmer Press, Sussex.

Centre for the Development of Nursing Policy and Practice (CDNPP) (2003) *Report on an Evaluation Study of the Leading and Empowered Organisation Programme (LEO) for Clinical Nurse Managers 1*, Office for Health Management, Dublin.

Coghlan D. & Brannick T. (2001) *Doing Action Research in your Own Organization*. Sage Publications, London.

Coghlan D. & Casey M. (2001) Action research from the inside: issues and challenges in doing action research in your own hospital. *Journal of Advanced Nursing* 35 (5), 674–682.

Coghlan D. & McAuliffe E. (2003) *Changing Healthcare Organisations*. Blackhall Publishing, Dublin.

Cohen L., Manion L. & Morrison K. (2000) *Research Methods in Education*, 5th edn. Routledge Falmer, London.

Cooper S. (2003) An evaluation of the leading an empowered organisation programme. *Nursing Standard* 17 (24), 33–39.

Council for Excellence in Management and Leadership (CEML) (2002) *Managers and Leaders: Raising our Game*. Available at: http://www.managementandleadershipcouncil.org, accessed on 21/3/03.

Davidhizar R. (1995) The seven S's for successful management. *Health Care Supervisor* 13 (1), 65–70.

Department of Health and Children (2001) *Quality and Fairness: a Health System for you*. Department of Health and Children, Dublin.

Department of Health and Children/Dublin City University (2003) *Nurses' and Midwives' Understanding of Empowerment in Ireland*, Final report. Department of Health and Children, Dublin.

Duffield C. (1991) Maintaining competence for first–line managers: an evaluation of the use of the literature. *Journal of Advanced Nursing* 16 (1), 55–62.

Eraut M. (1994) *Developing Professional Knowledge and Competence*. The Falmer Press, London.

Flanagan J. (1998) Achieving partnership: the contribution of nursing education and the production of a flexible workforce. *Journal of Nursing Management* 6 (3), 129–136.

Fox S. (1997) From management education and development to the study of management learning. In *Management Learning: Integrating Perspectives in Theory and Practice* (J. Burgoyne & M. Reynolds eds), pp. 21–37. Sage, London.

French P., Anderson J., Burnard P. et al. (1996) International comparison of baccalaureate nursing degrees: collaboration in qualitative analysis. *Journal of Advanced Nursing* 23 (3), 594–602.

Government of Ireland (1998) *Report of the Commission on Nursing a Blueprint for the Future*. The Stationery Office, Dublin.

Howley B. (1997) *An analysis of the continuing education/training needs of ward sisters 'a timely study'.* Unpublished MSc (Econ) Management of Care thesis. University of Wales College, Newport.

Jennings E. (1996) *Perceptions and evaluations of management courses by Irish nurses.* Unpublished MEd thesis. Trinity College, Dublin.

Joyce P. (2002a) Nursing management—an Irish perspective: challenges in the 3rd millennium. *All Ireland Journal of Nursing and Midwifery* 2 (5), 40–41.

Joyce P. (2002b) Shaping the future of nurse education in Ireland. *Nurse Educator* 27 (2), 68–70.

Lewin K. (1946) Action research and minority problems. *Journal of Social Issues* 2 (1), 34–46.

McCormack B., Kitson A., Harvey G., Rycroft-Malone J., Titchen A. & Seers K. (2002) Getting evidence into practice: the meaning of 'context'. *Journal of Advanced Nursing* 38 (1), 94–104.

McNiff J. (2000) *Action Research in Organisations.* Routledge, London.

Malby R. (1997) Developing the future leaders of nursing in the UK. *European Nurse* 2 (1), 27–36.

Margerison C. (1988) Action learning and excellence in management development. *Journal of Management Development* 7 (5), 43–53.

Mintzberg H. (1975) The manager's job: folklore and fact. *Harvard Business Review* July–August, 49–61.

Neubauer J. (1995) The learning network: leadership development for the next millennium. *Journal of Nursing Administration* 25 (2), 23–32.

Nursing Research and Development, Eastern Health Board (EHB) (1997) *Continuing Research Education Development (CRED).* Eastern Health Board, Dublin.

Office for Health Management (1998) *Stocktaking Results.* Office for Health Management Newsletter, Issue 5, p. 4.

Office for Health Management [on behalf of The High Level Group on Empowerment of Nurses and Midwives] (2002) *Guidance on the Commissioning of Nursing Management Development Programmes.* Front line and middle level managers, Office for Health Management, Dublin.

Pedlar M. (1996) *Action Learning for Managers.* Lemons and Crane in Association with Learning Company Project, London.

Reason P. & Bradbury H. (eds) (2001) *Handbook of Action Research.* Sage, London.

Revans R. (1980) *The Origins and Growth of Action Learning.* Chartwell-Bratt, London.

Schon D. (1983) *The Reflective Practitioner: how Professionals Think in Action.* Temple Smith, London.

Sullivan P., Baumgardner C., Henninger D. & Jones L. (1994) Management development: preparing nurse managers for the future. Part 1: Program model. *Journal of Nursing Administration* 24 (1), 32–38.

Williams S. (2002) *Characteristics of the Management Population in the UK: Overview Report for the Council for Excellence in Management and Leadership (CEML),* Available at: http://www.managementandleadershipcouncil.org, accessed on 21/3/03.

Williamson G. & Prosser S. (2002) Illustrating the ethical dimensions of action research. *Nurse Researcher* 10 (2), 38–49.

Zuber-Skerritt O. (1992) *Professional Development in Higher Education: a Theoretical Framework for Action Research.* Kogan Page, London.

Correspondence
Pauline Joyce
Faculty of Nursing and Midwifery
Royal College of Surgeons in
Ireland
123 St Stephens Green
Dublin 2
Ireland
E-mail: pjoyce@rcsi.ie

15

Triangulation as a Qualitative Research Strategy

*T*riangulation is an approach to research that uses a combination of more than one research strategy in a single investigation. Navigators use the term *triangulation* to describe a technique of plotting a position using three separate reference points. Navigators must know the exact location of a ship or plane at any given time. However, navigation is not an exact science, particularly when the vessel is moving. Imagine the difficulty of describing the exact location of a ship when it is in the deep ocean far from shore. The ship navigator takes a compass reading between the boat and one reference point, often a star. This reading makes it possible for the navigator to draw a line on a map. The navigator knows the position of the ship is somewhere on the line drawn; however, the position on the line is far from accurate. To increase accuracy, the navigator then takes a compass reading between the boat and a second reference point, often a second star. This reading makes it possible for the navigator to draw a second line on a map that intersects with the first. The intersection of the two lines, still not an exact point, provides a more accurate location of the boat. This second location is inaccurate because both the first compass reading and the second compass reading have a margin of error. To decrease the margin of error, the navigator takes another compass reading from a third reference point. The line from this reading intersects the previous two lines at the location of the boat, providing a more exact location. Just as the navigator increases the accuracy of the location of a boat by adding different compass readings, the researcher applying principles of triangulation to a study design adds new confidence to the reliability and validity of data.

Campbell and Fiske (1959) were the first to apply the navigational term *triangulation* to research. The metaphor is a good one because a phenomenon under study in a qualitative research project is much like a ship at sea. The exact description of the phenomenon is unclear. To gain clarity about the phenomenon, researchers study the phenomenon from a particular vantage point, from which they learn additional information about the phenomenon. However, the information at this point is not precise. Like navigators, researchers then move to a different vantage point to study the phenomenon. Information from the second vantage point provides additional data about the phenomenon, hence making the description clearer. A third vantage point makes the description of the phenomenon far clearer than either of the first two vantage points. As in compass readings, techniques of qualitative research have their margins of error. The goal in choosing different strategies in the same study is to balance them so that each counterbalances the margin of error in the other (Fielding & Fielding, 1989).

Proponents of triangulation recognize that application of multiple approaches to an investigation can improve reliability and validity of data because the strengths of one method may help to compensate for the weaknesses of another. The ultimate goal of triangulation is to "overcome the intrinsic bias that comes from single-method, single-observer, and single-theory studies" (Denzin, 1989, p. 313). Four types of triangulation for qualitative research have been described: (1) data triangulation; (2) investigator triangulation; (3) theory triangulation; and (4) method triangulation (Denzin, 1989). This chapter examines the four types of triangulation described by Denzin (1989). Mitchell (1986) and Denzin (1989) have also suggested a fifth type, multiple triangulation, whereby combinations of triangulation strategies are used. This is a complex approach, using a combination of two or more triangulation techniques in one study. For example, using multiple triangulation, the study design may include more than one data source as well as more than one researcher (Denzin, 1989; Polit, Beck, & Hungler, 2004).

CHOOSING TRIANGULATION AS A RESEARCH STRATEGY

Qualitative investigators may choose triangulation as a research strategy to ensure completeness of findings or to confirm findings (Campbell & Fiske, 1959; Miles & Huberman, 1989; Patton, 1983, Polit et al., 2004; Risjord, Dunbar, & Moloney, 2002). Ensuring complete and thorough findings provides breadth and depth to an investigation, offering researchers a more accurate picture of the phenomenon (Denzin & Lincoln, 1994). Further, triangulation approaches reveal the varied dimensions of a phenomenon and help to create a more accurate description (Fielding & Fielding, 1989). The metaphor of a group of visually impaired people describing an elephant based on the area they touch provides a good description of completeness. The person touching the trunk describes the elephant based on what that person feels. The person touching the foot provides a different description because of what he or she feels. The person touching the tail provides a third description. The most accurate description of the elephant comes from a combination of all three individuals' descriptions. None of the three alone is complete or accurate. Combining data from the vantage point of all three people results in a more complete and holistic description of the elephant.

Researchers might also choose triangulation to confirm findings and conclusions. Any single qualitative research strategy has its limitations. By combining different strategies, researchers confirm findings by overcoming the limitations of a single strategy (Breitmayer, Ayres, & Knafl, 1993). Confirmation occurs when investigators compare and contrast the information from different vantage points. Uncovering the same information from more than one vantage point helps researchers describe how the findings occurred under different circumstances and assists them to confirm the validity of the findings.

TYPES OF TRIANGULATION

*I*nvestigators have the option of using several different types of triangulation to confirm or ensure completeness of findings. The triangulation approach selected depends on the research question asked and the complexity of the phenomenon under study. When planning a study, researchers carefully consider the research methodology necessary to adequately answer a research question. Qualitative researchers may choose to use triangulation as a strategy in any investigation in which their goal is to provide understanding or to obtain completeness and confirmation. In designing their study, researchers may use data triangulation, methodological triangulation, investigator triangulation, and theory triangulation, or a combination. Each type of triangulation possesses both strengths and weaknesses. Table 15.1 illustrates the strengths and weaknesses of each approach. A discussion of each triangulation type follows.

Data Triangulation

Using data triangulation, researchers include more than one source of data in a single investigation. Denzin (1989) described three types of data triangulation: (1) time; (2) space; and (3) person. Researchers choose the type of data triangulation that is relevant to the phenomenon under study. Using *time triangulation*, researchers collect data about a phenomenon at different points in time. Time of day, day of week, and month of year are examples of times researchers would collect data for triangulation. Studies based on longitudinal designs are not considered examples of data triangulation for

TABLE 15.1 • Strengths and Weaknesses of Four Types of Triangulation		
Type of Triangulation	*Strengths*	*Weaknesses*
Data Triangulation	Extensive data Data convergence and divergence	False interpretation due to overwhelming amount of data
	Increased confidence in the research data	Difficulty dealing with vast amounts of data
	Creative, innovative ways of phenomena	Fitting qualitative data into a quantitative mold
Investigator Triangulation	Expertise of more than one researcher in more than one methodology	Investigator bias Disruptive during interview Potential disharmony based on investigator biases
	Decreased potential for bias	
	Increased credibility of findings	
Method Triangulation	Exposing different types of information that contribute to overall understanding of the research problem	Multimethod research is expensive Difficulty meshing narrative and numerical data
	Unique findings	
Theoretical Triangulation	Broader analysis of findings	Adds to confusion if conflicts due to theoretical frameworks
		Lack of understanding as to why triangulation strategies were used

Adapted from Thurmond, V. A. (2001). The point of triangulation. *Journal of Nursing Scholarship, 33*(3), 253–258.

time because they are intended to document changes that occur over time, rather than specific time intervals for data collection (Kimchi, Polivka, & Stevenson, 1991).

Space triangulation consists of collecting data at more than one site. For example, a researcher might collect data at multiple units within one hospital or in multiple hospitals. At the outset, the researcher must identify how time or space relates to the study and make an argument supporting the use of different time or space collection points in the study. For example, a researcher studying decision making on a nursing unit might collect data on six different nursing units to triangulate for space. The researcher might also collect data on each shift and on weekdays and weekends to triangulate for time. The rationale for using the various collection spaces and times is to compare and contrast decision making at each time and in each location. By collecting data at different points in time and in different spaces, the researcher gains a clearer and more complete description of decision making and is able to differentiate characteristics that span time periods and spaces from characteristics specific to certain times and spaces.

Using *person triangulation*, researchers collect data from more than one *level of person*, that is, a set of individuals, groups, or collectives (Denzin, 1989). *Groups* can be dyads, families, or circumscribed groups. *Collectives* are communities, organizations, or societies. Investigators choose the various levels of person relevant to the study. In the previous example of studying decision making on a nursing unit, the level of person might be individual nurses, the staff working on a given shift, or the staff assigned to a given unit. Researchers use data from one level of person to validate data from the second or third level of person. Researchers might also discover data that are incongruent among levels. In such a case, researchers would collect additional data to reconcile the incongruence.

Reising (2002) conducted a grounded theory study to explore the early socialization of new critical care nurses. She used data triangulation in her research by interviewing both critical care nurses and their preceptors regarding the experience of socialization to the critical care area. The interviews with the preceptors were conducted following the conclusions of data collection with the critical care nurses. This was done "to help clarify the orientation process from the preceptors' points of view" (p. 21). Person triangulation added to the trustworthiness of Reising's findings by confirming and clarifying data. Kan and Parry (2004) used data triangulation to investigate the types of nursing leadership that are used to overcome resistance to change in the hospital setting. Data sources for this study included nonparticipant observation, informal/unstructured and formal/semi-structured interviews, document analysis, and the Multifactor Leadership Questionnaire. Data triangulation added to the breadth and depth of the findings in this grounded theory investigation.

When carried out responsibly, data triangulation contributes to the rigor of a qualitative study. When planning a study, investigators should consider their data carefully. They should decide if time, space, or level of person is relevant to the data. They should plan to collect data from all appropriate sources, at all appropriate points in time, and from all appropriate levels of person. The result will be a broader and more holistic description of the phenomenon under study.

Methodological Triangulation

Qualitative researchers use methodological triangulation when they incorporate two or more research methods into one investigation. Methods triangulation can occur at the level of design or data collection (Kimchi et al., 1991). Method triangulation at the design level has also been called *between-method triangulation*, and methods triangulation at the data collection level has been called *within-method triangulation* (Denzin, 1989). Design methods triangulation most often uses quantitative methods combined with qualitative methods in the study design. Sometimes triangulation design method might use two different qualitative research methods. For example, Wilson and Hutchinson (1991) described how researchers might use two qualitative research methodologies, Heideggerian hermeneutics and grounded theory, in qualitative nursing studies. They explained that using two unique methods in one study can explicate realities of the complex phenomena of concern to nursing that might remain illusive if researchers used either method alone. "Hermeneutics reveals the uniqueness of shared meanings and common practices that can inform the way we [nurses] think about our practice; grounded theory provides a conceptual framework useful for planning interventions and further quantitative research" (p. 263).

When researchers combine methods at the design level, they should consider the purpose of the research and make a cogent argument for using each method. Also, they should decide whether the question calls for simultaneous or sequential implementation of the two methods (Morse, 1991). If they choose *simultaneous implementation*, they will use the qualitative and quantitative method simultaneously. In *sequential implementation*, they will complete one method first, then, based on the findings of the first technique, plan and implement the second technique. Using simultaneous implementation, researchers must remember that they must limit interaction between the two data sets during data generation and analysis because the rules and assumptions of qualitative methods differ (Morse, 1991, 1994). For example, it is usually impossible to implement qualitative and quantitative methods on the same sample. Qualitative methods require a small, purposive sample for completeness, whereas quantitative methods require large, randomly selected samples. In simultaneous triangulation, the qualitative sample can be a subset of the larger quantitative sample, or researchers might choose to use different participants for each sample. An exception occurs if the quantitative measure is standardized. In this case, researchers would have the participants in the qualitative sample complete the quantitative measure and then would compare the findings with the standardized norms (Morse, 1994). If the measure is not standardized, then researchers must use a sequential triangulation technique as well as a much larger sample for the quantitative measure.

Combining quantitative and qualitative data can be particularly valuable in providing detailed descriptions of phenomena. Combining methods once again provided a more complete understanding and description of the problem. Cavendish, Konecny, Luise, and Lanza (2004) used method triangulation in their study dealing with prayer, empowerment, and performance enhancement. In contrast, researchers using a sequential triangulation technique begin by collecting either quantitative or qualitative data. If substantial theory has already been generated about the phenomenon, if the researchers can identify testable hypotheses, or if the nature of the phenomenon is amenable to objective study, the investigation would begin with a quantitative technique. If there is no theory, the theory is not well developed, or the phenomenon is not amenable to objective study, researchers would begin with a qualitative technique (Morse, 1991). Researchers who begin a study with a qualitative approach do so to further explore unexpected findings following the completion of a quantitative analysis. A study might begin with a qualitative technique to generate testable hypotheses that a researcher will then study quantitatively.

Im, Lee, Park, and Salazar (2004) used sequential methods triangulation at the design level in an investigation exploring the cultural meanings of breast cancer among Korean women. This descriptive, longitudinal study used methodological triangulation to gather both quantitative and qualitative data regarding Korean women's breast cancer experience.

When combining research methods, it is essential that investigators meet standards of rigor for each method. Using qualitative methods, researchers should ensure sampling is purposive and should generate data until saturation occurs. Using quantitative methods, researchers should ensure sample sizes are adequate and randomly chosen. Theory should emerge from the qualitative findings and should not be forced by researchers into the theory they are using for the quantitative portion of the study (Morse, 1991). Likewise, investigators should appropriately use validity and reliability measures to ensure rigor of quantitatively derived data. Analysis techniques should be separate and appropriate to each data set. The blending of qualitative and quantitative approaches does not occur during either data generation or analysis. Rather, researchers blend these approaches at the level of interpretation, merging findings from each technique to derive a cohesive outcome. The process of merging findings "is an informed thought process, involving judgment, wisdom, creativity, and insight and includes the privilege of creating or modifying theory" (Morse, 1991, p. 122). If contradictory findings emerge or researchers find negative cases, the investigators most likely will need to study the phenomenon further. If knowledge gained is incomplete and saturation has not occurred, additional data collection and analysis should reconcile the differences and result in a more complete understanding.

In another study, Dreher and Hayes (1993) used methods triangulation at the design level to study the effects of marijuana use during pregnancy and lactation on children from birth to school age. The researchers planned to study two groups of Jamaican women: marijuana users and non-marijuana users. However, the tool they had expected to use had been developed in the United States and, thus, was culturally inappropriate to Jamaican society. Instead, the researchers used ethnographic interview and observation of Jamaican women to revise the tool for culture appropriateness. The ethnographic data helped the researchers refine the language and relevancy of the instruments and modify the manner in which the tool was administered. By administering the tool in a culturally appropriate manner, the researchers were able to elicit valid and reliable responses.

Using methods triangulation at the level of data collection, researchers use two different techniques of data collection, but each technique is within the same research tradition. In a qualitative study, researchers might combine interview with observation or diaries with videotaping. The purpose of combining the data collection methods is to provide a more holistic and improved understanding of the phenomenon under study. When combining methods at this level, researchers must first carefully consider the advantages and disadvantages of each method. Then, they should combine methods so that each overcomes the weaknesses in the other. For example, observation is an excellent technique for qualitative data generation. However, using observation, researchers cannot determine the reasons behind actions observed. Interview is an excellent method for determining reasons behind behavior. However, researchers can never be sure that individuals' actions mirror what they say they would do in an interview. By combining the techniques, investigators can see behavior in action and hear the participants describe the reasons behind behavior.

Miles and Huberman (1989) described methods triangulation at the data collection level as a state of mind. They suggested that a rigorous qualitative researcher automatically checks and double checks findings and uses multiple data generation techniques to ensure accuracy and completeness of findings. For this reason, many qualitative researchers do not specifically identify their use of triangulation when combining data collection techniques. However, designing qualitative research with multiple data collection methods requires careful planning. Researchers must carefully incorporate each data collection techniques into the research design and state the rationale for the use of each technique. They also should delineate the strengths and limitations of each technique. Researchers may not always create the design *a priori*. A study may begin with two data generation techniques, each designed to overcome the weaknesses of the other. After collecting data, the researchers may realize an additional limitation in the data. At this point, the researchers may add a third data collection technique to the design. For example, an investigator studying a phenomenon using interview and observation might realize that participants have sketchy memories of past experiences. To get a more accurate view of experiences that have occurred over time, the researcher might decide to add diaries to the research design.

Carr and Clarke (1997) reported using methods triangulation at the data collection level in their study on the phenomenon of vigilance in families who stay with hospitalized relatives. The researchers used informal, semi-structured interviews and participant observation of the caregivers to confirm and complete the data. The interviews provided insight into the caregivers' perceptions of what it meant to have the day-to-day experience of staying with a hospitalized relative. The investigators also observed the family members as they interacted with their relative to gain insight into patterns of interaction. Participant observation allowed the investigators to observe the environmental aspects of the client unit, relationships, processes, and events. The observational data confirmed the interview data; that is, observations confirmed families' verbalized commitment to their hospitalized relative. In their report, the researchers indicated that the combination of interview and observation data resulted in a more complete and holistic picture of vigilance than either method would have provided alone.

It is not an easy task to use methods triangulation; it is often more time-consuming and expensive to complete a study using methods triangulation (Begley, 1996). The study design is more complicated, complex, and difficult to implement, and imprecise use may actually increase error and enhance the weaknesses of each method rather than compensate for weaknesses (Fielding & Fielding, 1989; Morse, 1991). Often a single researcher is not expert in using more than one technique; consequently, investigator triangulation is required.

Investigator Triangulation

Investigator triangulation occurs when two or more researchers with divergent backgrounds and expertise work together on the same study. To achieve investigator triangulation, multiple investigators each must have prominent roles in the study, and their areas of expertise must be complementary (Kimchi et al., 1991). Having a second research expert examine a data set is not considered investigator triangulation. Rather, all researchers need to be involved throughout the entire study so they may compare and neutralize each other's biases.

The choice of investigators depends on the nature of the phenomenon under study. Research method, data generation technique, data analysis, or theory may drive the choice. For example, the use of multiple theories in a study directs the choice of investigators when researcher experts in parenting and researcher experts in homelessness collaborate to study what parenting means to homeless women. In this example, each investigator brings theoretical expertise to the study. Or, using methods triangulation, research method drives the choice of investigators—investigators expert in each method used in the study participate in the study. When each investigator participates fully in the investigation, his or her expertise contributes to every aspect of the study. Each investigator ensures that he or she has properly implemented the research method, data generation technique, or theory to formulate the ultimate study outcome. Then, all the investigators discuss their individual findings and reach a conclusion, which includes all findings.

Use of methods triangulation usually requires investigator triangulation because few investigators are expert in more than one research method (Oberst, 1993). Researchers experienced in each method need to collaborate to design and implement the study, particularly when combining qualitative and quantitative methods because the philosophical orientation and the requirements for rigor are so different between the two methods. An understanding of the phenomenon under study will increase as each researcher combines his or her differing perspectives and approaches. Through these collaborations, the researchers will synthesize new understandings and theories. It is vitally important that researchers representing each discipline approach the investigation with open minds. Ideally, each will come with his or her discipline-specific biases but, simultaneously, will be open to hearing other investigators' approaches. Open dialogue with articulation and acceptance of biases will result in unique understandings.

Woodhouse, Sayre, and Livingood (2001) applied the principles of investigator triangulation in their study on tobacco policy and the role of law enforcement in preventing tobacco use. During data analysis, two researchers worked simultaneously and separately to analyze interview data. This approach strengthened the reliability and validity of the findings.

Theoretical Triangulation

Theory triangulation incorporates the use of more than one lens or theory in the analysis of the same data set (Duffy, 1987). In a quantitative study, researchers identify two theories *a priori* and articulate rival hypotheses. Through the investigation, the researchers test and compare the rival theories. The result might be accepting one theory over the other or merging the theories to form a new, more comprehensive theory. In qualitative research, more than one theoretical explanation emerges from the data. Researchers investigate the utility and power of these emerging theories by cycling between data generation and data analysis until they reach a conclusion. By considering rival explanations throughout analysis of qualitative data, researchers are more likely to gain a complete or holistic understanding.

Lev (1995) used theory triangulation to investigate efficacy in clients who were receiving chemotherapy. The researcher triangulated the Orem's self-care theory and Bandura's self-efficacy theory because she believed neither theory completely explained efficacy in this client population. From the combined theories, the researcher designed an efficacy-enhancing intervention that she applied to clients who were receiving chemotherapy. The researcher implemented a combination of qualitative and quantitative methods to investigate the effectiveness of the intervention, using a form of methods triangulation at the level of data collection. Because the researcher used both theory triangulation and methods triangulation, the study is also an example of *multiple triangulation*, the use of more than one method of triangulation in a single study (Mitchell, 1986). Cavendish, Luise, Russo, and Mitzeliotis (2004) used multiple triangulation to describe nurses' spiritual perspectives as they relate to education and practice. Multiple triangulation included two data sources, two methodological approaches, and none investigators.

In another example of theoretical triangulation, Boutain (2001) combined critical social theories, African-American studies, and critical discourse concepts in her qualitative study on hypertension in rural south Louisiana. Her rationale was related to the fact that multiple perspectives intersect in the development of knowledge about African-American health.

Clearly, each type of triangulation has both strengths and weaknesses. As Boutain (2001) noted, "Appropriately used, triangulation might enhance the completeness and confirmation of data in research findings of qualitative research. The use of both quantitative and qualitative strategies in the same study is a viable option to obtain complementary findings and to strengthen research results. However, researchers must articulate why the strategy is being used and how it enhances the study" (p. 257).

SUMMARY

*T*riangulation is essentially a combination of methodologies used to study a particular phenomenon. Triangulation can be a useful tool for qualitative as well as quantitative researchers. Used with care, it contributes to the completeness and confirmation of findings necessary in qualitative research investigations. As researchers plan and carry out investigations, they should strive to provide the most complete understanding possible, using triangulation only when appropriate in their search for understanding. Nursing phenomena are complex and multifaceted. Clearly there are times when a multidimensional perspective will provide rich, unbiased data that are reliable and valid. This chapter has explored the various types of triangulation strategies that may be applied to a research study, their disadvantages, and their benefits. Ultimately, the fundamental design of the study must be strong.

Qualitative researchers should approach investigations with openness to philosophic approaches. If different philosophical and research traditions will help to answer a research question more completely, then researchers should consider using triangulation.

References

Begley, C. M. (1996). Using triangulation in nursing research. *Journal of Advanced Nursing, 24,* 122-128.

Breitmayer, B. J., Ayres, L., & Knafl, K. A. (1993). Triangulation in qualitative research: Evaluation of completeness and confirmation purposes. *Image, 25,* 237-243.

Boutain, D. M. (2001). Discourse of worry, stress and high blood pressure in rural south Louisiana. *Journal of Nursing Scholarship, 33*(3), 225-230.

Campbell, D. T., & Fiske, D. W. (1959). Convergent and discriminant validation by the multitrait-multimethod matrix. *Psychological Bulletin, 56,* 81-105.

Carr, J. M., & Clarke, P. (1997). Development of the concept of family vigilance. *Western Journal of Nursing Research, 19,* 726-739.

Cavendish, R., Konecny, L., Luise, B. K., & Lanza, M. (2004). Nurses enhance performance through prayer. *Holistic Nursing Practice, 18*(1), 26-31.

Cavendish, R., Luise, B. K., Russo, D., & Mitzeliotis, C. (2004). Spiritual perspectives of nurses in the United States relevant for education and practice. *Western Journal of Nursing Research, 26*(2), 196-205.

Denzin, N. K. (1989). *The research act: A theoretical introduction to sociological methods* (3rd ed.). Englewood Cliffs, NJ: Prentice Hall.

Denzin, N. K., & Lincoln, Y. S. (1994). Entering the field of qualitative research. In N. K. Denzin & Y. S. Lincoln (Eds.), *Handbook of qualitative research* (pp. 1-17). Thousand Oaks, CA: Sage.

Dreher, M. C., & Hayes, J. S. (1993). Triangulation in cross-cultural research of child development in Jamaica. *Western Journal of Nursing Research, 15,* 216-229.

Duffy, M. E. (1987). Methodological triangulation: A vehicle for merging quantitative and qualitative research methods. *Image, 19,* 130-133.

Fielding, N. G., & Fielding, J. L. (1989). *Linking data.* Newbury Park, CA: Sage.

Im, E., Lee, E. O., Park, Y. S., & Salazar, M. K. (2004) Korean women's breast cancer experience. *Western Journal of Nursing Research, 24*(7), 751-772.

Kan, M. M., & Parry, K. W. (2004). Identifying paradox: A grounded theory of leadership in overcoming resistance to change. *Leadership Quarterly, 15*(4), 467-478.

Kimchi, J., Polivka, B., & Stevenson, J. B. (1991). Triangulation: Operational definitions. *Nursing Research, 40,* 364-366.

Lev, E. L. (1995). Triangulation reveals theoretical linkages and outcomes in nursing intervention study. *Clinical Nurse Specialist, 9,* 300-305.

Miles, M. B., & Huberman, A. M. (1989). *Qualitative data analysis.* Newbury Park, CA: Sage.

Mitchell, E. S. (1986). Multiple triangulation: A methodology for nursing science. *Advances in Nursing Science, 8*(3), 18-26.

Morse, J. M. (1991). Approaches to qualitative-quantitative methodological triangulation. *Nursing Research, 40,* 120-123.

Morse, J. M. (1994). Designing funded qualitative research. In N. K. Denzin & Y. S. Lincoln (Eds.), *Handbook of qualitative research* (pp. 220-235). Thousand Oaks, CA: Sage.

Oberst, M. T. (1993). Possibilities and pitfalls in triangulation. *Research in Nursing & Health, 16,* 393-394.

Patton, M. Q. (1983). *Qualitative evaluation methods.* Beverly Hills, CA: Sage.

Polit, D. F., Beck, C. T., & Hungler, B. P. (2004). *Nursing research: Methods, appraisal and utilization* (7th ed.). Philadelphia: Lippincott Williams & Wilkins.

Risjor, M. W., Dunbar, S. B., & Moloney, M. F. (2002). A new foundation for methodological triangulation. *Journal of Nursing Scholarship, 34*(3), 269-275.

Reising, D. L. (2002). Early socialization of new critical care nurses. *American Journal of Critical Care, 11*(1), 19-26.

Thurmond, V. A. (2001). The point of triangulation. *Journal of Nursing Scholarship, 33*(3), 253-258.

Woodhouse, L. D., Sayre, J. J., & Livingood, W. C. (2001). Tobacco policy and the role of law enforcement in prevention. *Qualitative Health Research, 11,* 682-692.

Wilson, H. S., & Hutchinson, S. A. (1991). Triangulation of qualitative methods: Heideggerian hermeneutics and grounded theory. *Qualitative Health Research, 1,* 263-276.

16

Writing a Qualitative Research Proposal

The research proposal is essentially a formal request to conduct a study. Before beginning any research project, the central components of the study must be articulated in such a way that appropriate application of the method is clear to all who read the proposal. This writing process begins with clear articulation of the question followed by the problem and purpose statements, a review of relevant literature, and a detailed description of the planned study methodology. The proposal must communicate, in a formal manner, the critical material necessary for a review panel to grasp the scope and significance of the investigation. Additionally, the proposal is essential for the conduct and possible funding of any research project. Sandelowski and Barroso (2003) note that writing a proposal for a qualitative research study presents a dual challenge: the emergent nature of qualitative research design, along with the notion that methodology is very often a description of a process, to produce a process, can challenge the best researchers' writing skills (Sandelowski & Barroso, 2003).

This chapter explores issues related to development of a qualitative research proposal, elements of the research report, and challenges facing qualitative researchers. A discussion of the essential elements and philosophical underpinnings relevant to a qualitative research proposal are emphasized. An example of a funded qualitative proposal is included at the end of the chapter.

SELECTING AN AREA OF RESEARCH

Beck (1997) emphasized that "[a] productive research program for nurse scientists in both academic and clinical settings is critical to career advancement" (p. 265). Given the significance one's scholarly work can potentially have on a professional career, selecting an area of research must be guided by several factors. More important, one's career will be affected negatively if qualitative research is "poorly valued in university communities, where researcher prestige is given according to the number of research dollars obtained, not by the worthiness of the completed research and the impact it has on the discipline" (Morse, 2003a, p. 834). First and foremost, the researcher must be immersed enough in the nursing research literature to know what areas of research are more fully developed and where research is still needed. Because research in nursing is still evolving, many opportunities exist to select an area of interest and develop a research agenda that is relevant and that will make a meaningful contribution to nursing's substantive body of knowledge. Second, it is critical to select an area of research that is meaningful not only to the discipline but also to the researcher. One's research agenda should complement one's professional career in nursing practice, education, or administration. The effort needed and the significant amount of time required to develop a research agenda demand that the researchers become immersed in and feel connected to what they are doing. Boyd and Munhall (2001) articulate this position skillfully:

> On some level, most researchers settle on a research topic because of some personal reason. Even for the opportunistic researcher with an eye on funding priorities, personal interest is usually aroused with ties to the researcher as person. For the qualitative researcher, personal interest is a strategic tool in the research project; it provides the energy and the motivation to persevere with the challenges and tedium inherent in any scholarly work. More importantly, however, personal interest can position the researcher to attend to the phenomenon under study in a certain way; it establishes figure and ground for the research endeavor in what can be highly personalized ways that make the research a passion, a preoccupation, an intimate companion. (p. 615)

Additionally, establishing an area of research requires that the investigator confirm the significance of the problem and articulate not only why the study needs to be done but also why the study requires a qualitative format. This stage is complex and requires diligence and clarity of thought. The process is one that takes time and requires an ongoing process of evaluation. Reading, sharing ideas with colleagues, writing, and rewriting are all necessary aspects of the refinement of one's research agenda. When conducting a qualitative study for the first time, investigators inexperienced in this methodology should consider enlisting the help of a seasoned qualitative researcher to serve as a mentor during the development of a new project.

GENERAL CONSIDERATIONS

*I*dentifying a research agenda requires that the researcher clarify the problem or phenomenon of interest to be studied. Articulating the need for a particular study and articulating one's purpose will provide the appropriate direction needed to proceed with proposal development. Ideas must be logically developed and conceptually linked.

Determining scientific merit and quality of the proposal is guided by the researcher's ability to communicate the research paradigm and method. The conduct of any research study requires precision and rigor. The proposal must be clear, concise, and complete (Dexter, 2000). Knowledge of qualitative methodology, prior experience with the methodology, and availability of appropriate resources to successfully complete the study are important considerations. The extensiveness of a research proposal is essentially determined by its ultimate purpose. Variation exists depending on whether you are preparing a proposal for a dissertation, a grant, or an individual research project. For academics, guidelines can generally be obtained from the office of research services. If you are writing a grant proposal, then the granting agency's requirements determine how you prepare your materials. The content of the proposal must address all the stipulations set forth in enough depth to be meaningful, clear, and educational. To begin, it is helpful to prepare a basic outline or plan for the research idea. The detailed plan will then develop into a research proposal as each step in the outline is narrated and gaps are filled to illustrate logical and consistent expansion of an idea from question to answer (Brink & Woods, 2001).

Very often, members of Institutional Review Boards are grounded in quantitative research approaches. Therefore, the composition of the board may result in qualitative research proposals that face unnecessary obstacles. Qualitative research cannot be evaluated from a quantitative paradigm. This should be clear at this point in the textbook. The abstract nature of many qualitative approaches is so different from a qualitative worldview that the proposal will require excellent rationale and explanation of qualitative method applications. The proposal should be written in such a way that it provides enough theoretical support for the research paradigm so as to answer the questions of individuals reviewing the project who may not be familiar with qualitative approaches. The content of any proposal must always be written with the interest and expertise of the reviewers in mind. Morse (2003a) delineates criteria that could be used to evaluate qualitative proposals in terms of relevance, rigor, and feasibility. According to Boyd and Munhall (2001), when the *"guardians of the dominant paradigm"* (p. 614) are reviewing your qualitative research proposal, the readers should be provided with the following:

- Education about and description of the method from its aim to its outcome. Such detail also enhances confirmability by leaving a decision trail.
- Justification for using the method through a logically developed explanation of why the researcher has chosen to use it
- Translation of language unique to the method in terms that are likely to be understood by readers (p. 614)

The overall appearance of the proposal is an additional consideration. It is expected that the work is completed professionally. Therefore, in addition to clear and accurate content, the writer must also ensure that there are no spelling, punctuation, or grammatical errors. The document must be aesthetically appealing in addition to being described clearly (Dexter, 2000).

The reader will now be provided with an overview of the essential components of the research proposal. The detail needed to complete a written account of each aspect of the proposal can be found in method-specific chapters.

ELEMENTS OF THE RESEARCH PROPOSAL

*T*he purpose of the research proposal is similar for both quantitative and qualitative research paradigms; however, evaluation criteria used by review boards must be significantly different. The document must communicate to the reviewers the essential elements of the study in such a way that the study's purpose, method, data generation, and treatment strategies are clear and methodologically precise. Further, the document must communicate to the reader that the participants in the project will be protected from harm. An overview of each component of the proposal follows. Box 16.1 lists the elements that should be included in a complete proposal. As with any document, the writer should begin with an introduction and overview of the project.

Introduction and Overview of the Project

All research must begin with a judgment regarding the importance of the project to the development of knowledge in the discipline. Introducing the study requires identification of the *phenomenon of interest, the problem statement,* and *purpose.* The researcher must clearly describe the background

Box 16.1

Elements of the Research Proposal

The Introduction

1. Identification of the phenomenon or problem of interest
2. Statement of purpose
3. Rationale for research approach
4. Significance of the phenomenon to nursing

The Literature Review

1. Review of relevant theoretical and research literature
2. Discussion of literature review and how it will be used in the qualitative investigation

The Research Design

1. Introduce the research design (phenomenology, grounded theory, ethnography, action research, historical research)
2. Describe the philosophical underpinnings
3. List the procedural steps
4. Describe strengths and potential limitations of the design

Methodology

1. Researcher's role and credentials
2. Participant selection/sample
3. Gaining access, entering the setting for data generation
4. Protection of participants and ethical considerations relevant to qualitative inquiry
5. Data generation and treatment (process, data collector's training, data management, data analysis)

Discussion of Communication of the Findings

1. Within the proposal, briefly address how the findings will be addressed within the context of the literature review
2. Address rigor in relationship to the method
3. Discuss implications for nursing practice, education, and administration
4. What are the implications for future research?

References

Appendices

1. Consent forms
2. Any other relevant supporting documents

and significance of the project. Linking the proposed investigation to the current body of nursing knowledge adds to the development of the significance of the research for the discipline of nursing and verifies that what is currently known about the topic is insufficient, requiring additional investigation. The researcher must identify where gaps in the literature exist, how the study will potentially contribute to scientific understanding, and ultimately how our substantive body of knowledge regarding the topic will be advanced. "The onus is on the investigator to convince the reviewers that the project is vital for the advancement of their disciplinary goals" (Morse, 2003a, p. 837).

The *literature review* refines the questions and builds the case for the conduct of the study. It is important to prepare the literature review in a way that will familiarize the reader with the selected area of study. Additionally, this section of the proposal should clarify what is known about the phenomenon under investigation and the rationale for selecting a qualitative approach. Chapter 2 addresses issues related to the conduct of the literature review in a qualitative investigation. The discussion addresses the fact that often qualitative researchers do not begin with an extensive literature review to reduce the likelihood that researchers might bias their data collection or analysis through development of preconceived notions about the topic under investigation. Should the qualitative researcher choose to maintain this standard, then rationale should be provided for the reviewers. In any case, the researcher should include a cursory review of the literature. The goal of the literature review is the development of an argument backed by adequate evidence to create and support a clear purpose statement. The writing style must be compelling and convince reviewers that the study is critically needed (Penrod, 2003).

Research Approach

Following the study's introduction, it is important to discuss the rationale for selecting a qualitative format and the philosophical underpinnings that support the approach. Qualitative research approaches vary, and consequently the conceptual foundations that support the approaches vary as well. The underlying assumptions relevant to the qualitative approach selected must be described in detail. See Chapter 2 for a detailed discussion of how different qualitative approaches may be used to study particular phenomena.

Method

Once the phenomenon of interest has been fully described and the research approach selected, the investigator should then proceed with a detailed discussion of the actual application of the design. This is an essential component of the proposal, and it is critically important that this section "flow from the developed background and significance and that the methods be congruent with the desired product of the project" (Penrod, 2003, p. 825). Often, research methods are grounded in specific philosophical perspectives such as feminist inquiry or critical theory. When developing the method section, the researcher must make clear to the reader the philosophical underpinnings of the work. Discussion of the research protocol will ensure consistent application of the method. Decisions made related to method application are essential to the overall cohesiveness of the project. They culminate in a road map of how the study will be conducted. The method section should also address resources needed to conduct the study, such as time, money, and personnel.

Within the section addressing method, the strengths and weaknesses of the research design must also be addressed. A level of expertise in the application of qualitative methods is expected from the researcher and should be evident in a description of the researcher's credentials. If the individual is not a skilled qualitative researcher, then the mentor's credentials should be included. The emerging nature of a qualitative investigation also should be addressed. Explicit description of the philosophical stance guiding method application will enhance the credibility of the proposal. The researcher should also address the possibility that the study may need to be modified for implementation. The rationale for potential modifications must be provided (Sandelowski, Davis, & Harris, 1989).

In addition to the researcher's credentials, the proposal must include how participants will be selected, how the researcher will gain entry into the setting where data will be collected, and once there, how the rights of participants will be protected. "Threats to validity are addressed as potential limitations of the study to demonstrate the researcher's attention to methodological rigor" (Penrod, 2003, p. 825). For a detailed discussion of protection of human subjects and the ethical issues facing qualitative researchers, the reader is referred to Chapter 4.

Data generation and treatment in a qualitative investigation generally consist of in-depth interviewing. Often the interviews are tape-recorded and can range from very open-ended to very structured interviews. Data analysis techniques should be discussed along with issues related to how the researcher will ensure authenticity and trustworthiness of the data (see Chapter 4).

Protection of Human Subjects

Protection of human subjects is without question a critical component of any research study and must be addressed completely in the proposal. "The government's system for regulating research involving human subjects was born out of fear that researchers might, whether wittingly or not, physically or mentally injure the human beings that they study" (American Association of University Professors, 2001, p. 55). This report further notes that "IRB's, in carrying out their responsibilities, too often mistakenly apply standards of clinical and biomedical research to social science research, to the detriment of the latter" (p. 56). Protection of human subjects essentially ensures that participants are informed, that they consent to participation in the study, and that they are aware that they may withdraw from the study at any time. Although generally low risk, qualitative studies pose unique concerns for participants. These concerns are discussed in detail in Chapter 4. Because of the open-ended process of data collection used in qualitative research, interviews and observations may move in unanticipated directions. Therefore, informed consent takes on a new and different meaning when applied to qualitative studies as opposed to clinical or biomedical research. For this reason, Boyd and Munhall (2001) have suggested that qualitative researchers address the idea of *process consent* as opposed to *informed consent.* This essentially involves renegotiating informed consent throughout the study as data emerge and the research evolves. If the proposal author plans to use process consent, then this type of consent should be explained fully to proposal reviewers in terms of its definition and application.

Qualitative Research Findings

The proposal is prepared to gain permission to conduct a formal study and in some cases obtain funding for the research. Although the results cannot be addressed in the proposal, a brief discussion of why the findings will be important and how they will be used may be helpful in adding a sense of completeness to the proposal. Addressing how the results will ultimately be disseminated will strengthen the value of the research and its potential ability to contribute to nursing's substantive body of knowledge. Again, the writer must be sure to address the specific guidelines provided as they relate to the type of proposal being written.

Appendices and References

Appendices and references of the proposal should include an example of the consent form to be used as well as any other supplemental material to be included in the research. For example, if participants will be asked to write detailed responses to open-ended questions, the format and items to be included should be placed in the appendix. The reference list provided will verify the need for the study and will substantiate the researcher's expertise in the research area as well as the methodology planned.

SUMMARY

*T*he researcher completing a funding proposal for a qualitative study for the first time should be aware that despite precise attention to all the elements of the proposal, qualitative research is often reviewed by unqualified individuals (Morse, 2003b). Seasoned qualitative researchers continue to raise their voices about the injustices in a system that values measurement over understanding. To improve one's chances for funding, it is essential to search for organizations and agencies that have demonstrated a commitment to fund qualitative proposals so as not to spend protracted periods of time developing proposals that will not be supported.

This chapter has addressed issues related to the development of a qualitative research proposal. The fundamental elements necessary for proposal development are highlighted, along with some suggestions for avoiding roadblocks with Institutional Review Boards. Detailed discussions of all elements of the proposal are included within individual chapters of this book. Further, application is addressed in the sample grant found at the end of this chapter.

References

American Association of University Professors. (2001). Protecting human beings: Institutional review boards and social science research. *ACADEME* (May-June), 55-67.

Beck, C. T. (1997). Developing a research program using qualitative and quantitative approaches. *Nursing Outlook, 45*, 265-269.

Boyd, C. O., & Munhall, P. L. (2001). Qualitative research proposals and reports. In P. L. Munhall (Ed.), *Nursing research: A qualitative perspective* (3rd ed., pp. 613-638). Boston: Jones and Bartlett.

Brink, P. J., & Woods, M. J. (2001). *Basic steps in planning nursing research: From question to proposal.* Boston: Jones and Bartlett.

Dexter, P. (2000). Tips for scholarly writing in nursing. *Journal of Professional Nursing, 16*(1), 6-12.

Morse, J. M. (2003a). A review committee's guide for evaluating qualitative proposals. *Qualitative Health Research, 13*(6), 833-851.

Morse, J. M. (2003b). The adjudication of qualitative proposals. *Qualitative Health Research, 13*(6), 739-742.

Penrod, J. (2003). Getting funded: Writing a successful qualitative small-project proposal. *Qualitative Health Research, 13*(6), 821-832.

Sandelowski, M., & Barroso, J. (2003). Writing the proposal for a qualitative research methodology project. *Qualitative Health Research, 13*(6), 781.

Sandelowski, M., Davis, D. H., & Harris, B. G. (1989). Artful design: Writing the proposal for research in the naturalist paradigm. *Research in Nursing and Health, 12*(2), 77-84.

Funded Grant Proposal

Critical Care Air Transport Team (CCATT) Nurses' Deployed Experiences

Principal Investigator: Dremsa, Theresa L., Lt. Col., USAF, NC

Introduction

The Critical Care Air Transport Team (pronounced "c-cat") was designed to function as a component of the Aeromedical Evacuation System and extend the capabilities of aeromedical transportation of critically ill or injured patients (AFTTP-3, 2001). A typical CCATT mission consists of three to four hours of flight time and four hours of preparation (i.e. ground transportation, equipment checkout). The CCATT concept was developed as a result of transporting critically ill patients during Operation JUST CAUSE and DESERT STORM. In 1996, Wilford Hall Medical Center in San Antonio, Texas supported 25 "live patient" CCATT missions in the peacetime setting (Topley, et al, 2002). Now that our country is at war, since President Bush's declaration of war on terrorism (Cowley, 2001) the CCATT mission has changed. For the first time ever, CCATT team members are performing nursing care during war. Deployed locations include Southwest Asia in support of Operation Enduring Freedom, northern and southern Iraq, the former Yugoslavia and Afghanistan (Correll, 2002), exposing team members to a combat environment. The Critical Care Air Transport Teams (CCATT), composed of one critical care physician, one critical care nurse and one respiratory technician are designed to provide emergent and rapid transportation of the injured troops out of the combat areas and are attached to the deployed units. Throughout history nurses have shared accounts of the experience of combat exposure, but most have been anecdotal and acquired long after the exposure. Tapping into the knowledge gained from the experience of nurses performing patient care in the combat environment provides an opportunity to capture the experiential knowledge offered by nurses with this unique life experience. A previous research study captured the unique experience of CCATT nurses, contributing to the empirical knowledge base of the CCATT experience and delineated the scope of care and the knowledge necessary to provide In-flight patient nursing care for the critically ill and injured (Topley, et al, 2002). The current study extends the previous study to address the experience of nurses on the CCAT Teams deployed in support of troops taking part in armed conflict. This study will document the knowledge gained from the experience of providing patient care during war. As a result of knowledge gained, a Self-Assessment Measure to evaluate self-perceptions of readiness for deployment can be developed in future studies.

SPECIFIC AIMS

Purpose:

The purpose of this study is to describe Critical Care Air Transport Teams (CCATT) nurses' experiential knowledge when assessing and treating critically ill patients during transportation by fixed wing aircraft (Aeromedical Evacuation) in a forward deployed location with a potential risk for exposure to combat.

The specific aims of this study are to:

1) Describe CCATT nurses experiential knowledge in the care of patients when in a combat environment;
2) Distinguish salient features of CCATT nurses' knowledge of care of patients when in a combat environment and compare to critical care nursing during pre-war conditions,
3) Describe the collaborative relationships involved in providing nursing care in combat environment.

Research Questions

Collecting and analyzing these data will enable us to answer the following questions:

1) What are the characteristics of the combat environment?
2) How does the combat environment affect care?
3) What aspects of providing nursing care to critically ill patients are particular to this situation?
4) What do Air Force nurses do as part of their peacetime healthcare duties that they will also be required to do in a combat environment?
5) To what extent does traditional critical care nursing knowledge translate to the AE environment when exposed to combat conditions?

SIGNIFICANCE AND BACKGROUND

There is a paucity of literature available that addresses the experience of flight nurses during armed conflict. Therefore, excerpts of nurses' experience throughout history during armed conflict are provided as a means to provide examples of nurses' lived experiences while deployed. Nurses' deployed experiences provide a rich base for knowledge development on ways to best prepare personnel for

PHS 398/2590 (Rev. 05/01)

worldwide tasking. Numerous studies are available addressing nurses' experience in support of declared war (Barger, 1991; Concannon, 1992; Holm, 1982; & Norman, 1986). However, the great majority of nurses' experiences in the literature consist of anecdotal accounts or case histories (Martin, 1967; Holm, 1982; McVicker, 1985; Odom, 1986; Marshall, 1987; & Kassner, 1993). An increase in international conflict requires that Air Force nurses be prepared to deploy in support of any worldwide tasking at a moment's notice. Many fears and concerns come to the forefront of one's mind when faced with the practice of nursing in a foreign environment, an environment that lacks most of one's usual support systems such as family and friends. The following literature review is based on historical literature addressing nurses' military experiences since the Crimean War.

Historical Chronology

Crimean War. Florence Nightingale (1935) the mother of modern nursing addressed the shortage of supplies during her wartime experience in the Crimean war with letters addressed to her home country. She requested a colleague send "A Mackintosh sheet for a patient soiling the bed: - obtain one if you have not one - but send something immediately" (letter dated 17/7/77, Edwards, 1935). Nightingale appreciated a nurse's ability to improvise through her request to send "something" if unable to locate the desired item. Nurses' ability to adapt is a central theme throughout their wartime experiences. Nurses' accounts during the Civil War further portray this adaptability.

Civil War. Culpepper & Adams (1988) related nurses' versatility in the ability to provide nursing care in any situation. Nurses converted schools, churches, and makeshift structures into field hospitals. Corn shucks and stacks of straw were made into mattresses to provide a soft surface for their patients. Techniques were devised to avoid crawling insects by "placing the legs of the bed in cans of water" (p. 982). Nurses continued to have opportunities to adapt while serving in the military during World Wars I and II.

World Wars I and II. During World War I, nurses' assignment extended beyond the field hospital to serving on "troop trains and transport ships" (Holmes, 1982, p. 10). In World War II, forward thinking resulted in development of new postoperative care concepts that saved "countless lives" (Holm, 1982, p. 91). The inception of flight nursing added another dimension of nursing care during World War II. "As flight nurses, they provided care on air evacuation flights, a concept employed for the first time in World War II" (Holm, 1982, p. 149). The flight nurse experience provided a unique knowledge base for Barger (1991) to study nurses' coping strategies. Barger (1991) interviewed 25 flight nurses who served in World War II to identify coping behaviors and specific situations that necessitated coping. Specific situations identified were: (a) demands of living conditions, including communication, food, hygiene, living quarters, weather, insects, snakes and lizards; (b) care of sick and wounded patients on air evacuation missions with lack of supplies and equipment, patient safety, (c) demands of training, appearance and inactivity, (d) demands of spirit, personal concerns for family members back home and for those missing in action and the death of patients and colleagues. The overall response of women interviewed was a perception of their role during the war as a challenge, which allowed them to feel more confident in their abilities, less emotionally overwhelmed by their situation and more able to draw on available resources. This study provided some valuable data about those who successfully cope with great stress and yet, emerge with a sense of accomplishment and confidence. The stress nurses experienced during wartime taskings was even more profound during the Korean and Vietnam conflicts.

Korean and Vietnam Wars. Holm (1982) found the adage 'sink or swim' often applies to military nurses in operational field settings. She found that nurses were caring for battle casualties "within four days after the first U.S. troops landed in Korea" (p. 225). This was necessary the day after they arrived in country. Involvement in Southeast Asia continued to overwhelm nurses with horrifying experiences. Holm (1982) identified it was necessary for nurses to set up and operate field equipment. In addition, nurses were unprepared for what they would experience "nothing in training or experience of military nurses could have preconditioned them for the casualties encountered in the Vietnam War" (p. 226). McVicker (1985) described the horror of war during the Vietnam era, noting that nurses were largely unprepared for the kind of combat carnage they would witness. In addition, they were faced with an extreme lack of resources and limited supplies to provide nursing care. Odom (1986) addressed operational requirements and living conditions. He described the typical portable field hospitals provided by the military:

> we are practicing setting up and taking down expandables, which are metal boxes that become lab, OR, and x-ray facilities, and inflatables that make up the receiving area, postop ward, and holding units . . . We cleaned them up, hooked up the generator and got a latrine from the engineers . . . we have to carry all our water in"... most of the seven nurses assigned to the 18th are new to Vietnam... (p. 1035).

Marshall (1987) provided an introduction that revealed the horror facing young, inexperienced nurses tasked to care for soldiers injured in the Vietnam War:

> 60% of the Army nurses had less than two years of nursing experience; of this 60%, most had less than six months. Nor did the Army, or any branch of service, adequately prepare nurses for the carnage they would see in Vietnam... The country was small, and because Americans had an enormous number of hospitals, and because helicopters could transport the wounded to base camps in a matter of minutes, soldiers lived who, in earlier wars, would have died enroute. Even nurses with backgrounds in trauma surgery were unprepared for the kinds of injuries they saw. Traumatic amputations of one or more limbs were routine" (p. 7).

Norman (1989) did a qualitative study using phenomenology to examine the experiences of military nurses during the Vietnam War. Interviews were conducted with 50 women who served in Vietnam in the Army, Navy and Air Force Nurse Corps. Experiences shared by these nurses related to: (a) reasons for volunteering, (b) professional stresses and moral dilemmas or wartime nursing, and (c) positive aspects of service in the Vietnam War. Major factors that differed between groups of nurses were the year in which the nurse served in the war and the branch of service in which they served. "Flight nurses in the Air Force Nurse Corps had an experience different from that of Navy nurses who worked on hospital ships or Army nurses who worked in evacuation hospitals" (Norman, 1989).

Scannell (1992) used a phenomenological approach to study the lived experience of female military nurses who served in Vietnam. A constant comparative technique was used to extrapolate metathemes related to nurses' experiences. Seven metathemes were identified: (a) facing moral and ethical dilemmas, (b) giving of oneself, (c) improvising, (d) feeling out-of-place, (e) lacking privacy, (f) recreating home, and (g) bonding. This qualitative study provided a significant contribution to the developing body of knowledge about nurses during war and identified specific categories where educational preparation and supportive care for nurses was needed. Kassner (1993) reiterated the need for educational preparation and supportive care in Operation DESERT STORM.

Desert Storm/Desert Shield. Operation DESERT STORM in 1991 also generated stories of lived experiences. Kassner (1993) published, in a journal format, her story of deployed life in the desert. She related day-to-day occurrences from the initial tasking for deployment, through the lived experience of being stationed at a field hospital during the war, through her exuberant return home. She summarized by stating:

> Now two years later I am home and safe. I can say Desert Shield/Desert Storm was a positive experience. Going to Saudi Arabia gave me the opportunity to learn about field nursing, deployment and survival. Military nursing is a twenty-four hour commitment, with staffing shortages that seldom allow for extended participation in field problems. As part of Desert Shield/Desert Storm, I was able to learn first-hand the logistics and technicalities involved in deploying a hospital. I learned how to live and adapt to a field environment, how to shower in the cold and dark and how to wash sandy, filthy clothes in small pails of water...I became a stronger person; I witnessed a cohesiveness seldom seen in the modern world. I and the others in my unit (sic) had to depend on each other and work together as a team to survive in that frightful, desolate situation (pp. 87-88).

Concannon (1992) used a grounded theory approach to study nurses deployed in support of Operation Desert Shield/Desert Storm. Categories identified in her work included: camaraderie, mortality issues, patriotism, technical preparations, leadership, personal growth, morality, loss of identity, spiritual support, information seeking, support from home, military concerns, waiting, and feeling alone. The central themes of camaraderie, patriotism, and personal growth emerged as key concepts for a theory of the deployment experience. The categories are placed within the key themes and are related to central concepts of physical dimension, emotional dimension, and psychological dimension. Concannon's (1992) work is a very good initial effort toward development of a theory for a deployment experience. The work is limited by the small sample size and lack of diverse experiences.

West and Clark (1995) seized the opportunity to conduct oral histories of individual experiences from nurses redeploying from Operation Restore Hope in Somalia. The authors conducted 90 oral history interviews with Army Medical Department (AMEDD) personnel assigned or Professional Filler System (PROFIS) to the 86th Evacuation Hospital (Fort Campbell, KY) who served during the bloody urban operation in Somalia. They described the necessity for deployed ANC officers to adapt to the filth, difficult living conditions, blowing sand, and lack of supplies, discomfort and danger. They found that the need for flexibility and innovation was clear to the deployed nurses. Expecting that everything one has in peacetime will be there in an austere theater of operations is unrealistic. The authors concluded their synthesis of the oral histories by stating that, "An Army Nurse who deployed to the field must know basic soldier skills, such as use of weapons, personal defense, field craft, and how to provide nursing care to people of different culture with different values" (p. 183).

As well as physical problems, there are psychological concerns. Britt and Adler (1999) contributed an understanding of responses to deployment during Operation Provide Hope in Kazakhstan. Responses included stress, isolation, and the use of a variety of coping mechanisms. Well known for their work in the psychological literature, Rosen, Weber, and Martin (2000) studied 1,060 male and 305 female soldiers in Army support units, investigating the experience of deployment. Respondents in their study voiced operational stress, job stress, and the influence of organizational unit climate in moderating the operational and job stressors.

Conclusion of the Review of Literature. Holm (1982) recounted nurses' experiences on the battlefield throughout history. Holm's (1982) work is an excellent historical presentation of nurses' comments related to war. As presented, several authors address nurses' recapitulation of experiences in Vietnam and Desert Storm. All are related to nurses' experiences during wartime scenarios. Unfortunately, outside of the anecdotal accounts, the literature reveals limited research studies pertaining to nurses' experience with deployment. Central themes that emanate from the anecdotal accounts throughout history as a result of nurses' experience during war include adaptability under stress, ability to improvise with limited resources, flexibility, resilience, versatility, and ability to perform under intense pressure. Similar themes in addition to new responses related to the present operational environment are expected in the current study.

Current Aeromedical Evaluation System

The current study will specifically focus on nurses' experience with deployment as a member of a CCATT. The CCATT members are attached to Aeromedical Evacuation units for transport of the critically ill patients to definitive care. The Aeromedical Evacuation (AE) mission provides air transport to a broad spectrum of patients under medical supervision, while delivering optimal care in a dynamic environment. A typical aeromedical evacuation crew consists of two flight nurses and three medical technicians. This crew is responsible for up to 113 patients on some types of aircraft. The majority of patients transported on routine aeromedical evacuation flights are ambulatory and stable litter patients who need little in the way of specialized or critical care. The CCAT Teams were established to provide specialized care to the critically ill when needed. The American Association of Critical Care Nurses (AACN) has defined flight nursing as a critical care component, supporting the same aspects of critical care as stated by AACN's scope of practice in the areas of patients, environment, and practice (Bader, Terhorst, Heilman, & DePalma, 1995). Dyer (1990) states that the mission of a critical care transport team is to "assess, stabilize, and prepare the patient for transport while in the referring hospital promoting and uneventful transfer". The ultimate goal of patient transfer is to move a patient to a facility that will be able to provide more extensive care or additional services that will enhance patient care (Connolly, Fetcho, & Haheman, 1992).

Critical Care Air Transport Team Concept

Since its inception in 1994 the CCATT has met the ever-changing requirements of this dynamic patient care environment. The CCATT, designed to function as a component of the Aero-medical Evacuation System, extends the capabilities of aeromedical transportation of critically ill or injured patients. The Air Force shift to an expeditionary warrior frame of mind and creation of the Aerospace Expeditionary Forces (AEFs) resulted in rotational deployment of teams on operations in support of national military strategy (Air Force Link, 2002). Fifteen (15) CCATT Teams deployed between October 2001 to March 15 2002 and 11 CCAT Teams were deployed from April to June 2002. The role of CCATT members is to prepare the patient for flight, monitor and intervene as necessary during flight, and maintain continuity of care. Each team consists of a physician, a nurse and a respiratory therapist. Experienced physicians and nurses from the emergency department and critical care units are eligible for CCAT Teams.

Wilford Hall Medical Center continues to take the lead on the implementation of the CCATT concept for the active duty, Air Force Reserve and Air National Guard. There remains little literature describing the CCATT experience due to the unique nature of the CCATT concept, especially related to deployment in the current operational environment following the declaration of war or terrorism. As a result, developing the role of the CCATT nurse is difficult. The nurses' role as a team member deployed to forward locations during armed conflict clearly extends beyond that of a typical critical care unit nurse or a flight nurse. Thus it is extremely important to study the skills, knowledge and scope of care provided in this unique wartime practice environment.

Scope of Care

Specific standards of care and certification examinations have been developed for flight nurses over the last 30 years. The National Flight Nurses Association has published practice standards, recommendations, and essential topics to be included in flight training programs (Stanley, 1987; Holleran, 1996). The flight nurse continuously assesses the patient's airway, breathing, and circulation and intervenes if indicated when transporting critically ill or injured patients. Environmental conditions such as noise, vibration, decreased humidity, extreme temperature changes and lack of light challenge the nurse's assessment skills. Such an environment can hinder a critical care nurse in giving patient care, if that nurse has not been trained to function in a transport environment. The previous research study on the experience of the CCATT nurse generated several studies contributing to recommendations for practice (Topley, D., Schmeiz, J., Henkensius-Kirshbaum, J. & Horvath, K; 2002).

Qualifications/Training

As a CCAT Team member deployed to forward locations exposed to armed conflict, the critical care nurse must perform at a level higher than in the typical peacetime CCATT missions or critical care environment. In addition to exceptional clinical expertise, a CCATT nurse must demonstrate extraordinary leadership and decision-making skills. Flexibility, adaptability, resilience to undue stress and sensitivity to team communication are vital to a successful transport team when deployed in a forward location that has the potential for exposure to armed conflict.

Due to the current international climate, with conflicts occurring simultaneously throughout the world, deployments in support of the war on terrorism occur frequently, and are very much a part of the future for Air Force nurses. It is imperative that a study of nursing experiences be accomplished to guide recommendations that will better prepare nurses to deploy at a moment's notice. Phenomenology, a qualitative research methodology, is the ideal technique to study the lived experience of CCATT nurses on deployment. This research method "focuses on describing subjects' lived experience as they interact with their environment" (Beyea & Nicoll, 1997, p. 323). Knowledge gained from nurses' lived experience of CCATT nurses in the deployed setting during a real world war experience will be used to develop a tool for self-assessment of readiness for deployment in addition to clarification of core competencies for CCATT nurses.

The participant becomes a co-researcher in phenomenology, and must engage in "cooperative dialogue" with the researcher (Knaack, 1984, p. 110). The truth exists in the context of the environment in which it occurs for each individual (Kikuchi, Simmons, & Romyn, 1996). The researcher seeks to discover this truth through research questions that encourage individuals to describe their everyday lived experience. "Typically, this information is collected through long interviews with informants ranging in number from 5 to 25" (Creswell, 1998, p. 54). Benner's (1994a) method for analysis of qualitative data is ideal for obtaining experiential knowledge of CCATT nurses in the care of critically ill or injured patients in a deployed setting at risk for exposure to combat conditions. The strength of Benner's method is the opportunity to identify competencies from actual practice situations while CCATT nurses are in the deployed setting rather then obtaining information from experts who set up training but may not have the experience so uses hypothetical situations. Interview transcripts are read several times, reinforced with field notes and group discussion of narrative by participants. There is a systematic attempt to go between parts and the whole of the experience for clarification. The advantage of this method allows actual performance demands, resources and constraints to be described and results in a rich description of nursing practice as a CCATT nurse deployed to a real world war time environment. The previous study on the CCATT nursing experience, which compared the CCATT experience to usual critical care nursing in a hospital setting, also employed Benner's method of qualitative analysis. Therefore, the research team will be able to compare findings of the current study with that of the previous study of the CCATT nursing experience in a non-deployed setting.

PRELIMINARY STUDIES/PROGRESS REPORT

LtCol Dremsa has extensive experience in instrument development and psychometric evaluation of reliability and validity. Her Development and Psychometic Evaluation of the Readiness Estimate and Deployability Index Short Form (READI-R-AFN [SF]) was a result of rigorous development and testing. LtCol Dremsa expanded Reineck's (1996) qualitative approach, which involved focus group methodology to clarify the concept of individual readiness (IR). The original process of conceptualization involved use of three expert focus groups comprised of Army nurses from a broad range of duty positions, readiness experience and geographical locations were included to discuss the meaning of individual readiness. Six dimensions of individual Readiness are as follows: Clinical Nursing Competency, Operational Competency, Soldier/Survival Skills, Personal/Psychosocial/Physical Readiness, Leadership and Administrative Support and finally Group Integration and Identification. Specific subsections of the READI (Reineck, 1998) were revised with the assistance of nurses experienced in Air Force deployment missions. The instrument was modified to produce an instrument that appropriately samples the content domain of the construct of interest (in this case, 'perceived state of readiness in Air Force nurses'), and which was found acceptable in terms of its language and physical characteristics. Items in several dimensions were expanded and standardized for uniformity as part of the ongoing development process of the READI-R-AFN. Phase I (Pilot Study) of the READI-R-AFN was based on responses from 181 active duty Air Force nurses. A confirmatory factor analysis of the READI-R-AFN through structural equation modeling techniques (Stevens, 1996) showed every subscale had internal consistency reliability ≥ 0.71 and factor loadings $> .45$ for all items. Based on evaluation of reliability and validity estimates the original 83-item READI-R-AFN was revised to a more efficient 40-item READI-R-AFN Short Form [SF] version, which was tested, based on responses of 205 active duty Air Force nurses. Results of the READI-R-AFN [SF] (Collins-Dremsa, 2001) 40-item version of the READI-R-AFN [SF] show that the initial 6 subscales identified in the READI (Reineck, 1998) were confirmed in this sample of active duty AF nurses. Phase III of the study was conducted to evaluate the READI-R-AFN for its sensitivity to intervention and further add to the construct validity of the measure by administering it to nurses attending the CCATT and EMEDS courses conducted at Brooks AFB, TX. Resulting Change scores were significant in all subscales except the Personal/Physical/

Psychological (PPP) in both groups and the Group Identification and Integration (GII) subscale in the CCATT group. This previous work of LtCol Dremsa shows an increased awareness and expertise in assessing readiness for deployment which lead to the current study of raising questions pertaining to the experience of CCATT nurses in the deployed setting during wartime. LtCol Dremsa has not previously been involved in qualitative work, therefore the current study will provide the opportunity to participate in the conceptual phase of instrument development through conducting the qualitative approach to item generation. In support of this process, LtCol Dremsa has built a research team with experience in the proposed method, expertise in qualitative research and an understanding of the CCATT team preparation and readiness mission. The proposed qualitative study represents personal development in the initial process of instrument development. In addition the revised READI-R-AFN [SF] which is shown to be a reliable and valid instrument for assessing nurses' readiness for deployment will be used for construct validation of an instrument to be developed as a self-assessment of CCATT nurses' readiness for deployment.

The current study is an extension of the original study conducted of CCATT nurses under non-wartime conditions. Dr. Schmelz was a key investigator in the original descriptive, exploratory design using qualitative methods to interview CCATT nurses to describe the practical knowledge possessed by registered nurses that are part of the Air Force's Critical Care Air Transport Team (CCATT). He brings the expertise in the use of Benner's (1996a) qualitative method to distinguish salient features of CCATT knowledge as compared to critical care nursing in the hospital. In the previous study, four major themes developed from the data. The knowledge embedded in CCATT nursing included: Preflight Preparation, In-flight Assessment and Environment, Characteristics of CCATT Nurse and Hospital vs In-flight Nursing Practice. CCATT nurses improvise, and provide nursing care based on past experiences using a broad critical care knowledge base. This has led to the development of a unique body of knowledge for nursing care in peacetime operations (Schmelz, Bridges, Duong, & Ley, 2002; Bridges, Schmelz, & Mazer, 2002; Schmelz, Stone, Johnson, Sylvester, Bridges, O'Toole, & Meade, 2000; Bridges, Schmelz, Stone, Sylvester, O'Toole, E., & Johnson, 2000). The areas of assessment and preparation described by the CCATT nurses can serve as a template for the Air Force's CCATT training program and CCATT orientation checklists. The current study represents a replication of the previous study with additional components to capture the wartime mission.

LTC (Ret) Agazio has specialized in primarily qualitative methods and triangulation. Past research activities and publications include her qualitative descriptive research of families receiving home care nursing for technology-dependent children and with Korean-American families to identify childrearing practices and beliefs. She recently completed two funded studies using integrated methods of survey and interviews on health promotion in active duty women and the effects of separation upon families during hospitalization. LTC (Ret) Agazio broadened her qualitative experience with a more recent study that used a combination of individual interviews and focus groups to describe nursing in a

TriService environment. While her previous research has primarily used content analysis, her most recent involvement as a co-investigator in a grounded theory study of e-mail as a management tool in Army nursing provided more expertise in qualitative research. She has received training in the use of Ethnograph and Atlas-ti, qualitative analysis software programs, and with added QSR Nudist expertise in the e-mail study. Additionally, due to her previous integrated methods studies, she is well-versed in National Computer System and Teleform packages for design, scanning, and form management for exporting into SPSS for Windows.

LtCol Evers is currently the Director of the Critical Care Air Transport Team (CCATT) Course at the USAF School of Aerospace Medicine at Brooks AFB, Texas. LtCol Evers has taught the CCATT Team since 2001 and is well-versed in preparations required for all CCATT Missions. LtCol Evers expertise on this study will contribute to the interpretation of findings with ongoing data analysis following interviews with the participants and focus groups.

LtCol Schaffer is on location at Keesler AFB MS to facilitate the process of individual and focus group interviews at that site since Keesler is second to Wilford Hall in providing Critical Care nurses for CCATT missions.

In summary, this research project team has considerable experience in the content area and methods required for carrying out this proposed project and have demonstrated that they are able to develop a critical idea into a credible program of research. Additionally, they have received the support of key positions in the Air Force Nurse Corps to facilitate the conduct of this project.

RESEARCH DESIGN AND METHODS

This study is exploratory and descriptive using Benner's (1994a) Interpretive Phenomenological Method. In a practice discipline such as Nursing, the distinction and relationship between theoretical and practical knowledge is indispensable (Benner, 1983; Dreyfus & Dreyfus, 1986; 1996). Theory, which strives for generalizability in context-free situations, cannot fully explain phenomena where human meaning is a concern. Interpretive phenomenology (Benner, 1994a) is a research method that recognizes the social embeddedness of knowledge in the realm of human experiences and concerns. It provides a means to understand subjects' perceptions, concerns, and judgments in the practical (experimental) world of context-specific situations (Benner, 1994b). The intent is to describe the practical knowledge of expert nurses in the care of critically ill patients as a member of the CCATT deployed to a forward location, with potential exposure to armed conflict. The outcome desired by this study is to develop items to use in conjunction with the current checklist designed prepare CCATT nurses to deployment. The thematic analysis uses low-inference descriptors, often verbatim statements, that capture in particular aspects of experiential knowledge that can serve as item statements. The items will be incorporated into a Self-Assessment CCATT Deployment Survey that will be refined and tested in future studies to systematically identify areas of strength and areas in need of change of the preparation of the CCATT nurse for deployment to forward combat locations.

PHS 398/2590 (Rev. 05/01)

The Commanders and Chief Nurse Executives in selected Medical Centers and Medical Treatment Facilities (MTFs) will be consulted for access to their organization for this research. Upon approval of the study by the institutional review boards (IRB) at WHMC and Keesler AFB, an estimated 12 participants will be recruited from a list of nurses who have deployed with CCAT Teams to forward deployed locations since the declaration of war on terrorism, September 11, 2001. Phenomenology results in rich, thick, contextual descriptions of experiences illuminate the desired phenomenon (Moustakas, 1994). "Data generation or collection continues until the researcher believes saturation has been achieved" (Streubert & Carpenter, 1995, p. 44). Data saturation is realized when there is repetition of data elements. For purpose of this study and requested funding, rich descriptions from 12 to 25 participants will provide the foundation for the study of experiences of nurses deployed as a member of the CCATT Teams to forward combat locations. Twelve to twenty-five participants will provide comprehensive descriptions to study the phenomena of a CCATT forward-deployed experience. Participants must be able to speak English, and be willing to share their experience in a tape-recorded interview. The Flight Commander from the Critical Care Units at each facility will assist with identification of participants who have experienced deployment as a CCATT member to a CCATT member to a forward-deployed location and would be willing to share their experience.

Demographic information about the sample will be collected in order to assist the reader to make a judgment about the transferability of results (Sandelowski, 1986). In addition to individual Interviews, a methodology outlined by Benner (1985; 1987; 1994a, b) will be incorporated. Since this study is intended to describe Nursing expertise or knowledge (not role function), it is not appropriate to include other members of the team (e.g. physicians).

Ethical Considerations Ethical considerations are of primary importance when doing qualitative research, since data will be collected through tape-recorded interviews. Anonymity for informants is not an option, thus, all efforts to maintain confidentiality are essential. In addition, Informants will be reassured audiotapes and videotapes are destroyed once the interview is transcribed and verified by the principal investigator. Another consideration pertains to the culture of the military environment, since the principal investigator is a field grade military officer, informants may feel 'coerced' to participate. It will be stressed with informants that participation is strictly voluntary. It will be stressed that the researcher does not fall in their chain of command, so they have no obligation to participate if they do not wish to do so. The researcher will accomplish data collection wearing civilian clothing during the data collection process, introducing herself using her civilian title to avoid any sense of coercion by informants. Also, the researcher will stress the study is designed to gain information that will help improve future deployment preparation procedures.

Data Collection Data will be collected via five methods: group interviews where nurses describe the written narratives and other incidents in the care of critically ill patients during air transport in forward deployed locations; individual interviews of CCATT nurses who have deployed to forward locations on CCATT missions; written narratives by CCATT nurses who have returned from a deployment; participant observations of at least four (3) CCATT nurses in a deployed location; and review of in-flight documentation of care. Multiple methods of data collection will help to correct for the threats to validity posted by any one of the above methods, such as observer bias or individual preconceptions (Mitchell, 1986; Duffy, 1987). Unobtrusive measures such as review of documentation can add to the understanding of the phenomena without placing additional strain on either patients or nurses.

At the time of each interview, willingness to participate will be reaffirmed and a written and verbal explanation of the procedure will be provided. All participants will be assured that their identities will not be disclosed in any reports. The procedures will be explained to each informant and consent forms will be signed. Demographic data will be completed prior to the tape-recorded interview. Each participant will then be asked: What was your experience while on deployment? Each interview will be tape-recorded for approximately 60 to 90 minutes. The researcher's role is to be an active listener, nodding or using "ahs" to encourage the participant to continue to explicate the meaning of the experience for them. The goal is to discover the reality of the subjective experience for each individual. "Reality exists only in the context of a mental framework (construct) for thinking about it" (Guba, 1990, p. 25).

A professional transcriptionist (preferably a court reporter) will record and transcribe all interviews. A tape-recording will serve as back up for transcribing within 24 hours of each interview, if necessary. The researcher will listen to each tape and match it up with transcribed notes for verification of the transcription. Once transcription is verified, the audiotapes will be destroyed and transcribed interviews will be maintained in a locked filing cabinet located in the researcher's office.

Narratives or stories provide a means for the participant to get situated in the context of an actual patient situation (Benner, 1994a). The participant structures his/her own account of the clinical situation and can tap into the immediate experience rather than use hypothetical cases or non-specific generalizations. In addition, individual case studies have been suggested as the most valid and ethical means of investigating problems in the patients at high risk of complications (Watson, 1993). Each participant will be asked to write one narrative following the guidelines shown in Appendix A, which are intended to help the participant explore all aspects of the clinical situation. The participant will be told that this written narrative will be shared in a group discussion with other experienced nurses where this and other stories will be shared. The text of each subject's narrative will be read into the recording equipment during the group interview stage that the information will be included in the transcripts for consideration during data analysis.

Sharing the narratives in a group interview provides a naturalistic setting similar to the dialogue nurses might have on a unit when engaged in patient care. Through the discussion, nurses can confirm common perception and challenge each other's understanding of the situation. As nurses respond to each other with similar and dissimilar accounts, a discourse in practical reasoning is worked out (Benner, 1994b). The group format helps to correct interviewer and individual preconceptions of what is salient and thus provide clarity and confidence in the practical knowledge of the participant. The investigator takes a stance of active and open listening, soliciting specific details to get a thick description of the nurses' practice.

For the purpose of sharing the narratives, participants will be divided into two groups. Each group will meet three times for two hours each session. The investigators and an expert in focus group interviews will facilitate group discussion. The principal investigator will attend all sessions. Subsequent discussion of the group facilitation among the investigators will provide a means to validate impressions and observations of non-verbal behavior. The discussion will be taped for later transcription and data analysis by the four investigators. Data analysis for the first group will begin prior to collecting data from the second group in order to identify themes or lines of inquiry that need more exploration.

Participant observations will be conducted in order to identify practices that are so commonplace they may go unnoticed by the nurses themselves. A sub sample of three nurses in a deployed location will be observed in their practice on one occasion each. The same process noted above will be followed in the deployed setting. It is critical that interviews be conducted in the Theater of Operations to provide an opportunity to observe what is taking place in the field. The principal investigator will collect the data during the participant observation section. All CCATT missions are considered emergencies. Following the observation period, the investigator will conduct a 30-minute individual interview to corroborate both the observation and earlier data. Previous studies have found these time frames to be both sufficient and realistic (Benner et al, 1992; Topley, Schmelz, Henkensius-Kirshbaum, & Horvath; 2002). The questions on the interview guide were developed from practice issues identified in the literature. The interview guide will be piloted prior to use in the study. In addition, as the data are analyzed, revisions in the interview guide will be made as needed in order to explore particularly relevant themes or issues that were not recognized initially.

The individual interview provides an opportunity to ask additional questions that might have been missed in the group interviews and therefore the observation will commence after the completion of data collection from the second series of group sessions. Repeated engagement enables the researcher to correct misinterpretations and to feel more confident that the data collected are representative of the phenomena of concern.

The following diagram (next page) illustrates how the data collection will proceed using the following procedure.

Data Analysis

Data analysis will begin concurrently with collection of data from second session of each group, allowing an opportunity to follow-up on inadequately explored issues and concerns from the first session. Interpretive phenomenology, also known as Heideggerian hermeneutics, will be employed to identify recurring themes and patterns of meaning (Benner, 1994; Diekelmann, 1992). This method has been used successfully in other studies of expert nurses' practical knowledge (Brykczynski, 1989). The investigators will conduct the interpretation. Utilization of

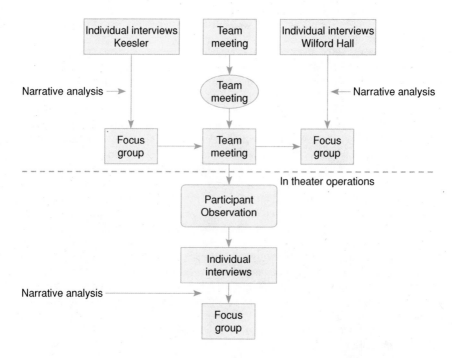

Co-investigators allows peer checking to occur as the interpretation evolves, thus helping to identify potential biases and to confirm interpretations (Lincoln & Guba, 1985; Benner, 1994). In addition, examples of the interpretation will be shared with the CCATT nurses who meet the inclusion criteria but who do not participate in the study in order to provide further validity for the data interpretation (Goodwin & Goodwin, 1984; Lincoln & Guba, 1985). The QSR (NVivo) software program will be used for technical assistance (Diekelmann, Schuster & Lam, 1994).

The following diagram (next page) illustrates the iterative nature of the data analysis process. The process is described in detail below.

Three narrative strategies will be used as the basis for identifying and describing nurses' practical knowledge: paradigm cases, thematic analysis and exemplars (Benner, 1985; Benner, 1994). A paradigm case is a strong instance of a pattern of meanings that illustrates well the themes it encompasses. Working from the whole, the investigators will get a global understanding of the story and grasp the contextual meaning before identifying topics, issues and concerns in more detail. Systematic moving from the parts back to the whole allows for understanding incongruities and unifying concerns that were repeatedly expressed by the expert nurse participants. The investigators will note the stories that are frequently told because they convey important meanings and lessons, but because they also

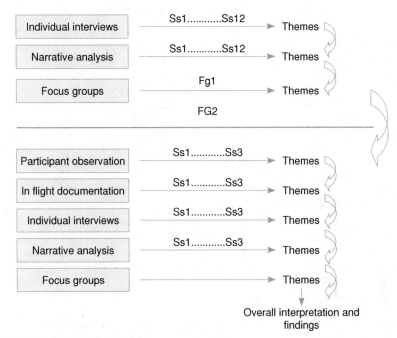

convey multiple layers of social constructions, they will be distinguished from the first-told stories that are closer to the lived experience. The researchers will also clarify why they chose a particular case as a paradigm, e.g. one they understand well or one that is puzzling or unsetting.

As subsequent paradigm cases are discussed, the following questions are posed by the investigators to extend the interpretation of the data (Benner, 1994): How would the event unfold in another situation?" "What would happen if the context were different?" "Would the same issues and concerns show up for two different cases?" "What events, concerns and issues show up in some paradigms that do not show up in others?"

Thematic analysis is done across cases to clarify common meanings and qualitative distinctions. The interpreter moves back and forth between themes in the text and the evolving analysis and from themes to paradigm cases to uncover inconsistencies and new questions. Low-inference descriptors will be used to stay close to the textual data, to avoid theoretical preconceptions, and to enable the reader to better judge the transferability of results to other settings.

An examplar is "a strong instance of a particularly meaningful transaction, intention, or capacity" (Benner, 1985, p. 10). Exemplars are excerpts of the data text that convey aspects of a paradigm case or a thematic analysis. They allow the researcher to demonstrate intentions and concerns within context where objective attributes of a situation might be different. For example, this study is exploring nurses' practical knowledge of critical care during air transport while in a forward-deployed location caring for patients injured in combat. The investigators to reveal the evolution in their understanding of the phenomena will identify exemplars. In the research report, a range of exemplars will allow the reader to recognize the distinctions the investigators are making and to judge the credibility of the interpretation and transferability to other settings.

Comparison to other, formal texts will be undertaken after the thematic analysis and identification of exemplars. Following the analysis of the text for paradigm cases, recurring themes and exemplars, the interpretation will be compared with the nursing and allied health literature on critical care during air transport or related topics.

Using the recurring themes and patterns of meaning, items will be formed to use in conjunction with the current deployment preparation checklist to develop the CCATT Pre-Deployment Survey which will be tested in future research studies.

In summary, qualitative research, with its emphasis on discovery, exploration, and description, utilizes a different set of criteria to ensure rigor than quantitative methods (Sandelowski, 1986; 1993). The following techniques will be used to ensure credibility, confirmability, transferability and audibility (Benner, 1994; Linclon and Guba, 1985).

Credibility, analogous to validity, will be achieved through thick description of the phenomena, repeated engagement with respondents, concurrent data collection/data analysis, group discussions and member checking. Transferability (fittingness, external validity or generalizability) is achieved through demographic description of the sample and method of selection of respondents, comparisons with other extant literature, the use of low inference descriptors and verbatim excerpts from the text that enables readers to determine if the findings will apply to their own setting. Confirmability (objectivity) is achieved through peer checking, triangulation of the data sources and data collection methods, and checking the representativeness of the data as a whole by asking questions such as: How would the event unfold in another situation? Would the same issues and concerns show up for two different cases? Audibility (reliability) will be ensured through the maintenance of a paper trail documenting decisions and their rationales so another investigator could review the conclusions and determine if they would arrive at similar or comparable (but not contradictory) conclusions.

Human Subjects

The proposal will be submitted to the Institutional Review Boards* at the study sites and the Uniformed Services University as exempt research based on the following criteria:

1. This research will be conducted in an established or commonly accepted educational setting, involving normal educational practices,

Study Timetable*

Year 1	Activity	J	A	S	O	N	D	J	F	M	A	M	J
	IRB Approval				X								
	Hire study personnel			X	X	X							
	Develop blueprint for study				X	X	X						
	Train focus group interviewers							X					
	Subject recruitment								X	X	X	X	X
Year 2	Activity	J	A	S	O	N	D	J	F	M	A	M	J
	Subject Recruitment	X											
	Conduct Interviews	X	X	X	X								
	Data Analysis		X	X	X	X	X						
	Interpret Findings					X	X	X	X	X			
	Preparation of final report										X	X	
	Present Findings												X

*Assuming funding in July 03

2. This research involves the use of educational tests (cognitive examination, and simulation lab performance) and survey procedures

AND

1. The nature of the information obtained in this study does not reasonably place the subjects at risk of criminal or civil liability or be damaging to the subject's financial standing, employability, or reputation should any disclosure of the participant's response outside the research occur.

All Institutional Review Boards (IRB) will review and approve this research prior to any data collection. Informants will read an informational letter that fully describes the study. The information letter will include the telephone number of the researcher, a statement reminding the participant they can withdraw from the study at any time, and that they may request results of the study. The only known benefit from participating in this study is the opportunity to share deployment experience with the researcher. The shared experience can contribute to improvements in future deployment procedures. There are no known risks, but if sharing the experience

PHS 398/2590 (Rev. 05/01)

creates emotional distress for any participants, referrals will be made to Wilford Hall Medical Center (WHMC) or Keesler Medical Center mental health counselors to provide needed support. Participants will be reassured that all information shared with the researcher will remain confidential. Code numbers will identify audiotapes, videotapes and demographic data only. A codebook containing code numbers and names and addresses of informants will be stored in a locked file cabinet separately from all other data. Participants will be assured that their superiors will not be aware that they have chosen to participate in this study. Any publications resulting from data generated will not contain identifying information.

Sources of data:

Data will be obtained through subject interviews and surveys. These data will be obtained specifically for research purposes. Data will not be available to anyone outside the study team. Each subject will be given a code and subject names will not be entered into the database. Additionally, military members of the study team are not supervisors of any of the participants in the study. All participants will be given the option of withdrawing from the study at any time.

Vertebrate Animals: N/A

Literature Cited:

Air Force Medicine (1996). HQ USAF, pamphlet on Air Force Medical Service Strategic Plan. USAF: Publishing Distribution Office.

Air Force Link (2002). An introduction to the Expeditionary Aerospace Force. USAF: [online], Available: http://www.af.mil/eaf/intro.shtml. Accessed 9 July 2002.

Bader, G.B., Terhorst, M., Heilman, P., & DePalma. J.A. (1995). Characteristics of Flight Nursing Practice. Air Medical Journal, 14(4), 214–218.

Barger, J. (1991). Coping behaviors of U.S. Army flight nurses in World War II: an oral history. Aviation, Space, and Environmental Medicine, 2(1), 153–157.

Benner, P. (1985). Quality of life: A phenomenological perspective on explanation, prediction and understanding in nursing science. Advances in Nursing Science, 8(1), 1–14.

Benner, P. (1987). A dialogue with excellence. American Journal of Nursing, (9), 1170–1172.

Benner, P. (Ed.). (1994a). Interpretive phenomenology: Embodiment, caring and ethics in health and illness. Thousand Oaks, CA: Sage.

Benner, P. (1994b). The tradition and skill of interpretive phenomenology in studying health, illness, and caring practices. IN P. Benner (Ed.) Interpretive phenomenology: Studying embodiment, caring and ethics in health and illness. Sage Publications

Benner, P., Tanner, C. & Chesla, C. (1992). From beginner to expert: Gaining a differentiated clinical world in critical care nursing. Advances in Nursing Science, 14(3), 12–28.

Beyea, S.C., & Nicoll, L.H. (1997). Qualitative and quantitative approaches to nursing research. AORN Journal, 66, (2), 323–325.

Bridges, E., Schmelz, J. & Mazer, S. (Submitted). Skin interface pressure associated with the NATO litter. Military Medicine

Bridges, E., Schmelz, J., Stone, K., Sylvester, J., O'Toole, E., and Johnson, A. (2000). "Endotracheal suctioning at altitude: Implications for practice". American Journal of Critical Care; 9(3), 218.

Britt, T. & Adler, A. (1999). Stress and Health during Medical Humanitarian Assistance Missions. *Military Medicine, Vol 164* (4), 275.

Brykczynski, K. (1989). An interpretive study describing the clinical judgment of nurse practitioners. *Scholarly Inquiry for Nursing Practice, 3*(2), 75–104

Cohen, M.Z., & Omery, A. (1994). Schools of phenomenology: Implications for research. In *Critical issues in qualitative research methods*, J.M. Morse (ed.) Thousand Oaks, CA: Sage, 136–156.

Concannon, K.O. (1992). The experience of Desert Storm Nurses (unpublished Master's Thesis). Tucson: University of Arizona.

Connolly, H.V., Fetcho, S., & Hageman, J.R. (1992). Education of personnel involved in the transport program. *Critical Care Clinics, 8*(3), 480–490.

Correll, J.T. (2002). The EAF in Peace and War. *Air Force Magazine, 85,* (7): 24–31.

Cowley, G. (2001). Bush's battle cry. *Newsweek.* October 1: 24–26.

Creswell, J. W. (1998). *Qualitative inquiry and research design: Choosing among five traditions.* Thousand Oaks, CA: Sage.

Culpepper, M.M., & Adams, P. G. (1988). Nursing in the Civil War. *American Journal of Nursing, 7*(7), 981–984.

Department of Defense (1995). Medical Readiness Strategic Plan 2001 [online], Available: http://www.ha.osd.mil/hmrfr2.html.

Diekelmann, N. (1992). Learning-as-testing: A Heiddeggerian hermeneutical analysis of the lived experiences of students and teachers in nursing. *Advances in Nursing Science*, 14(1), 72–83.

Diekelmann, N., Schurter, R. & Lam, S. (1994). Martin, a computer software program: On being able to find the meaning in the text. In P. Benner (Ed.). *Interpretive phenomenology: Studying embodiment, caring and ethics in health and illness.* Sage Publications.

Dillman, D. (2000). *Mail and telephone surveys: The total design method.* New York: Wiley-Interscience.

Dremsa-Collins, T.L. (2001). Readiness Estimate and Deployability Index Revised for Air Force Nurses (READI-R-AFN) and READI-R-AFN Short Form [SF]: Psychometric Evaluation. (Doctoral dissertation). Baltimore: University of Maryland.

Duffy, M. (1987). Methodological triangulation: A vehicle for merging quantitative and qualitative research methods. *Image, 19*(3), 130–133.

Dyer, L.L. (1990). Training and development of the ICU nurse for critical care transport. *Critical Care Nurse*, 9(4), 74–80.

Goodwin, L. & Goodwin, W. (1984). Are validity and reliability "relevant" in qualitative evaluation research? *Evaluation & The Health Professions, 7*(4), 413–426.

Guba, E.G. (1990). *The paradigm log.* Newbury Park, CA: Sage.

Hacker, P. (1994). US National Security Strategy. *Challenge and Response.* Maxwell AFB, AL: Air University Press.

Holleran, R.S. (Eds.). (1996). *Flight nursing principles and practice.* St. Louis: Mosby.

Holm, J. (1982). *Women in the Military.* Novoto, CA: Presidio.

Holter, I.M. (1988). Critical Theory: A foundation for the development of nursing theories. *Scholarly Inquiry for Nursing Practice: An International Journal, 2*(3), 223–232.

Joint Publication 3-07 (1995). *Unified Action Armed Forces (UNAAF)*, USAF: Publishing Distribution Office.

Kassner, E. (1993). *Desert Storm Journal: A nurse's story.* Lincoln Center, MA: Cottage Press.

Kikuchi, J.F., Simmons, H., & Romyn. D. (1996). *Truth in nursing inquiry.* Thousand Oaks, CA: Sage.

Knaack, P. (1984). Phenomenological research. *Western Journal of Nursing Research, 6* (1), 107–114.

Lauer, Q. (1965). Edmund Husserl: Phenomenology and the crisis of philosophy. New York: Harper & Row.

Lefebvre, R.C., & Sandford, S.L. (1985). A multi-model questionnaire for stress. *Journal of Human Stress, 11,* 69–75.

Lincoln, Y. & Guba, E. (1985). *Naturalistic inquiry.* Beverly Hills, CA: Sage.

Magyar, K.P. (1994). The emerging post-cold-war international order and changing conflict environment. *Challenge and Response.* Maxwell AFB, AL: Air University Press.

Marshall, K. (1988). *In the combat zone: An oral history of American women in Vietnam.* Boston: Little, Brown & Co.

Martin, L.G. (1967). Angels in Vietnam. *Today's Health, 8,* 17-22 & 60–62.

McVicker, S.J. (1985). Invisible veterans: The women who served in Vietnam. *Journal of Psychosocial Nursing, 22*(2), 26–28.

Mitchell, E. (1986). Multiple triangulation: A methodology for nursing science. *Advances in Nursing Science, 8*(3), 18–26.

Morgan, D.L. (1988). *Focus groups as qualitative research.* Newbury Park, CA: Sage.

Moustakas, C. (1994). Phenomenological research methods. Thousand Oaks, CA: Sage.

Norman, E.M. (1986). A study of female military nurses in Vietnam during the war years 1965-1973. *Journal of Nursing History, 2*(1), 43–60.

Odom, J.D. (1986). The Vietnam nurses can't forget. *American Journal of Nursing, 86*(10), 1035–1037.

Parse, R.R. (1996). Building knowledge through qualitative research: The road less traveled. *Nursing Science Quarterly, 9*(1), 10–16.

Reineck, C. (1996). Individual medical readiness: Concept clarification. *TriService Nursing Research Program, [online]: http://www.usuhs.mil/tsnrp/awards/fy96/reineck.html.*

Reineck, C. (1998). Readiness instrument psychometric evaluation. *TriService Nursing Research Program, [online]: http://www.usuhs.mil/tsnrp/awards/fy98/reineck.html.*

Reineck, C. (1998). *[Readiness instrument psychometric evaluation].* Unpublished proposal obtained from author.

Reineck, C. (1999). Individual readiness in nursing. *Military Medicine, 164*(4), 251–255.

Reineck, C., Finstuen, K., Connelly, L.M, & Murdock, P. (2001). Army Nurse Readiness Instrument: Psychometric Evaluation and Field Administration. *Military Medicine, 166*(11).

Richards, L.E. (1935). *Letters of Florence Nightingale.* Yale Review: University Press.

Rosen, L., Weber, J., and Martin, L. (2000). Gender-related personal attributes and psychological adjustment among U.S. Army soldiers. *Military Medicine, Vol 165*(1), 54.

Sandelowski, M. (1986). The problem of rigor in qualitative research. *Advances in Nursing Science, 8*(3), 27–37.

Scannell, E. (1992). *The lived experience of women military nurses in Vietnam during the Vietnam War.* Unpublished doctoral dissertation, Georgia State University, College of Health Sciences, Atlanta, GA.

Schmelz, J., Bridges, E., Duong, D., & Ley, C. (Accepted for publication). Care of the Critically Ill Patient in a Military Unique Environment: A Program of Research. *Critical Care Clinics of North America*

Schmelz, J., Stone, K., Johnson, A., Sylvester, J., Bridges, E., O'Toole, E., and Meade, D. (2000). "Preventing suctioning-induced hypoxemia at altitude". *American Journal of Critical Care*; 9(3), 218.

Topley, D., Schmelz, J., Henkensius-Kirshbaum, J. & Horvath, K (Accepted for publication). Critical care nursing expertise during air transportation. *Military Medicine*

Spiegelberg, H. (1976). *The phenomenological movement (Vols I & II)*. The Hague: Martinus Nijhoff.

Stanley, T. (1987). Flight nursing- trend for the future. *Imprint, 34*(4), 22–24.

Streubert, J., & Carpenter, D.R. (1995), *Qualitative research in nursing: Advancing the humanistic imperative.* Philadelphia: J.B. Lippincott.

Strickland, O.L. (1999). Selecting instruments for construct validity assessment. *Journal of Nursing Measurement*, 7(2), 99–100.

Topley, D., Schmelz, J., Henkensius-Kirshbaum, J. & Horvath, K (2002). (Accepted for publication). Critical care nursing expertise during air transportation. *Military Medicine.*

West, I., and Clark, C. (1995). The Army Nurse Corps and Operation Restore Hope. *Military Medicine Vol 160*, 179–183.

h. Consortium/Contractual Arrangements:
Attach any letters of collaboration here.
i. Consultants Letters and Biographical Sketches for consultants are attached.

Appendix A

CCATT Nursing Interview Guide

Begin the interview by clarifying any concrete details of the participant observation. The following questions may be focused on an individual patient(s) that was observed or may be asked in a more general way.

1. Prior to picking up a critically ill patient in the forward-deployed location, what process do you go through to prepare for the transport?
2. Is there information, which you find particularly important to know about each patient prior to pickup?
3. Is there equipment and supplies you find particularly important to have?
4. What do you look for in a patient prior to departing on a flight?
5. Have you ever discovered something prior to flight, which changed your plan of care?
6. During the course of the flight:
   a. What type of plan of care do you typically use?
   b. What are the common problems patients experience during CCATT missions in the forward deployed location?
   c. What heightens your suspicion that someone is having trouble during flight? What are the cues you look for?
   d. If you suspect a patient is having trouble, what actions do you typically take?
   e. What and how do you share your concerns about patients with your team members? Aerovac medical team? Flight crew?
   f. How have your CCATT training and preparation courses helped you during these periods when patients have trouble in-flight?
   g. How has your previous critical care experience helped you during these periods when patients have trouble in-flight?
7. Is there equipment or supplies you think should be added to CCATT operations?
8. Is there additional education and training that should be added to the CCATT program?
9. What do you think the qualifications of a CCATT nurse should be?
10. Compared to critical care nursing on a typical CCATT peacetime mission, what aspects of care are unique to CCATT missions in forward deployed locations?
11. What do you discuss with members of your team?

Appendix B

Guidelines for Writing Clinical Narratives

Write a story about a patient you cared for during a CCATT mission. The account should be written in narrative or story form, rather than as an analytical, condensed case study or report. Fill in as much detail as you think others will need in order to understand your intentions, feelings, and concerns during the incident. Also, include significant information about others involved in the incident.

A clinical narrative can be a situation:

- where you feel you made a difference in the outcome, directly or through others
- that went unusually well
- where there was a breakdown
- that is ordinary and typical
- that you feel reflects the essence of nursing practice transporting the critically ill in a forward deployed location
- from which you learned something
- that stands out in your mind for any reason

Include in your narrative the context of the incident (time, place, people involved, circumstances) and a description of what happened that is as close to "actual" as possible, not a summary, condensation or analysis.

You might want to ask yourself the following questions either in the body of the narrative or at the end:

- Why is this incident important to you?
- What were you thinking and feeling before, during, and after the incident?
- What, if anything, was particularly demanding or satisfying about the incident?

(Adapted from Benner 1984 & 1987)

APPENDIX C

<u>Please place an [X] or fill in the blank in each item below to indicate your response</u>

Demographic Data

1. What is your current component? (Check one)
- ❏ Active Duty
- ❏ Air National Guard
- ❏ Air Force Reserve
- ❏ Other _____
2. What is your primary AFSC? (Check one)
- ❏ 46S3 Operating Room Nurse
- ❏ 46M3 Nurse Anesthetist
- ❏ 46F3 Flight Nurse
- ❏ 46N3E Critical Care Nurse
- ❏ 46N3F Neonatal ICU Clinical Nurse
- ❏ 46N3J Emergency Room Nurse

---

3. How many years of nursing experience do you have (include military and RN or LPN civilian experience) [in years and months]?

_____

4. Do you have prior technical medical experience (i.e. medical technician)?
❑ yes ❑ no

5. Are you male or female?
❑ Male ❑ Female

6. What is your military rank?
❑ 01 2nd Lieutenant
❑ 02 1st Lieutenant
❑ 03 Captain
❑ 04 Major
❑ 05 Lieutenant Colonel
❑ 06 Colonel

7. What is your highest education level?
❑ Bachelors in Nursing
❑ Bachelors other than nursing
❑ Masters in Nursing
❑ Masters other than nursing

8. Are you currently assigned to a mobility platform (i.e. Unit Type Code (UTC) such as Expeditionary Medical Support/Air Force Theater Hospital (AFTH) or Aeromedical Evacaution?
❑ yes ❑ no

9. Have you ever deployed before? **(if No, proceed to question 15)**
❑ yes ❑ No

10. How many times have you deployed? _____

11. What was the length of your deployment (longest, if more than one)?
❑ 2 weeks ❑ 90 days
❑ 30 days ❑ 120 days
❑ 60 days ❑ 179 days

12. What were the dates of your most recent deployment (months and year)?
From _____ To _____

13. What is your age? (fill in blank) _____

14. How frequently do you exercise?
❑ at least 3–5 times a week
❑ twice a week
❑ once a week
❑ less often than once a week

15. Check the box that represents how long ago it was that you had a physical exam.
❑ 1–12 months ago
❑ 1–5 years ago
❑ longer than five years ago

_____

PHS 398/2590 (Rev. 05/01)

16. Are you up to date on routine gender specific (i.e. mammogram for women/prostate for men), health related exams?

❑ Yes   ❑ No   ❑ not sure

17. Which of the following would you use to help you in coping with stress? (Check ALL that apply)

❑ Tobacco   ❑ Alcohol
❑ Physical Exercise   ❑ Reading
❑ Relaxation/Meditation Techniques   ❑ Music
❑ Talking with Friends   ❑ Religious Faith
❑ Eating   ❑ Sleeping
❑ Other _____

Critique of Funded Grant

Department of Defense
Triservice Nursing Research Program
Proposal Number: NO3-014
Principal Investigator: Lt. Col. Theresa L. Dremsa
Title of Proposal: CCATT Nurses' Deployed Experience

Primary Reviewer's Evaluative Comments

ABSTRACT

The Critical Care Air Transport Teams (CCATT) "pronounced c-cat", were established to extend the Air Force's Aeromedical Evacuation (AE) capabilities when transporting critically ill or injured patients. Air Force Aeromedical Evacuation of patients with combat related injuries began immediately following the President's declaration of war on terrorism. As a result, numerous CCATT teams were deployed to the combat environment. Critical Care nurses function as key members on CCATT missions that are tasked to transport injured soldiers. Transporting the injured out of the combat environment places all team members at risk for exposure to ongoing combat. The purpose of this study is to describe knowledge gained by CCATT nurses while providing patient care when in a combat environment. The specific aims of this study are to: 1) describe CCATT nurses' experiential knowledge in the care of patients when in a combat environment; 2) distinguish salient features of CCATT nurses' knowledge of care of patients when in a combat environment and compare to critical care nursing during pre-war conditions; and 3) describe the collaborative relationships involved in providing nursing care in a combat environment. This exploratory, descriptive study will use interpretive phenomenology by means of individual interviews, written narratives, group interviews, participant observation and review of in-flight documentation of care. Using purposive sampling, at least 12 nurses who deployed with CCATT missions, will be recruited to share their recent experience as a CCATT nurse in a combat environment. Data will be transcribed and entered into a qualitative research computer program. Data analysis will begin concurrently with data collection. The investigators will identify recurrent themes and patterns of meaning, using verbatim statements and low-inference *descriptors, which will facilitate item statements for instrument development. Items developed from the thematic analysis of qualitative data can then be converted to a self-assessment scale for future deployments, which will be further developed and tested in future studies.*

Evaluation Criteria

Scientific Approach and Technical Merit

The purpose of this project is to describe Critical Care Air Transport Team (CCATT) nurses' experiential knowledge when assessing and treating critically ill patients during transportation by fixed wing aircraft in a forward deployed location with a potential risk for exposure to combat. It is a replication of a study of the CCATT nursing experience in non-combat conditions, which compared the CCATT experience to usual critical care nursing in a hospital setting. This proposal has many strengths related to the scientific approach and technical merit. First, this study is carefully linked to the literature base related to military nursing and the critical care air transport team concept. The literature review is thorough and well synthesized. The historical perspective and the careful consideration of empirical studies in the area make the purpose of the study understandable and thoroughly enjoyable to read. The background section provides a very nice justification of the use of the method chosen and is logically linked to the research question and the methods section. This makes the proposal internally consistent which is very helpful for the review. Second, the preliminary studies section addresses the strengths and experience of the research team and provides convincing evidence that the team can conduct this study and findings from this study will be useful and will contribute to improving nursing practice. Third, the research design and methods section is equally well developed. There is a nice description of the method and the section describing interpretive phenomenology demonstrates knowledge as well as experience. There is justification provided for almost all of the methodological decisions including sample size, subject selection criteria, the group analysis of the narratives, and participant observation. Careful attention is paid to the "science" of the project and appropriate attention is paid to issues related to trustworthiness. Multiple sources of data are being collected and that is a strength of the design. In addition, careful attention is also given to the ethical issues related to the project. The analysis section is very nicely done and accurately reflects the interpretive phenomenological technique being used.

While few, there are some points of confusion in the text. First, it isn't clear to me if the nurses who are involved in the individual interviews will be the same individuals who also write narratives and participate in the group analysis of the narratives. Second, although the investigators will review in-flight documentation of care, how the data will be analyzed is not specified. Specific Aim 3 is being addressed in some ways in the questions being asked, but is not very prominent. The investigator might want to be more specific about collecting data related to this aim. Overall, however, these weaknesses are minor.

Originality And Innovative Nature of the Proposal: Applicability of Previous Findings

This study is very innovative while closely linked to the literature and consistent with previous research of one of the team members.

Qualifications, Expertise and Research Experiences of the Principal Investigator and Staff

Theresa L. Dremsa, Principal Investigator, is a nurse researcher in the active military who completed her PhD at the University of Maryland in 2001. Her expertise lies in the area of instrument development and testing. Her previous research includes the development of the Readiness Estimate and Deployability Index. She was co-investigator on a grounded theory study of nurses during deployment to Croatia. Dr. Dremsa's publications are eclectic and include a recent publication on absenteeism among care seeking Gulf war veterans with ill-defined medical conditions and musculoskeletal disorders. Joseph O. Schmelz, co-investigator, is currently Director, Nursing Research, Clinical Investigation Directorate, Wilford Hall. He received his PhD from Boston College in 1996. His publications focus on critical care nursing during air transport. He is currently involved in a research study focusing on computerized lung sound analysis. He brings expertise in the use of Brenner's method and conducted the original study on which this project is based. He has a publication on that project accepted for publication in <u>Military Medicine</u>. Janice B. Agazio, co-investigator, is an Assistant Professor at the Graduate School of Nursing, Uniformed Services University of the Health Sciences. Dr. Agazio is currently funded by the TSNRP to study nursing practice in operations other than war. Her publications focus on health promotion of active duty women. Her research expertise focuses on qualitative methods and triangulation. She also has expertise in computer applications for qualitative research. Karen G. Evers is Director, Critical Care Air Transport Team Course at Lackland AFB. She completed her MSN in 1994. She has no publications and no previous research. Her expertise for this study is to contribute to the interpretation of findings with on-going data analysis. Judith Schaffer, co-investigator, is nurse researcher at Keesler AFB. She completed her MSN in 1989 and her MPA in 1993. She is currently enrolled in the doctoral program at the University of Utah. She has one publication in press on flight physiology and has two projects in progress. Her role is to facilitate interviews at Keesler. Lorraine S. Gravley, co-investigator, is Patient Movement Clinical Coordinator and Instructor Flight Nurse. She has no previous experience in research or publications, but she has technical expertise that will be used in data analysis and interpretation and will receive mentoring as a new investigator. The consultant for the project is Kathy J. Horvath, Associate Director, Education and Program Evaluation, Geriatric Research Education and Clinical Center in Bedford, MA. Dr. Horvath has expertise in Brenner's method and she has previously worked with Dr. Schmelz.

Overall this team is well formulated. The team reflects expertise in the method as well as the substantive area. In addition, the consultation identified is appropriate. It is quite likely this team can accomplish the project aims in a credible fashion. As a whole, however, the team needs to be more aggressive in publishing their research as a strategy for evolving as scientists.

Availability of Institutional Resources and Adequacy of the Environment to Support the Project

There is an adequate description of the resources available at Wilford Hall Medical Center. There is no similar description about Keesler, the other performance site. The resources appear adequate to support the project, but there is no description of the environment and how that acts to support scholarly inquiry.

Significance and Relevance to Nursing Research

This investigator makes some very important points about the effects on nurses of being unprepared for what is expected under wartime conditions. Identifying ways to ameliorate some of these effects and better prepare nurses are extremely important for retention as well as quality of care. In addition, this study has potential to offer new knowledge about critical care nursing and the models that undergird expert nursing in these situations.

Reasonableness of the Budget and Duration of the Project in Relation to the Proposed Research

There doesn't appear to be anything out of line in the budget and for the most part the justification is adequate. It is difficult to understand how the budget for travel, however, squares with the work plan for interviewing subjects. The year 1 budget involves travel of 3 nurses. Dinners for focus groups involves 10 sessions at 3 sites (9 sessions total). How these square with an anticipated sample size of 12 to 25 isn't clear. In addition, the time commitment of the investigative team (15% + 5% for **6** investigators) seems very skimpy given the scope of the project.

Summary

This project is designed to describe knowledge gained by CCATT nursing while providing patient care when in a combat environment. Data, from 5 different sources, will be collected and analyzed using interpretive phenomenology. The participants will include nurses who have experienced deployment on a CCAT Team. The ultimate goal is to better prepare nurses for service on CCAT Teams in combat situations. The findings from this study have the potential to better inform our understanding of critical care nursing and models of expert clinical care in combat situations.

Strengths

- This study is carefully linked to the literature base related to military nursing and the critical care air transport team concept.
- The literature review is complete, well synthesized and thoroughly enjoyable to read.
- The background section provides a very nice justification of the use of the method chosen and is logically linked to the research question and the methods section.
- The preliminary studies section addresses the strengths and experience of the research team and provides convincing evidence that the team can conduct this

study and findings from this study will be useful and contribute to improving nursing practice.

- The research design and methods section is equally well developed.
- The description of interpretive phenomenology is accurate and demonstrated knowledge as well as experience.
- There are rationale for almost all of the methodological decisions.
- Careful attention is paid to the "science" of the project and appropriate attention is paid to issues related to trustworthiness.
- Multiple sources of data are being collected and that is a strength of the design.
- Careful attention is also given to ethical issues related to the project.
- The analysis section is very nicely done and accurately reflects the interpretive phenomenological technique being used.
- The study is original and innovative. It has the potential to contribute to our understandings about military nursing and civilian critical care nursing.
- The research team has appropriate expertise in research and methods as well as substantive expertise. Appropriate consultation has been identified.
- The resources appear adequate to support this project, but there is no description of the research environment or the resources at Keesler AFB.

Weaknesses:

- The recruitment plan isn't clear.
- No information is provided about what data will be collected from the in-flight documentation of care or how the data will be analyzed.
- Specific Aim 3 is being addressed in some ways in the questions being asked, but it is not very prominent.
- The research team needs to focus more attention on publishing their results.
- The budget is not as understandable as it could be, but the problem begins with lack of specificity in the recruitment plan.

I am very enthusiastic about this project. Overall the proposal is very well written and clear. The description of the phenomenological method is well done and attention to the science of the project is more than adequate. The idea of the project is also appealing and important.

Department Of Defense
Triservice Nursing Research Program
Proposal Number: N03-014
Principal Investigator: Lt. Col. Theresa L. Dremsa
Title of Proposal: CCATT Nurses' Deployed Experience

Secondary Reviewer's Evaluative Comments

Evaluation Criteria

Scientific Approach and Technical Merit

Strengths
- Appropriate mix of expertise in project team.
- Strong qualitative methodology.
- Well-organized research plan.

Weaknesses
- None.

Originality and Innovative Nature of the Proposal: Applicability of Previous Findings

Originality
This project will provide new knowledge about the lived experiences of CCATT nurses in combat conditions. Such knowledge has not been collected previously.

Innovation in Translation or Applicability of Previous Findings
This project will build on the PI's prior experience in developing and evaluating the Readiness Estimate and Deployability Index Short Form, which was designed to assess readiness among Air Force nurses generally. This project will also extend work done by Associates Investigator Schmelz to gain experiential knowledge from CCATT nurses under non-combat conditions.

Qualification, Expertise and Research Experience of the Principal Investigator and Staff

Lt. Col. Dremsa holds a MSN in cardiovascular nursing from the University of Alabama at Birmingham and a Ph.D. in nursing research methodology from the University of Maryland at Baltimore, the latter granted in 2001. Her military record includes considerable management experience in critical care nursing and flight nursing, some in a deployed position. For her dissertation she successfully developed a valid and reliable self-assessment instrument for CCATT nurses although not for those being deployed into combat positions. This will be her first experience with qualitative research, but other team members have substantial experience with that methodology. Her publication record is adequate for an investigator whose career has been military, not academic, and who has recently attained the doctorate. She had a TriService grant for her dissertation research.

Lt. Col. Evers has knowledge of current course content and is well qualified to judge the degree to which the knowledge gained about lived experiences of CCATT nurses in combat extends beyond what is currently taught. She is also in a position to identify former students who can be invited to participate in the study. Her background and experience are appropriate for her role in the project.

Lt. Col. Schaffer will assist with data collection at the second study site, where most of the formerly deployed CCATT nurses are based. Her experience as a flight nurse and as a doctoral student in nursing prepare her for this role. She will be learning the qualitative methodology.

Dr. Schmelz was an associate investigator in the qualitative study of CCATT nurses' experience that led to the assessment tool for non-combat conditions. He will help to train team members in individual and group interview techniques and qualitative data analysis.

Dr. Agazio has experience with both qualitative and quantitative research methods and a long-standing interest in readiness. She is well prepared for her role, helping to train the team in interview techniques and narrative analysis methods.

Capt. Gravley's experiences as an Aero Medical Evacuation Flight Nurse and as a CCATT nurse will provide useful insights as she assists with data collection and analysis.

Dr. Horvath has a number of published reports of clinical nursing knowledge derived from qualitative studies. She is qualified to train the investigators in the methods of the project.

Availability of Institutional Resources and Adequacy of the Environment to Support the Project

Strengths
- Access to sample of informants (CCATT nurses currently or formerly deployed to combat areas).
- Expertise of colleagues in sites where CCATT nurses are based.
- Facilities of Wilford Hall Medical Center.

Weaknesses
- None.

Significance and Relevance to Nursing Research

This project will use qualitative methods (analysis of data from interviews and focus groups) to clarify necessary core competencies for CCATT nurses in combat conditions. These identified core competencies will form the basis for a self-assessment tool for deployment readiness, to be developed subsequent to the currently proposed project. By formalizing knowledge from the lived experiences of critical care air evacuation nurses in combat, the proposed work will fill an important gap in knowledge. When eventually translated to the self-assessment tool, the new knowledge will help to assure that deployed CCATT nurses are at the peak of readiness.

Reasonableness of the Budget And Duration of the Project in Relation to the Proposed Research

The budget is quite reasonable for the work to be done. Travel to Seeb AB in Oman for interviews with deployed nurses is necessary to get the views of these participants. If policy permits coverage of the full cost of air fare ($2400 per person), that would be justified.

Summary

This project will collect and analyze qualitative data from CCATT nurses who have been deployed to combat sites. The intent is to discover knowledge from their lived experiences to improve the definition of readiness and to serve as the basis for a self-administered readiness assessment to be developed in a subsequent project. The design and methods are appropriate for the aims. This research will provide important knowledge for the eventual improvement of readiness. As a team, the investigators are qualified to conduct the study.

Strengths

- Appropriate mix of expertise in project team.
- Strong qualitative methodology.
- Well organized research plan.
- Access to sample of informants (CCATT nurses currently or formerly deployed to combat areas).
- Expertise of colleagues in sites where CCATT nurses are based.
- Facilities of Wilford Hall Medical Center.

Weaknesses

- None.

Support the project at the funding level requested; increase funding for air travel if policy permits.

Department of Defense
Triservice Nursing Research Program
Proposal Number: N03-014
Principal Investigator: Lt. Col. Theresa L. Dremsa
Title of Proposal: CCATT Nurses' Deployed Experience

Military Reviewer's Evaluative Comments

Evaluation Criteria

Military Feasibility

The PI describes 5 data collection methods (page 36) and procedures to gain access to the participants. She has anticipated the difficulties associated with interviewing participants while deployed and has letters/emails of support from the appropriate authorities. Recruiting for the study is well described and poses no problems, however, clarification is needed for the number of nurses to be observed in the deployed setting ('3' pages 36 and 37, '4' page 36). Further explanation addressing the 4th requirement ("means and ways to mitigate or eliminate any potential security or classification issues") noted in Col. Maul's email.

Military Relevance

CCATT teams are an integral part of the airevac system and the AEF concept of operations. This study has the potential to identify the areas of strength and areas in need of change for CCATT nurses preparing to deploy to combat locations. These deployment issues can then be explored in further studies with associated improvements in predeployment preparations. Expert nurses caring for critically ill patients in a combat environment are important for all members of the military who are deployed.

Stability of the Research Team

The highly capable research team is composed of active duty nurses, retired nurses and a civilian. The potential dates for rotation range from June '03 to Sept '04. The tasks associated with the study are not tied to any particular base. The associate investigators have a wide range of experience and should be able to continue the study even if the AD nurses are deployed.

Summary

Strengths

- There are 5 data collection methods (page 36) and procedures to gain access to the participants.
- The difficulties associated with interviewing participants while deployed have been anticipated and the PI has obtained letters/emails of support from the appropriate authorities.

- Recruiting for the study is well described and poses no problems, however, clarification is needed for the number of nurses to be observed in the deployed setting ('3' pages 36 and 37, '4' page 36).
- CCATT teams are an integral part of the airevac system and the AEF concept of operations.
- Areas of strength and areas in need of change for CCATT nurses preparing to deploy to combat locations may be identified.
- These deployment issues can then be explored in further studies with associated improvements in predeployment preparations.
- Expert nurses caring for critically ill patients in a combat environment are important for all members of the military who are deployed.
- The research team is composed of highly capable active duty nurses, retired nurses and a civilian.
- Potential dates for rotation range from June '03 to Sept '04.
- The tasks associated with the study are not tied to any particular base.
- The associate investigators have a wide range of experience and should be able to continue the study even if the AD nurses are deployed.

Weaknesses

- Further explanation addressing the 4th requirement ("means and ways to mitigate or eliminate any potential security or classification issues") noted in Col. Maul's email.

This study is a significant beginning in understanding the experience of CCATT nurses. The methods chosen promise an answer to the research question. There is support at every level for gaining access and implementing the research plan. Increased **ops** tempo may require the rapid preparation of CCATT nurses. This study may help to identify factors critical to their preparation and thus expedite the process.

Level of Enthusiasm for this proposal: Highest

TriService Nursing Research Program
FY2003 Programmatic Review Discussion Summary

Proposal Number: N03-014
Principal Investigator: Lt. Col. Theresa L. Dremsa
Title: CCATT Nurses' Deployed Experience
Programmatic Review Score: 1.5

Discussion: This is a well-conceived study with a strong research team. The potential problem identified by the SRP concerning the timeline of the interviews should be easily remedied. The qualitative methodology is sound. Particularly with the threat of bioterrorism, the study has additional relevance to the civilian population, which may be involved in transport of critically ill patients. The project is both unique and relevant to the military and the cost-benefit ratio appears reasonable.

With clarification of the timeline for completion of interviews for this ambitious study, it is recommended that it be funded.

TriService Nursing Research Program
FY 2003 Scientific Review Discussion Summary

Proposal Number: N03-014
SRP Score: 1.50
Principal Investigator: Lt. Col. Theresa L. Dremsa
Title: CCATT Nurses' Deployed Experience

Discussion: The primary reviewer pointed out many strengths of the proposal related to nurses assigned to CCATT (Critical Care Air Transport Team), which evacuates patients with combat-related injuries. The purpose is clearly presented, the background is well justified, the preliminary studies supply convincing evidence of the team's ability to conduct the study, and the research design and methods section demonstrates knowledge as well as experience. The multiple sources of data collected are a strong point. Careful attention is paid to ethical issues. It's not clear how data will be analyzed or how data to undergird Aim 3 (team interaction) will be collected. Team members could be more aggressive in publishing their strategy; resources are not described for Keesler Medical Center. The reviewer considered these to be minor weaknesses in a very innovative study that's closely linked to the literature, related to previous research of a team member, and has the potential to provide new knowledge about critical care nursing.

The secondary reviewer concurred. Formalizing knowledge from lived experience to critical care evacuation nurses will fill an important gap. When translated to a self-assessment tool, it will help ensure that CCATT nurses are at peak readiness to deal with personnel injured in combat.

The military reviewer found the recruitment plan well described, and the study important to all members of the military who are deployed. The number of nurses to be observed needs to be clarified, and ways to eliminate or mitigate classification or security issues need to be addressed. Because the tasks associated with the study aren't tied to a particular base, team members should be able to continue to study even if active-duty nurses are deployed. Overall, the military reviewer expressed a very high level of enthusiasm for this project.

The panel had questions about the sequence and timeline (e.g., page 36, data collection). If investigators begin recruiting in February, recruit for 6 months, and start to interview nurses only at the end of the 5th month, what will they do with people recruited early on? Who will write the narratives, and who will be involved in individual interviews? Some concern was expressed that a baccalaureate-prepared project director, the only paid person, will do everything, including interviews. The panel members suggested that three different groups of nurses be used. Multiple methods of data collection will correct for bias in any one method. Neither the hours allocated nor the budget reflects the complete involvement of the PI and AIs in data collection, as stated in the proposal. The proposal needs an assessment of the time involved in conducting the interviews and who will do them.

Budget: Although the costs requested are modest for the work to be done, several budget issues were mentioned. The time commitment of the team seems inadequate. Reviewers could not match travel and dinners for participants with the budget and found the plan for expenditures unclear.

Brief Summary: Panel members acknowledged the military relevance of the topic but noted the extremely ambitious amount of work to be done for the timeline and budgetary expenditures proposed. They also noted a lack of consistency in the timeline on pages 36 and 41 and requested clarification of who will participate in the interviews, narratives, and focus groups. Will subjects be the same for all activities or different for each? Will data be collected from different subsets or from the same sample at different points in time?

A Practical Guide for Sharing Qualitative Research Results

*T*he completion of a qualitative research study is only the beginning of the nurse investigator's work. The value of the research will never be fully appreciated unless it is shared. Dissemination of qualitative research can be invigorating, particularly when the investigator has the opportunity to share the richness of the data. Telling the story of participants invites a dialogue between professional colleagues. It also provides the researcher with the privilege of offering insights into previously unknown areas of participants' lives. Sharing the results of a qualitative research study is an exciting opportunity to provide insights, receive thoughtful critiques, and learn from others who have related experiences.

Once qualitative researchers develop a degree of comfort with research activities involved in the conduct of a qualitative project, they may become interested in developing a grant proposal using qualitative approaches. Grant writing requires qualitative researchers to develop additional skills, an effort well worth the time, especially when researchers' ideas are validated through the receipt of grant funds.

This chapter informs qualitative researchers about the differences in presentation style when a researcher submits a qualitative manuscript for publication, offers suggestions on how to submit a qualitative proposal for grant funding, and shares creative strategies for presenting qualitative research findings.

PUBLICATION PREPARATION

*T*he completion of a research study invites the opportunity to share the findings with a professional audience. The findings of an inquiry have no real value unless they are offered to the larger nursing community Publication is one of the ways that researchers can disseminate the results of their work. To be successful in sharing one's research, the qualitative investigator must be prepared for the nuances of publishing qualitative research. The following section is offered as a guide to those who are interested in sharing their work in the form of a journal article.

Identifying an Audience

When qualitative researchers begin their work, they should have an idea of what they will do with the results at the conclusion of the investigation. A report of some type generally is shared. To prepare a report in the form of a manuscript, researchers must be aware of their audience. If the audience is composed primarily of qualitative researchers, the manuscript will read differently than if the audience is made up of nurse clinicians, educators, or administrators without expertise in qualitative methodologies. Identify the audience clearly from the start. By reviewing current journals, the researcher can begin to identify which journals support the publication of qualitative research and which do not. Some nursing journals include more qualitative research studies on average than others. Regular review of major research journals will alert investigators to these journals. Journals that publish qualitative studies on a regular basis include *Advances in Nursing Science, Nursing Inquiry, Journal of Nursing Scholarship, Nursing Science Quarterly, Qualitative Health Research, Research in Nursing and Health,* and *Western Journal of Nursing Research.* This list is not exhaustive, nor is it offered to suggest that other journals do not publish qualitative studies. The purpose is to share the names of journals that have demonstrated a sustained and ongoing commitment to the publication of qualitative research.

In addition to identifying a journal that will be receptive to qualitative research approaches, it is essential to identify a journal with a focus on the content area of the study. For instance, the purpose of *Qualitative Health Research* is to disseminate qualitative research; however, the journal focuses on practice issues in health care and does not usually publish nursing education research articles. Therefore, an education study that utilizes qualitative methods would best be reported in an education journal such as the *Journal of Nursing Education* or *Nurse Educator*.

Once researchers have identified the potential journal, it is essential that they obtain a copy of the journal's guidelines for authors. This document assists researchers to develop a manuscript that meets the editorial expectations of the selected journal. Most guidelines for authors do not offer specific recommendations for the presentation of qualitative findings. Reading qualitative studies published in journals is the best way to develop an understanding of how to meet editorial guidelines when submitting results of a qualitative study for publication. Regardless of the journal in which the findings will be published, qualitative researchers should follow certain guidelines.

Each journal's readership has a specific purpose in reading a particular journal. Therefore, researchers must speak to the important facets of the research as they relate to the audience. These facets should reflect the purpose of the journal. For example, if researchers are writing for a scientific journal such as *Nursing Research*, detailing methods and data analysis will be as important as sharing the findings. In contrast, if they plan to publish in *Home Health Care Nurse*, the findings and implications for practice will be more important to the readership than the actual methods for conducting the study.

Most novice scholars are educated to submit query letters. A query letter tells the editor about what the author wishes to write. Many journal editors now report that query letters are unnecessary and may prolong the editorial process because of the time from submission of the query letter to response by journal staff. Often a phone call or e-mail will suffice to confirm whether the topic is of interest to the readership of a particular journal. Remember that, when developing a manuscript, you must be certain to present the research well. Poorly prepared manuscripts can set the stage for a rejection letter even if the study has significant merit.

Once researchers have submitted a manuscript, editorial staff will review the new submission and decide whether the content reflects the journal's purpose and is well written. If not, they will return the manuscript. Researchers are then responsible for identifying a more suitable periodical. Authors should expect to receive a postcard or letter within a few weeks of submission reporting on the status of the manuscript. The time from submission to publication may be more than 1 year. However, if, after 3 or 4 months, authors have not received a progress report on the disposition of the manuscript (i.e., whether it has been accepted or rejected), they should follow up with a phone call, e-mail, or letter.

Developing the Manuscript

The most difficult thing about writing is getting started. This statement is not intended to suggest that qualitative researchers have not been writing. However, documenting field notes and analyzing interviews are much different forms of writing than writing for publication. Documenting field notes or interviews is personal in nature and is not usually read or analyzed by others. Researchers usually learn through the implementation of their studies that it is easy and even fun to write notes for themselves, but it is more difficult to transfer those personal ideas to paper for others to read.

The very nature of data collection and analysis requires that researchers write. Documenting feelings, perceptions, observations, theoretical directions, or insights is part of the implementation of the qualitative research investigation. Transforming diaries, field notes, memos, or transcripts into a publishable manuscript requires rigor and determination, as well as keen synthesis, writing, and organizational abilities.

The most important point that a qualitative researcher must remember when beginning to write is to be clear. Qualitative research generates a large amount of raw data. In raw form, the data are interesting but unusable for research reporting. Qualitative researchers must condense, analyze, and synthesize for readers the importance of the research while not losing the richness of the findings. This effort can be a significant challenge because of the prolonged and intimate involvement of researchers with participants. It is also important to include evidence to support that the information included in the study was obtained from appropriates sources. In addition, it is essential to include relevant data to defend the interpretations made (Lambert, Lambert, & Tsukahara, 2002).

One way to focus on research for publication in a journal is to break the study into parts. Researchers often can develop more than one manuscript from a qualitative research study. If, for example, a researcher studies the culture of an open heart surgery unit over a 1-year period, he or she can develop a manuscript to examine the access and ethical considerations in this type of setting. The researcher may develop another manuscript that focuses on nurses, their activities, and artifacts that were discovered during the inquiry. Still another article might look at the interactions among clients, their families, and institutional structures. In addition, the researcher may develop a description of the process of conducting the inquiry into yet another manuscript. Ideally, a book or several chapters of a book would provide researchers with the best opportunity for presenting an entire qualitative research study. As Morse and Field (1995) point out, a book-length manuscript is best when researchers wish to share a description of the research process. However, time, commitment, and opportunity may limit publication in this format.

If researchers are uninterested in publishing the study in parts, then they can certainly develop the report so that it will be of greatest interest to readers. For instance, using the open heart surgery unit example, the researcher can present findings in the context of practice implications in critical care journals. A manuscript for publication in a practice journal would not require a great deal of emphasis on method or analysis but would require significant attention to findings and implications.

The most difficult obstacle to overcome in developing a qualitative manuscript for publication is the need to report the study in 12 to 15 pages, as required by most journals. With this limitation, it is critically important to be concise, focused, and logical rather than to try to report the entire study.

Once researchers have identified the journal and determined the focus, the next step is to logically develop the ideas they wish to convey. "An outline provides guidance in writing" (Field & Morse, 1985, p. 130). The purpose of the outline is to keep the writer directed. It is easy to drift away from the focus of the manuscript without an outline. Depending on the preference of the author, the outline may be more or less detailed.

When beginning to write, the author should be clear about the research questions and the audience for whom the publication is being prepared (Devers & Frankel, 2001). In addition to reporting on the steps of the qualitative research process, it is important to tell the story by using the participant's own words. It is equally important to be "cognizant of the differences between description and interpretations" (Choudhuri, Glauser, & Peregoy, 2004, p. 445). Interpretation moves beyond description to address what is going on in the setting.

Upon completion of the manuscript, authors should ask colleagues to critique the ideas presented. Too often, novice qualitative researchers make the mistake of believing that, because they have spent much time immersed in the data, writing about the data is merely a minor point. Qualitative research manuscripts are subjected to rigorous review. It is essential that the ideas be clear and demonstrate important findings to the nursing community. Review by knowledgeable colleagues will assist in ensuring the logic, organization, consistency, and importance of the findings.

Once the manuscript is submitted, researchers should be ready to revise as requested by the reviewers. Few manuscripts, qualitative or quantitative, sustain juried review without requests for revision. Morse (1996b) further suggests that, if researchers receive a request for revision in which reviewers' recommendations are contradictory, the researchers' responsibility is to attend to the most meaningful comments. Researchers should indicate why they did not use all of the reviewers' comments; however, when the comments do not reflect the truth of the study, researchers should not submit to revising based on those comments. Never be naïve, though, to the point of not considering reviewers' comments. Researchers have a great deal to gain in positive and negative comments. They need to ask, Why did someone read this in a particular way? When asked to revise, researchers must work quickly. The sooner they return the revised manuscript, the sooner the acceptance, and the earlier the manuscript will be queued for publication (Morse, 1996b).

If the unfortunate circumstance occurs—receipt of a rejection letter—do not throw away the manuscript. Look carefully at the critique, use the comments to improve the manuscript, and try another journal. It is acceptable also to use the comments, revise the manuscript, and resubmit it to the same journal. Quality research should be published. Sometimes, it takes a fair amount of tenacity to see ideas through to publication. But once published, researchers will enjoy the thrill of having the work available in print for readers interested in the topic and particular research approach.

CONFERENCE PRESENTATION

*S*atisfaction results from the publication of a manuscript that shares the results of intensive investigation. Manuscript publication is just one of researchers' responsibilities in their dissemination of the findings. In addition to getting ideas in print, which may take between 10 and 18 months, researchers should present the findings to the scholarly community using other forums. One way to share results in an efficient and effective way is through a formal conference presentation as a paper or poster presentation. Whether presenting findings in a paper or poster, qualitative researchers need to address important guidelines for sharing results in public forums.

Most formal presentations result from a *call for abstracts*, which requires investigators to submit a synopsis of the research in a few paragraphs, with an average limit of between 150 and 500 words. Guidelines for abstract submissions generally are available from the group sponsoring the research conference or workshop. It is essential that responses to the call reflect the theme of the conference and meet the criteria for presentation. The guidelines for abstract submission usually include the study purpose, the method the researcher used to conduct the inquiry, the sample, the findings, and the significance of the findings to nursing. Inclusion of the information requested will greatly improve the chances for abstract acceptance. However, because the results of a qualitative study are rich and dense, the question becomes, How do I demonstrate the richness of my work and the significance in 150 to 500 words when I have trouble writing it in 15 pages?

When submitting an abstract, be convincing. Illustrate for the reviewers that the work has been done well, will be interesting, and is significant to the profession. It is impossible to share the richness of the research in an abstract. What researchers should be striving for is to whet the reviewers' appetites so that they want to know more about the study.

A call for abstracts generally asks researchers to indicate the format in which they prefer to present: poster or paper. Novice qualitative researchers would be wise to indicate both. Podium presenters of a paper often have demonstrated their ability to successfully engage a group in their work through their ability to clearly articulate their ideas in the abstract. For individuals who have their abstracts rejected for podium presentation, poster presentations offer the opportunity to share the findings in a comfortable, relaxed atmosphere. A poster presentation provides new qualitative researchers with the chance to develop skill and confidence in presenting research findings. More important, in some conference formats, posters are the only opportunity to present findings because podium presentations may be reserved for keynote speakers.

Preparing for an Oral Presentation

If accepted for an oral presentation, researchers must keep in mind important aspects of sharing the results. They should present qualitative research so that they engage the conference participants in the work. Because the average length of podium presentation is between 20 and 30 minutes, be careful not to spend too much time discussing the method used to conduct the inquiry. Although the method is essential information, the audience will be most interested in the findings. Inform the audience about the method to give them the context and direction of the study, but do not share so much information that presentation of the findings is rushed. Presenters should not be hurried through the presentation of quotations from informants or the analysis of findings because these elements *are* the study results. Share the quotations and analysis thoughtfully, giving the audience time to absorb the words. Slides, overheads, or a computerized multimedia presentation can be used to provide a visual representation of the quotes, giving the audience additional time to assimilate the meaning of the words. Photographs and illustrations add to the presentation as well. Be sure to leave adequate time for questions. If the research has been presented well, the audience will want to know more because its interest has been aroused. During the question-and-answer period, a unique opportunity is available to share additional findings and anecdotal information.

Be aware that not all questions will be easy or fun to answer. At times, the audience can demonstrate interest in the trustworthiness or ethical considerations in the study. If you have executed a well-designed study, you can handle these questions. If you have not been insightful enough to predict questions and do not have ready answers, be honest. Use the critique questions shared in this text as a developmental learning experience. In this way, you, too, will have learned from sharing your results.

Preparing for a Poster Presentation

Presenting qualitative research in poster format is a unique challenge, but certainly one researchers can meet successfully. Many good articles are available on the mechanics of preparing and presenting a poster. Display poster presentations so that, in a glance, interested individuals can determine whether they want to know more or whether they prefer to move to the next poster. Anyone who has ever attended a poster session knows that the sheer volume of posters available limits interested parties from spending time with each poster presenter. Therefore, the poster must immediately capture the audience's attention. The title, color of the poster, size of print, and content should catch the passerby's interest first. However, the most important part of the poster is the title. It is essential to present a title that immediately informs readers of the topic and research approach. For instance, the title "Living in Fear" would attract individuals interested in the topic. Because the title is brief, passersby can decide in a moment whether they want to know more. Similarly, a title such as "Living with AIDS: A Cultural Examination" quickly informs people about the subject matter and research approach. Also of importance is the author's name and affiliation. There are situations in which the poster presenter may not be available to answer questions related to the research. If the consumer can jot down the presenter's name and affiliation or pick up a business card, then he or she can contact the poster author at a later time.

In addition, researchers should present the content in a visually appealing way. At a minimum, the poster should include the title of the research, the researcher's name, the purpose, the sample, the method used, the findings, a summary, and the implications. Not all of this information will fit on the poster, depending on the space provided. Therefore, it is up to the researcher to illustrate as much as possible and then indicate to the viewer the availability of additional information either on a handout or in a notebook. Pictures and illustrations capture the passerby's attention and give presenters an opportunity to verbally share results. For qualitative researchers, there is benefit in providing interested individuals with a handout of the abstract or handouts highlighting the important research findings or offering an exhaustive description, if appropriate. On the printed handouts, researchers should include their names and addresses so that nurses interested in the findings or the method may contact them for additional information. Russell, Gregory, and Gates (1996) suggest that researchers place a notebook on the table with the poster. In the notebook, the researcher can insert additional information, including narrative, pictures, and illustrations that are too cumbersome to place on the poster. The notebook provides people interested in additional information about the study an opportunity to get it "on the spot."

As well as using a matted poster format, some qualitative researchers have used audiovisual materials such as a multimedia projection system to give an added dimension to their presentations. The inclusion of sound and changing visuals connects consumers to the work. Presenting a poster using a multimedia system, however, requires access to electricity and additional space. Researchers interested in presenting a poster in this format need to contact the conference planners to see whether there is accessible electricity and adequate space.

Creativity is the key to the successful presentation of ideas. The nature of qualitative research supports creativity in presentation. Because of the type of data collected, the strategies used, and the rich narrative that results, researchers have much more to draw from in developing their poster. Nurses presenting a poster illustrating a qualitative research approach should take advantage of the possibilities open to sharing their findings and exploit those possibilities. However, remember to do so in a logical and appealing manner.

GRANT WRITING

*A*lthough some graduate students are successful in submitting proposals for funding of their dissertation work before they have a publication history, the more frequent scenario is for a researcher to submit a grant proposal after having had one or more research studies published. The development of a competitive research proposal requires researchers to construct the project so that they convince a panel of reviewers that they have the necessary knowledge, experience, and commitment to complete the proposed project. Reviewers will be looking at a researcher's credentials, the scientific merit of the project, and the potential contribution of the project to the profession.

Identifying Funding Sources

One of the first steps in developing a competitive proposal is to identify potential funding sources, a number of which are available to nurses interested in conducting a qualitative inquiry. Different organizations offer materials on the types of projects they fund and their submission guidelines. For researchers seeking their first funding dollars, small grants are the most useful and are generally easier to access. Examples of small grant programs include college or university funds, which are accessible through small grant proposals available on a competitive basis within institutions. The monies generally come from allocations to faculty development budgets, foundations, or alumni gifts.

In addition to college or university funding, several nursing organizations offer small grants. These organizations, among others, include Sigma Theta Tau International, National League for Nursing, American Nurses Foundation, American Association of Critical Care Nurses, and Association of Rehabilitation Nurses. Many corporations also offer small grants, including product companies such as infant formula manufacturers or durable medical equipment firms. Health care organizations, such as hospitals and community health organizations, frequently fund research as well.

Nurses interested in receiving funding need to identify the available resources. This effort will require a moderate amount of time to first determine the available funding sources and then select the source that will most likely be interested in funding the project. Nurses might use resource libraries found in universities that have established nursing research centers to identity potential funding sources. These institutions, where available and accessible, generally have a plethora of diverse materials and experienced staff to assist in locating the appropriate resources and developing the proposal. However, it is no longer necessary for potential grant writers to spend hours in the library: the Internet is a great source for identifying potential grant funds. If university-based nursing research centers are unavailable, researchers may log onto the Web sites of organizations such as the American Association of Colleges of Nursing (AACN), National League for Nursing (NLN), Sigma Theta Tau International (STTI), and American Nurses Association (ANA), which have resource materials on their sites, as well as links to other sites to help focus the search. In addition, sites such as http://fdncenter.org offer a starting point. This is a more general site and is not specific to nursing. It does, however, reference large foundations that provide funds for health-related projects, such as Kellogg and Coca Cola. If you choose to consider a non-nursing organization, look for the eligibility requirements, the organization's purpose and mission statement, and the compatibility with your project (Carey & Swanson, 2003).

Individuals interested in developing larger projects should have completed and published results of small, funded projects before seeking monies from organizations that offer larger funding support. Such organizations include the National Institute of Nursing Research (NINR), National Institutes of Health (NIH), American Education Association (AEA), Kellogg Foundation, Robert Wood Johnson Foundation, and National Science Foundation (NSF). In addition, many nonprofit organizations such as the American Heart Association, National Arthritis Foundation, and American Cancer Society provide moderate to large funding for projects. Critical to receiving larger sums of money and submitting a well-developed project is experience. Organizations that make large awards do not do so unless single researchers or research teams demonstrate significant, documented experience.

Developing the Proposal

Because Chapter 16 focuses on proposal development and grant writing, this section will not address the specific mechanics of developing a research proposal for funding. Instead, the section gives qualitative researchers ideas about the challenges and potential pitfalls in developing qualitative grant proposals. As Morse (1991) commented, "In comparison to the WYSIWYG (what you see is what you get) presentation of the quantitative application, the qualitative proposal is vague, obscure, and may even be viewed as a blatant request for a blank check" (p. 148). The idea of developing a proposal for funding, knowing beforehand that the ambiguities cannot be written out of the grant, presents a unique but not insurmountable challenge. Researchers interested in receiving funding for a qualitative study must convince reviewers not only of the merits of the project, which may seem obscure and undirected, but also of the researcher's experience. Carey and Swanson (2003) report that "the three major areas in common across most applications are identifying appropriate funding sources, developing a work plan and a team and writing the application" (p. 852). These should be carefully considered before moving forward.

There is inconsistency in the literature as to whether a pilot study is important for qualitative research funding. Clearly, quantitative research proposals require pilot work to demonstrate the potential design strengths and weaknesses. Connelly and Yoder (2000) offer that conducting pilot work enhances the qualitative researcher's chances for funding. Given the inconsistencies in the literature and strong possibility of review by quantitative researchers, qualitative researchers are well served to state why they did or did not conduct a pilot study.

In qualitative proposals, the number of participants is determined by data saturation, which can include as few as 5 or more than 50 people. In a quantitative study, the number of participants is determined by the design, projected outcome, and number of variables under study. Based on these parameters, researchers can establish a precise number of participants for inclusion in a study. In qualitative studies, data collection and analysis require flexibility. In quantitative studies, data collection and analysis are largely objective. The preceding comparisons focus on the precise and often predictable nature of a quantitative research proposal versus the often imprecise and unpredictable nature of a qualitative proposal.

Morse (1998) recommends, "the first principle of grantsmanship is to recognize that a good proposal is an argument—a fair and balanced one" (p. 68). Therefore, qualitative researchers must clearly and persuasively present evidence that will convince grant reviewers the proposal is worth funding. To facilitate a clear understanding of the researchers' ideas, proposal authors have the responsibility of explaining everything.

The second principle of grant writing offered by Morse (1998) "is that one should think and plan before starting to write" (p. 70). Planning before writing will give proposal authors an opportunity to clearly delineate the research plan, beginning with development of the research question and ending with the distribution of research results. In addition to assisting with writing the actual proposal document, planning conclusively before beginning to write allows authors time to draft a complete budget. Because the budget is the part of the proposal that provides researchers with the resources to fully operationalize a project, it is essential that researchers develop a strong budget detailing all expenses. Items to include in the budget are personnel, such as research assistants, transcription services, secretaries, and consultants; equipment, such as a computer, printer, video camera, and data analysis program; supplies, such as tape recorders, paper, printer cartridges, audiotapes or videotapes, and photocopies; and travel, including mileage between research sites, conference travel, presentation fees, and consultant travel. Carefully laying out the project will assist greatly in developing a proposal that is clear and succinct and can be funded.

Identifying Investigator Qualifications

The challenge in obtaining larger sums for qualitative research is for prospective grant recipients to convince reviewers they are a risk worth taking. Proposal authors need to illustrate for reviewers a track record in scholarly publication, presentation, consultation, and success in acquiring small awards. "Granting bodies must [be made to] recognize the process nature of the research and that they are funding the *investigator* rather than the *proposal* per se" (Morse, 1991, p. 149). Morse adds that "for major grant applications, evaluation of the *investigator* is critical and should be most heavily weighted" (p. 149). This is not to say that the research project does not need to have scientific merit and be described as fully as possible; rather, it illuminates the nature of the process that is decidedly imprecise when compared with a quantitative proposal.

In recent years, the NIH and other funding agencies have begun requiring that research proposals include a qualitative component (Morse, 1994). This situation is confusing: Does this requirement support the value of qualitative research and reflect the belief that qualitative research will be driven into the system, or is this a strongly misguided request that reflects a definite misunderstanding of research and the qualitative research process in general (Morse, 1994)? In either case, it is up to grant developers to clearly provide the reasons why they have selected one paradigm over another and indicate how the paradigm and, more specifically, the method will provide the answers to the questions asked.

Furthermore, Morse (1996a) points out that funding agencies have given the distinct impression that qualitative research is not an end but rather a means to an end. Based on the literature, qualitative researchers are led to believe that qualitative inquiry is a prelude to "good" quantitative design. This, too, may be a misguided belief. Researchers must make clear to funding agencies the project goal and clearly describe how the method selected is appropriate.

More than one researcher with expertise in quantitative methodology may be able to bring a dimension to an entire project that a qualitative researcher alone would be unable to do. It is up to the principal investigator to determine whether the study will be enhanced by the addition of a strong team with varied philosophical beliefs and interests. Based on experience with funded projects, grant reviewers are frequently viewing research teams more favorably, particularly if the teams are multidisciplinary.

A very serious problem identified by Morse (2003) is that many reviews of qualitative research proposals are not valid. She argues that rejection of proposals is often based on the inexperience of the reviewers with qualitative studies. Currently, the procedures for ensuring a meaningful evaluation of qualitative projects are limited at best. For instance, Morse explains that in one model, an external reviewer with qualitative expertise is invited to comment on the study. Depending on the reviewing agency, this can be in person or by phone. In some cases, the reviewer is permitted to be part of the discussion, and in others, the external reviewer is dismissed for the discussion. In another model, a token qualitative reviewer is added to the review panel (Morse, 2003, p. 741). Although this might at first glance seem a more responsible way to conduct the review, Morse explains that "proposals are funded using the average score obtained from the entire committee, not just the input from one advocate" (p. 741). It is important for qualitative researchers to be aware of the review process so that they can attempt to manage some of the ongoing questions relative to their work.

Identifying Mechanisms for Ensuring Participant Protection

Not only must qualitative researchers clearly demonstrate their expertise and qualifications, it is also essential that their qualitative research proposals conclusively identify the mechanisms for ensuring the protection of participants. One of the strengths of qualitative approaches is the unique opportunity to get to know individuals, groups, or communities over a long period. This strength creates its own potential hazards for participants' protection because the nature of the data—personal descriptions—precludes qualitative researchers from maintaining confidentiality, particularly when they publish quotes or use them as references in publications (Munhall, 1991). Nevertheless, qualitative researchers can ensure anonymity. It is essential that they demonstrate how they will protect informants' identities. In some cases, such as in ethnography or action research, participant identification may actually contribute significantly to the position of groups or their ability to access resources. In such cases, qualitative researchers must document that participants have agreed that researchers may make the informants' identities public. Audiotaping interviews and taking photographs are additional examples of potential violations of participants' rights. Researchers must document informants' permission for such activities.

Although developing mechanisms for ensuring confidentiality and anonymity contributes significantly to a grant proposal, it is also important to clarify for Institutional Review Boards and funding agencies that mechanisms are in place to deal with potentially sensitive outcomes. For example, if a researcher is living with a community and discovers that one of the group rituals involves physically isolating and abusing children who do not excel in academics, the researcher must be able to clearly define steps he or she will take to protect the vulnerable group (i.e., the children). It is essential to try to identify all the potentially sensitive situations and develop mechanisms to intervene or to have intervention available.

Qualitative research is unpredictable in its implementation. Often, the study moves in directions not originally planned. For this reason, it is important to describe for review panels the concept of process consent. "In process consent, researchers continuously renegotiate the consent, allowing participants to play a collaborative role in the decision-making process regarding their ongoing participation" (Polit & Beck, 2006, p. 93). Fully describing the necessity of process consent and the conditions under which it will be used gives reviewers a better understanding of the attention paid to protecting participants.

Other Considerations

Connelly and Yoder (2000) identify a number of common problems with qualitative research proposals that are worth noting. These authors share that researchers should clearly demonstrate an understanding of the assumptions of the research approach they are using. "It is critical to write from the perspective of the appropriate assumptions" (p. 70). Often the proposal author will slip from qualitative terminology to quantitative terminology, which is the second common problem identified. Qualitative researchers must be very careful to fully understand the philosophical foundations of qualitative research in general as well as the specifics of the particular method selected. Sharing methodological information is important. It is especially important when the reviewer is unfamiliar with the assumptions of the method, terminology, and techniques used to collect and analyze data. Connelly and Yoder (2000) state that qualitative researchers have a responsibility to respond to the outline presented for funding, albeit quantitative in orientation. It is the qualitative researcher's responsibility to explain why it is not possible to provide specific requested information.

Other common problems identified include no logical argument for why a qualitative research approach is warranted, no discussion of training data collectors, little or no discussion of methodological rigor, inadequate description of the unique nature of the researcher-informant relationship and its impact on human subjects' protection, inadequately developed significance of the research, inexperienced researcher without adequate consultation, and underestimating budget requirements (Connelly & Yoder, 2000). Any one or more of these common problems can lead to an unsuccessful grant proposal.

SUMMARY

Qualitative research is an exciting opportunity to create meaningful nursing knowledge from individuals' lives and experiences. To make the knowledge accessible, researchers must share the findings in a significant way. Presenting a qualitative project in an article, poster, speech, or grant proposal requires imagination and refined presentation skills. Qualitative researchers have a responsibility to their consumers and to developing qualitative scholars to present their ideas in a clear and meaningful manner. They should share their research in a way that illustrates the richness and value of conducting research using the approaches described in this text.

The development of qualitative research projects and the refinement of social sciences approaches to human inquiry that are appropriate to nursing science establish a major research focus for the profession. Nurses interested in these projects have a unique opportunity to be on the cutting edge of the developments. It is an exciting time for nurses and for research. There is a vast and expansive qualitative research landscape waiting for interested nurse researchers. This is a landscape of imagination that is colored by the lives and experiences of the individuals with whom nurses interact: clients, students, and other nurses. It is essential to document these unique experiences and share them to fully explore and describe the human experience. The challenge awaits those nurses who are willing to participate.

References

Carey, M.A., & Swanson, J. (2003). Funding for qualitative research. *Qualitative Health Research, 13*(6), 852-856.

Choudhuri, D., Glauser, A. & Peregoy, J. (2004). Guidelines for writing a qualitative manuscript for the *Journal of Counseling and Development, 82*, 443-446.

Connelly, M. L., & Yoder, L. H. (2000). Improving qualitative proposals: Common problem areas. *Clinical Nurse Specialist, 14*(2), 69-74.

Devers, K. J., & Frankel, R. M. (2001). Getting qualitative research published. *Education for Health, 14*(1), 109-117.

Field, P. A., & Morse, J. M. (1985). *Nursing research: The application of qualitative approaches.* Rockville, MD: Aspen.

Lambert, C. E., Lambert, V. A., & Tsukahara, M. (2002). Editorial: The review process. *Nursing and Health Science, 4,* 139-140.

Morse, J. (1991). On the evaluation of qualitative proposals [Editorial]. *Qualitative Health Research, 1*(2), 147-151.

Morse, J. M. (1994). Designing funded qualitative research. In N. K. Denzin & Y. S. Lincoln (Eds.), *Handbook of qualitative research* (pp. 220-235). Thousand Oaks, CA: Sage.

Morse, J. M. (1996a). Is qualitative research complete? [Editorial]. *Qualitative Health Research, 6*(1), 3-5.

Morse, J. (1996b). "Revise and resubmit": Responding to reviewers' reports [Editorial]. *Qualitative Health Research, 6*(2), 149-151.

Morse, J. M. (1998). Designing funded qualitative research. In N. K. Denzin & Y. S. Lincoln (Eds.), *Strategies of qualitative inquiry* (pp. 56-85). Thousand Oaks, CA: Sage.

Morse, J. M. (2003). Editorial: The adjudication of qualitative proposals. *Qualitative Health Research, 13*(6), 739-742.

Morse, J. M., & Field, P. A. (1995). *Qualitative research methods for health professionals* (2nd ed.). Thousand Oaks, CA: Sage.

Munhall, P. L. (1991). Institutional review of qualitative research proposals: A task of no small consequence. In J. M. Morse (Ed.), *Qualitative nursing research: A contemporary dialogue* (rev. ed., pp. 258-272). Newbury Park, CA: Sage.

Polit, D. F., & Beck, C. T. (2006). *Essentials of nursing research: Methods, appraisal, and utilization* (6th ed.). Philadelphia: Lippincott Williams & Wilkins.

Russell, C. K., Gregory, D. M., & Gates, M. F. (1996). Aesthetics and substance in qualitative research posters. *Qualitative Health Research, 6*(4), 542-552.

Glossary

Action Research A research method characterized by the systematic study of the implementation of a planned change to a system.

Actors Individuals within a particular cultural group who are studied by ethnographic researchers.

Analytic Induction A method of qualitative data analysis wherein the researcher seeks to refine a theory through the identification of negative cases.

A Priori Form of deductive thinking in which theoretical formulations and propositions precede and guide systematic observation.

Archives Contain unpublished materials that often are used as primary source materials.

Auditability The ability of another researcher to follow the methods and conclusion of the original researcher.

Authenticity Term used to describe the mechanism by which the qualitative researcher ensures that the findings of the study are real, true, or authentic. In historical research refers to assuring that a primary source document provides the truthful reporting of a subject.

Biographical History Studies the life of a person within the context of the period in which that person lives.

Bracketing A methodological device of phenomenological inquiry that requires deliberate identification and suspension of all judgments or ideas about the phenomenon under investigation or what one already knows about the subject prior to and throughout the phenomenological investigation.

Category Classification of concepts into broader categories following comparison of one category to another. Broader categories serve as an umbrella under which related concepts are grouped.

Chat Rooms A computer-mediated method of communication and data collection whereby individuals log on to the world wide web and can communicate back and forth in a synchronous manner.

Coding The process of data analysis in grounded theory whereby statements are grouped and given a code for ease of identification later in the study.

Conceptual Density Data generation that is exhaustive and comprehensive and provides the researcher with evidence that all possible data to support a conceptual framework has been generated.

Confirmability This is considered a neutral criterion for measuring the trustworthiness of qualitative research. If a study demonstrates credibility, auditability, and fittingness, the study is also said to possess confirmability.

Constant Comparative Method of Data Analysis A form of qualitative data analysis wherein the researcher makes sense of textual data by categorizing units of measuring through a process of comparing new units with previously identified units.

Core Variable The central phenomenon in grounded theory around which all the other categories are integrated.

Covert Participant Observation A method of data collection that involves observing participants however, the individuals are unaware that they are being observed.

Credibility A term that relates to the trustworthiness of findings in a qualitative research study. Credibility is demonstrated when participants recognize the reported research findings as their own experiences.

Critical Theory A philosophy of science based on a belief that revealing the unrecognized forces that control human behavior will liberate and empower individuals.

Cultural Scene An anthropological term for culture. It includes the actors, the artifacts, and the actions of the actors in social situations.

D

Deductive The process of moving from generalizations to specific conclusions.

Dependability This is a criterion used to measure trustworthiness in qualitative research. Dependability is met through securing credibility of the findings.

Dialectic A form of logic based on the belief that reality is represented by contradiction and the reconciliation of contradiction.

Dialectical Critique A form of qualitative data analysis wherein the researcher engages in dialogue with research participants to reveal the internal contradictions within a particular phenomenon.

Discipline of History Both a science and an art that studies the interrelationship of social, economic, political, and psychological factors that influence ideas, events, institutions, and people.

Dwelling A term used to demonstrate the degree of dedication a researcher commits to reading, intuiting, analyzing, synthesizing, and coming to a description or conclusion(s) about the data collected during a qualitative study. Also called immersion.

E

Eidetic Intuiting Accurate interpretations of what is meant in the description.

Embodiment (or Being in the World) The belief that all arts are constructed on foundation of perception, or original awareness of some phenomenon (Merleau-Ponty, 1956).

Epistemology The branch of philosophy concerned with how individuals determine what is true.

Essences Elements related to the ideal or true meaning of something that gives common understanding to the phenomenon under investigation.

External Criticism Questions the genuineness of primary sources and assures that the document is what it claims to be.

F

Field Notes Notes recorded about the people, places, and things that are part of the ethnographer's study of a culture.

Fittingness A term used in qualitative research to demonstrate the probability that the research findings have meaning to others in similar situations. Fittingness is also called transferability.

Free Imaginative Variation A technique used to apprehend essential relations between essences and involves careful study of concrete examples supplied by the participant's experience and systematic variation of these examples in the imagination.

G

Genuine When a primary source is what it purports to be and is not a forgery.

Grand Tour Question(s) General opening question(s) that offer(s) overview insights of a particular person, place, object, or situation.

H

History Webster's New International Dictionary defines history as "a narrative of events connected with a real or imaginary object, person, or career . . . devoted to the exposition of the natural unfolding and interdependence of the events treated." History is a branch of knowledge that "records and explains past events as steps in human progress ..." [it is] "the study of the character and significance of events." Barzen and Graff (1985) describe history as an "invention" and as an "art."

Historiography Historiography requires that historiographers study and critique sources and develop history by systematically presenting their findings in a narrative. Historiography provides a way of knowing the past.

Historian/Historiographer Balances the rigors of scientific inquiry and the understanding of human behavior; develops the skill of speculation and interpretation to narrate the story.

Historical Method Application of method or steps to study history systematically.

Holism A belief that wholes are more than the mere sum of their parts.

I

Immersion A term used to demonstrate the degree of dedication a researcher commits to reading, intuiting, analyzing, synthesizing, and coming to a description or conclusion(s) about the data collected during a qualitative study. Also called dwelling.

Induction The process of moving from specific observations to generalizations.

Inductive Theory Building Theory derived from observation of phenomena.

Informed Consent When engaging participants in a research study, ensuring that they have complete information, that they understand the information, and that they have freely chosen to either accept or decline participation in the investigation.

Intellectual History Studies ideas and thoughts over time of a person believed to be an intellectual thinker, or the ideas of a period, or the attitudes of people.

Intentionality Consciousness is always consciousness of something. One does

not hear without hearing something or believe without believing something.

Internal Criticism Concerns itself with the authenticity or truthfulness of the content.

Interpretive Phenomenology/Hermeneutics The interpretation of phenomena appearing in text or written word.

Intuiting A process of thinking through the data so that a true comprehension or accurate interpretation of what is meant in a particular description is achieved.

L

Life History A research method wherein the researcher listens to the telling of life story for the purpose of understanding a particular aspect of the individual's life.

Local Theory A theory that describes a particular group or sample that cannot be generalized to a larger population.

N

Narrative Picturing A data collection method whereby participants are asked to imagine or picture an event or sequence of events as a method of describing an experience.

Naturalistic Inquiry A research methodology based on a belief in investigating phenomena in their natural setting free of manipulation.

P

Participant Observation The direct observation and recording of data that require the researcher to become a part of the culture being studied.

Phenomenological Reduction A term meaning recovery of original awareness.

Present-Mindedness Use of a contemporary perspective when analyzing data collected from an earlier period of time.

Primary Sources Firsthand account of a person's experience, an institution, or of an event and may lack critical analysis; examples include private journals, letters, records.

Process Informed Consent Requires the same criteria as informed consent; however, is differentiated by the fact that this type of consent requires the researcher to reevaluate the participants' consent to be involved in the study at varying points throughout the investigation.

R

Reflexive This term refers to being both researcher and participant and capitalizing on the duality as a source of insight.

Reflexive Critique A form of qualitative data analysis wherein the researcher engages in dialogue with research participants to reveal each individual's interpretation for the meanings influencing behavior.

Reliability The consistency of an instrument to measure an attribute or concept that it was designed to measure.

S

Saturation Repetition of data obtained during the course of a qualitative study. Signifies completion of data collection on a particular culture or phenomenon.

Secondary Sources Materials that cite opinions and present interpretations from the period being studied such as newspaper accounts, journal articles, and textbooks.

Selective Sampling In a grounded theory investigation, selecting from the generated data those critical pieces of information relevant to the current investigation, and avoiding incorporation of material that is not connected to the current investigation.

Situated A term that reflects the position of the researcher within the context of the group under study.

Social History Explores a particular period of time and attempts to understand the prevailing values and beliefs through the everyday events of that period.

Social Situation The activities carried out by actors (members of a cultural group) in a specific place.

Symbolic Interactionism A philosophic belief system based on the assumption that humans learn about and define their world through interaction with others.

T

Tacit Knowledge Information known by members of a culture but not verbalized or openly discussed.

Theme Used to describe a structural meaning unit of data that is essential in presenting qualitative findings.

Theoretical Sampling Sampling on the basis of concepts that have proven theoretical relevance to the evolving theory (Strauss & Corbin, 1990).

Theoretical Sensitivity Personal quality of the researcher that is reflected in an awareness of the subtleties of meaning of data (Strauss & Corbin, 1990).

Transferability A term used in qualitative research to demonstrate the probability that the research findings have meaning to others in similar situations. Transferability is also called fittingness.

Triangulation Method of using multiple research approaches in the same study to answer research questions.

Triangulation of Data Generation Techniques The use of three different methods of data generation in a single research study for the purpose of generating meaningful data.

Trustworthiness Establishing validity and reliability of qualitative research. Qualitative research is trustworthy when it accurately represents the experience of the study participants.

V

Validity The degree to which an instrument measures what it was designed to measure.

Index

Note: Page numbers followed by *f* indicate figures; those followed by *t* indicate tables; those followed by *b* indicate boxed material.